P9-DXI-982

NOM NOM PALEO: FOOD FOR HUMANS IS A COOKBOOK THAT IS JUST PLAIN FUN—
IT'S PACKED WITH CREATIVE CARTOON GRAPHICS, TASTY FOOD PHOTOS, AND YUMMY RECIPES THAT
APPEAL NOT ONLY TO COMMITTED PALEO DIETERS, BUT TO ANYONE WHO LOVES GOOD FOOD.

BRUCE AIDELLS,
IACP Award-winning author of *The Great Meat Cookbook*

"WHAT'S FOR DINNER?" IS NO LONGER A STRESS-INDUCING CONUNDRUM,
AS **NOM NOM PALEO** PROVES THAT COOKING FOR YOUR FAMILY CAN BE
EASY, HEALTHY, AND FUN.

FEATURING DELICIOUS RECIPES AND LOTS OF KITCHEN SELF-HELP, THIS BOOK DETAILS
STEP-BY-STEP INSTRUCTIONS PERFECT FOR THE STOVETOP-CHALLENGED,
AND ENOUGH VARIATIONS TO INSPIRE THE BUDDING CHEF.

AND THE PHOTOS...OH, THE PHOTOS! WORTHY OF THEIR VERY OWN
COFFEE TABLE, THE PICTURES AND ORIGINAL ILLUSTRATIONS MAKE
THIS UNIQUE COOKBOOK PERFECT FOR THE VISUAL LEARNER.

MELISSA HARTWIG,
New York Times bestselling author of *It Starts with Food*

WITH ITS MOUTHWATERING PHOTOS, SASSY EXPLANATIONS, AND PLAYFUL
APPROACH TO FEEDING A FAMILY, THIS BOOK IS A MUST-HAVE FOR ANY KITCHEN, PALEO OR NOT.
PACKED WITH DELICIOUS INSPIRATION AND EASY-TO-FOLLOW RECIPES, IT MAKES BOLD,
INTERNATIONAL FLAVORS ACCESSIBLE TO COOKS OF ALL SKILL LEVELS.

MELISSA JOULWAN,
bestselling author of *Well Fed* and *Well Fed 2*

WITH THEIR CLASSIC BLEND OF CULINARY BRILLIANCE, GORGEOUS
IMAGERY, AND SHARP WIT, MICHELLE AND HENRY HAVE CREATED
A PALEO COOKBOOK THAT IS SECOND TO NONE.

WHETHER YOU'RE JUST STARTING OUT IN THE KITCHEN OR A DYED-IN-THE-WOOL
FOODIE, THIS BOOK WILL GIVE YOU BOTH THE INSPIRATION AND PRACTICAL ADVICE YOU NEED TO
TAKE YOUR PALEO COOKING TO THE NEXT LEVEL.

FROM KEY TIPS FOR NEWBIES TO DINNER RECIPES THAT WILL MAKE YOU LOOK
LIKE A SUPERSTAR, **NOM NOM PALEO: FOOD FOR HUMANS** HAS IT ALL.
IT HAS QUICKLY BECOME A FAVORITE IN OUR KITCHEN,
AND I'M SURE IT WILL BE IN YOURS, TOO.

CHRIS KRESSER,
acclaimed author of *Your Personal Paleo Code*

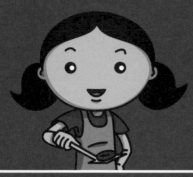

HELLO
my name is
MICHELLE

CHOCOHOLIC, GASTRO-TOURIST, TELLER
OF OFF-COLOR JOKES, NAP ENTHUSIAST

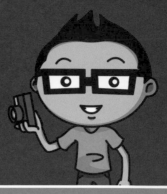

HELLO
my name is
HENRY

COFFEE ADDICT, DESIGN NUT, BIG NERD,
GARAGE GYM RAT, MAKER OF STUFF

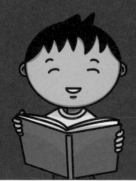

HELLO
my name is
OWEN

BASS GUITARIST, GHOST HUNTER, ROBOT
DESIGNER, STOP-MOTION ANIMATOR

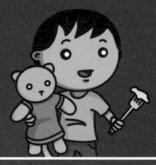

HELLO
my name is
OLLIE

AMATEUR SPY, MARTIAL ARTIST, PICKY
EATER, WRANGLER OF STUFFED CATS

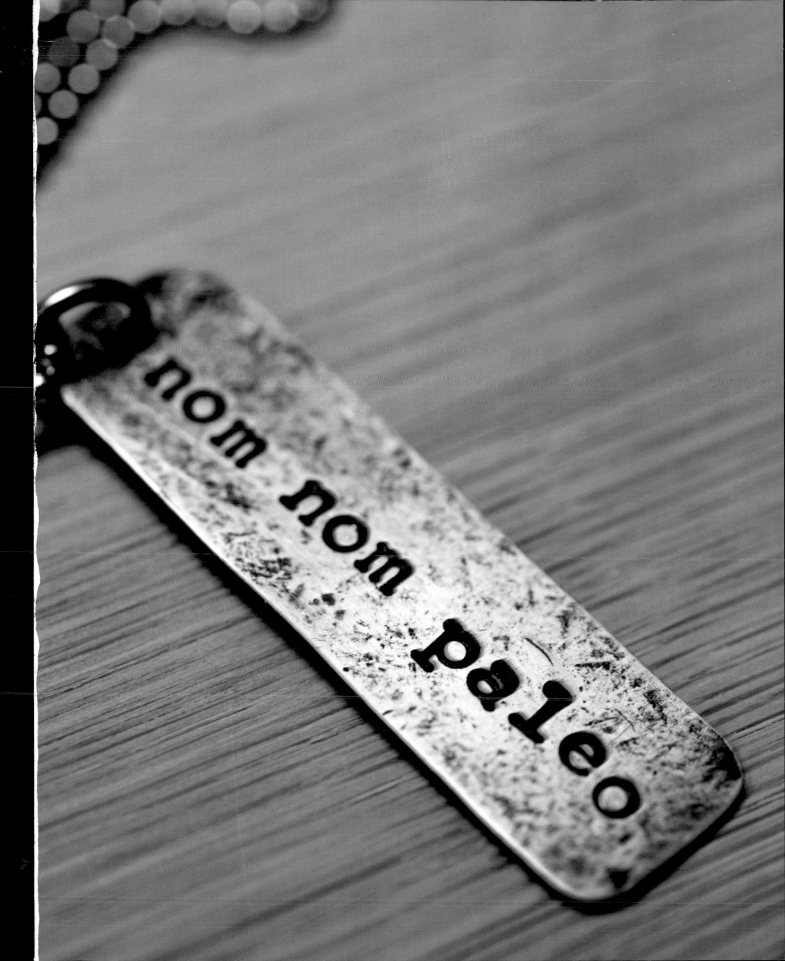

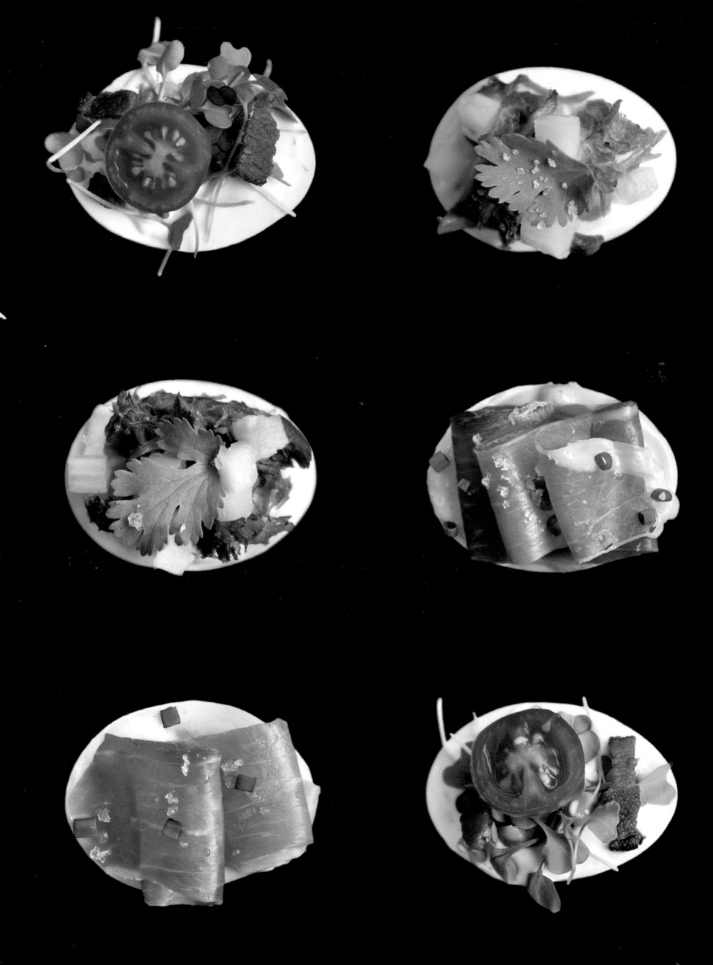

nom nom paleo

FOOD FOR HUMANS

MICHELLE TAM
+ HENRY FONG

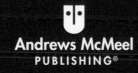

Andrews McMeel
PUBLISHING®

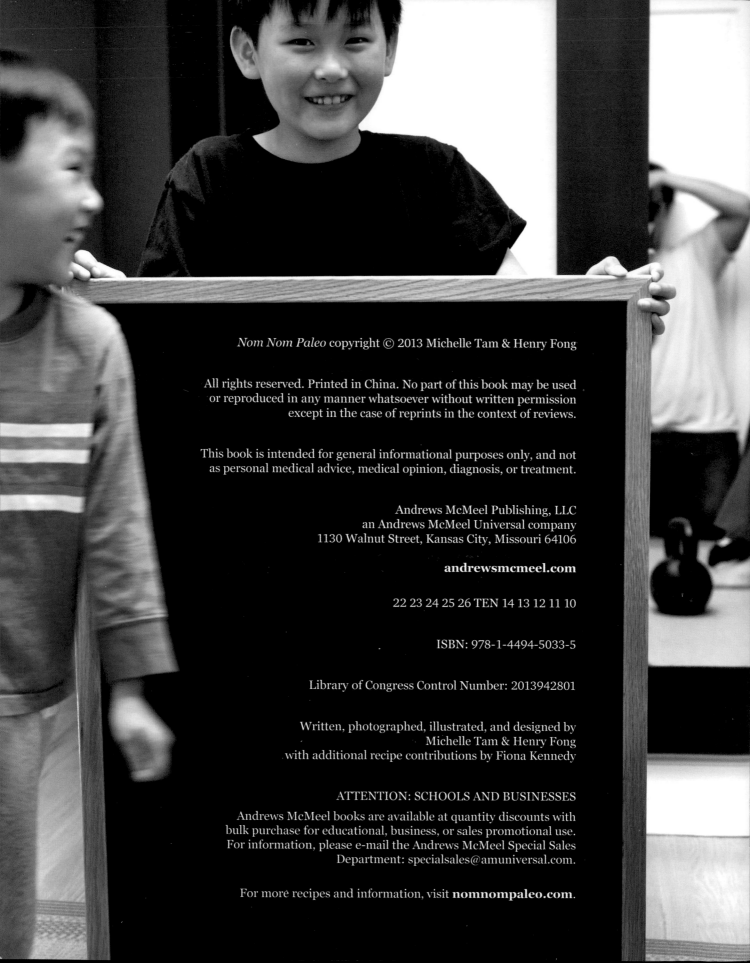

Nom Nom Paleo copyright © 2013 Michelle Tam & Henry Fong

All rights reserved. Printed in China. No part of this book may be used
or reproduced in any manner whatsoever without written permission
except in the case of reprints in the context of reviews.

This book is intended for general informational purposes only, and not
as personal medical advice, medical opinion, diagnosis, or treatment.

Andrews McMeel Publishing, LLC
an Andrews McMeel Universal company
1130 Walnut Street, Kansas City, Missouri 64106

andrewsmcmeel.com

22 23 24 25 26 TEN 14 13 12 11 10

ISBN: 978-1-4494-5033-5

Library of Congress Control Number: 2013942801

Written, photographed, illustrated, and designed by
Michelle Tam & Henry Fong
with additional recipe contributions by Fiona Kennedy

ATTENTION: SCHOOLS AND BUSINESSES

Andrews McMeel books are available at quantity discounts with
bulk purchase for educational, business, or sales promotional use.
For information, please e-mail the Andrews McMeel Special Sales
Department: specialsales@amuniversal.com.

For more recipes and information, visit **nomnompaleo.com**.

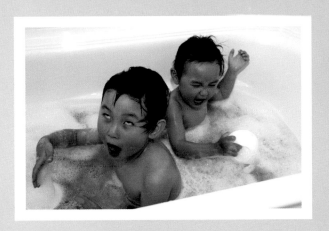

**FOR OWEN + OLLIE:
YOU ARE OUR EVERYTHING.**

(NOW GO FINISH YOUR VEGETABLES.)

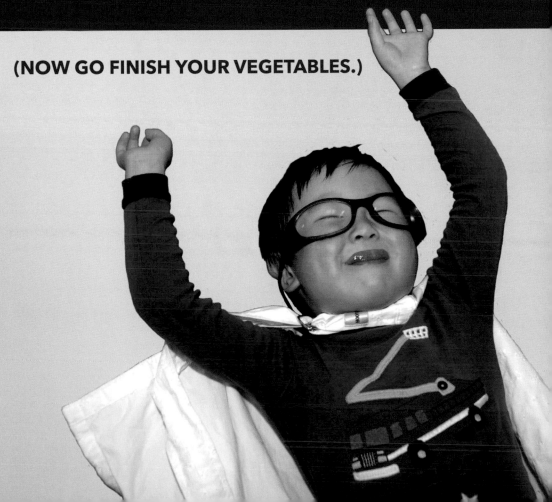

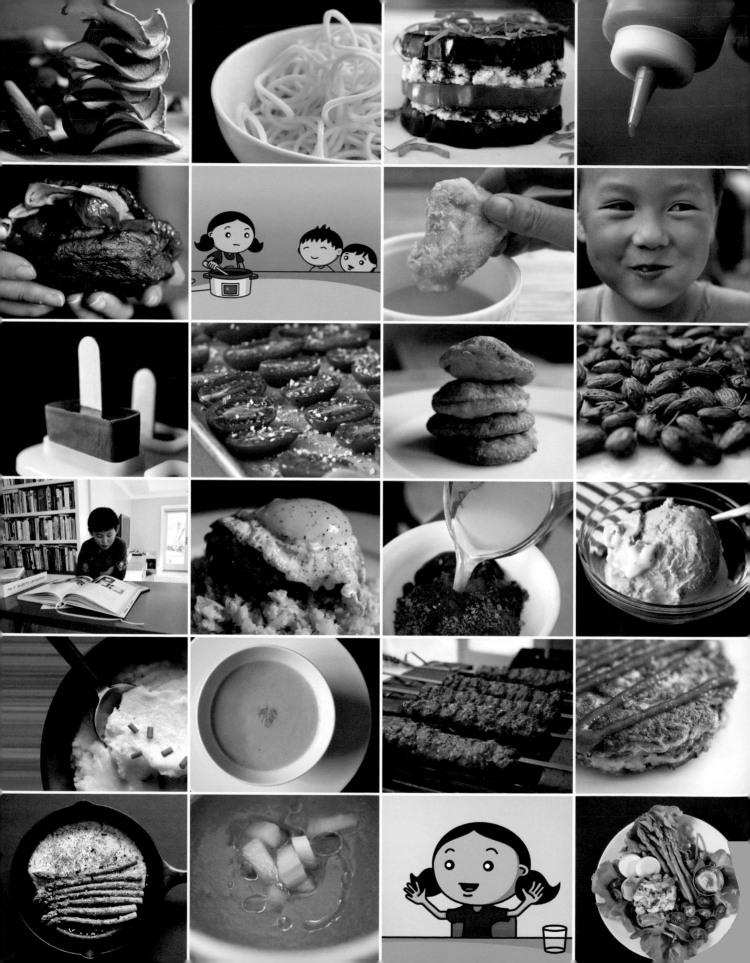

CONTENTS

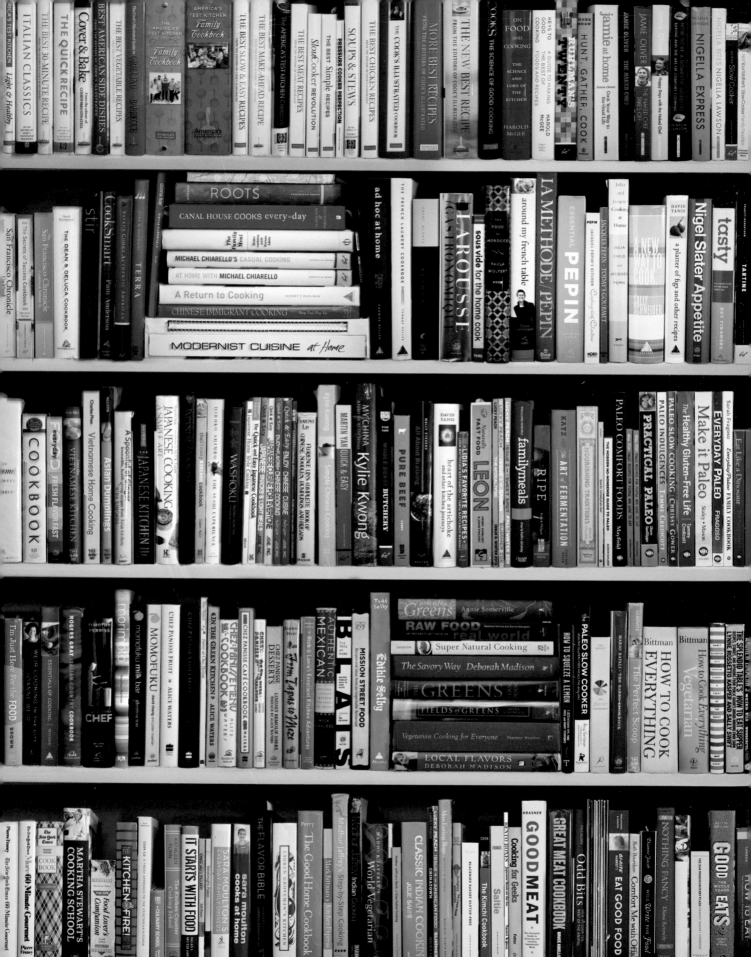

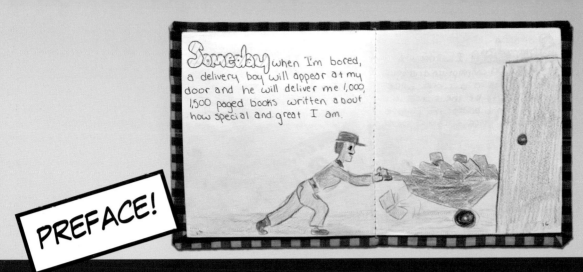

Someday when I'm bored, a delivery boy will appear at my door and he will deliver me 1,000, 1,500 paged books written about how special and great I am.

I'VE ALWAYS SECRETLY DREAMED OF WRITING A COOKBOOK.

Of course, I knew it was a preposterous notion, so I never gave it much thought—until I started receiving offers from book publishers. Naturally, I freaked out. "I don't know how to do this," I told my husband. "It was just a dumb dream."

Henry did his best to reassure me. "It's not a dream if you can do it," he said encouragingly. "It's a *goal*."

"Yuck!" I rolled my eyes. "The motivational poster store called, and it wants its clichés back."

As usual, my spouse was unfazed. "You should do it, Meech. Write the book. I'll help you. It'll be fun!"

I knew he wasn't kidding. When Henry's not working, he's forever throwing himself into creative endeavors: printing T-shirts in the garage, devising ways to make spicy jerky using toy blocks and a box fan, teaching himself photography, or renovating the entire house. I suppose I'm no slouch, either: for the past few years, I've been consumed with recipe development and food writing. Together, we created Nom Nom Paleo, a website that gradually evolved from a lark to a popular online destination for real food enthusiasts.

But a *cookbook*? We both have hectic careers: I'm a clinical pharmacist at a large hospital, and he's a busy lawyer. We have two young sons who need to be fed and watered (and hugged, too). Besides, the last book Henry designed was his high school yearbook, and the last book I penned was for a fourth-grade homework assignment. It was dreamily entitled *Someday*.

"Someday is *today*," Henry grinned. Yes, I married a cliché-spewing machine.

Now, after more than a few buckets of blood, sweat, tears, and very strong coffee, our cookbook is finally in your hands. I hope you dig it as much as we do.

To be crystal clear, this is a cookbook, not a textbook. In these pages, you won't find scholarly explanations of biochemistry or pages of citations to research studies. (Interested in the science behind ancestral eating? Visit the Resources page on nomnompaleo.com.)

Instead, I wrote this book to share my favorite flavor-packed, nutrient-rich recipes for demanding foodies and picky kids alike. As a busy working mom and unrepentant food geek, I wanted to create a book that focuses on three of the most important things in my life: food, family, and fun. That's why we crammed these pages full of photographs, cartoons, and tips for getting the clan back into the kitchen.

Frankly, I don't care if you're a committed Paleo eater or not—our goal is to get *everyone* excited to cook and savor meals made with real, whole, nourishing foods. So if you've ever dreamed of eating more healthfully but without sacrificing flavor, remember:

It's not a dream if you can do it. It's a goal.

And this book was written to help you achieve it.

Oh, *great*. Now he's got me doing it.

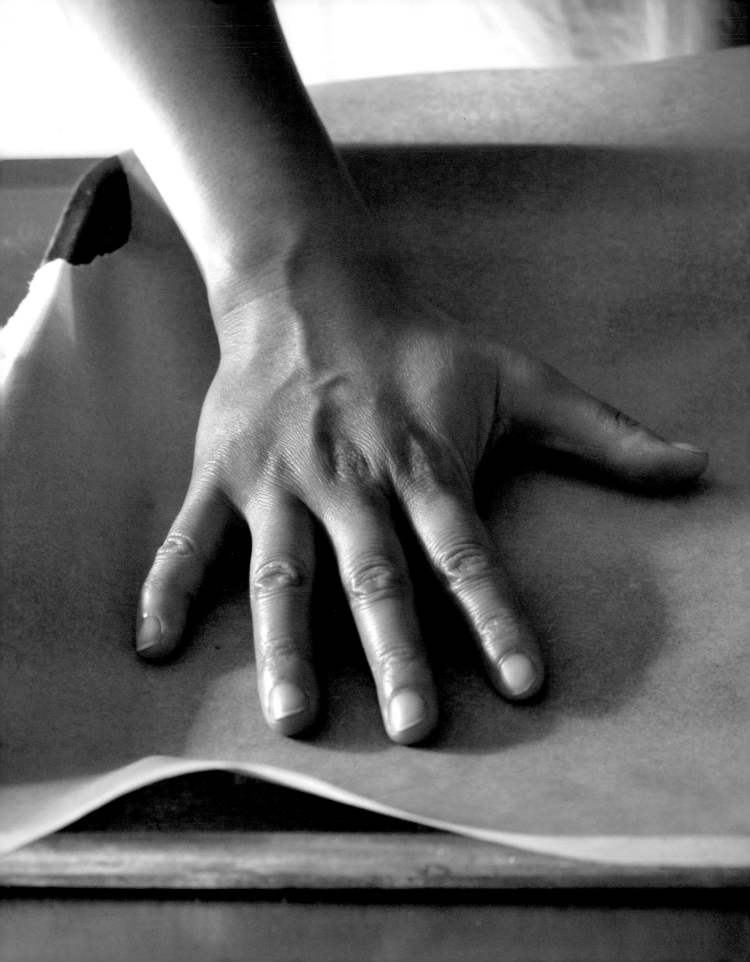

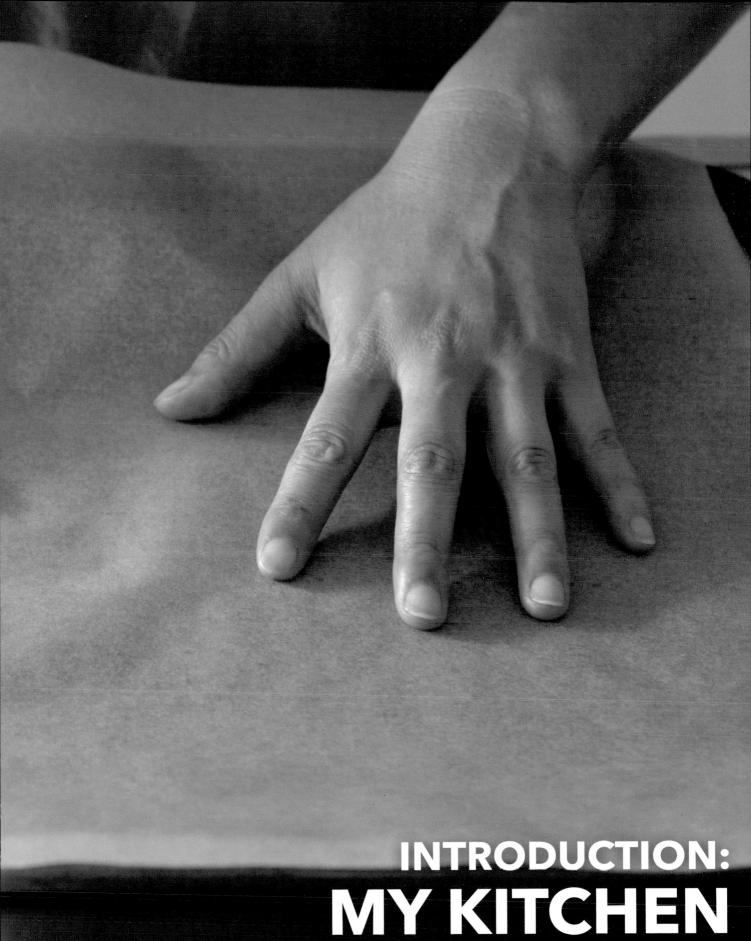

INTRODUCTION:
MY KITCHEN

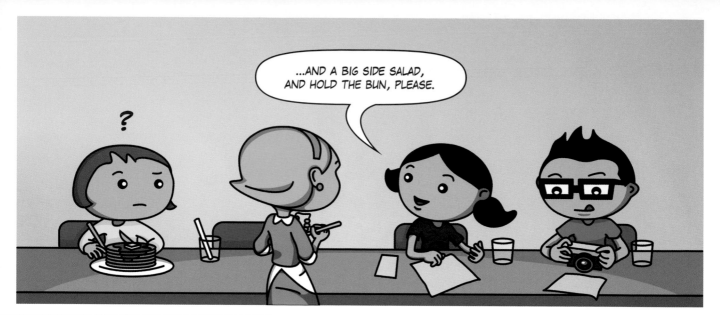

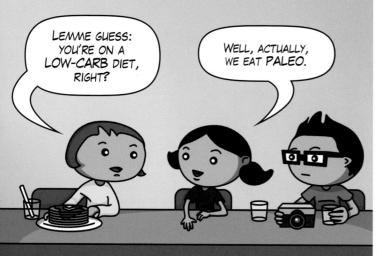

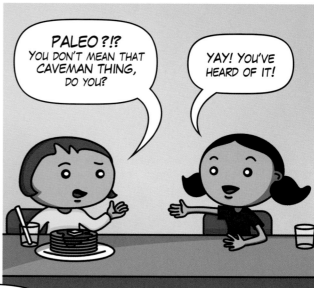

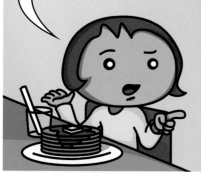

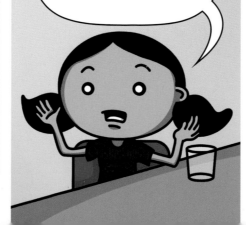

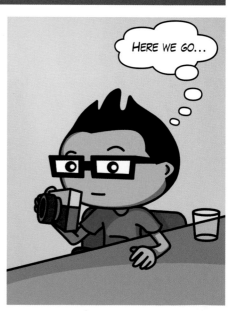

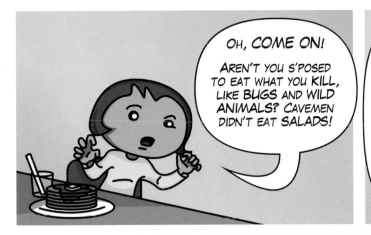

OH, COME ON!

AREN'T YOU S'POSED TO EAT WHAT YOU KILL, LIKE BUGS AND WILD ANIMALS? CAVEMEN DIDN'T EAT SALADS!

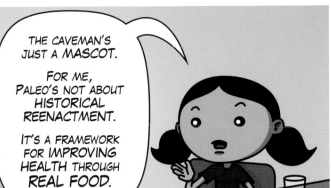

THE CAVEMAN'S JUST A MASCOT.

FOR ME, PALEO'S NOT ABOUT HISTORICAL REENACTMENT.

IT'S A FRAMEWORK FOR IMPROVING HEALTH THROUGH REAL FOOD.

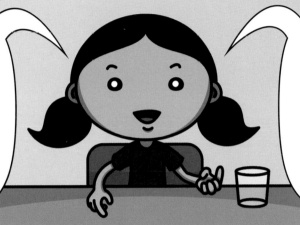

THE IDEA'S SIMPLE: EAT MORE WHOLE, NUTRIENT-RICH FOODS, LIKE VEGETABLES, MEAT, SEAFOOD, AND SOME NUTS AND FRUIT.

ALSO, TRY TO AVOID STUFF THAT TENDS TO BE MORE HARMFUL THAN HEALTHFUL, LIKE PROCESSED FOODS, ADDED SUGAR, SEED OILS, GRAINS, LEGUMES, AND DAIRY.

FROM THERE, YOU CAN GRADUALLY RE-INTRODUCE SOME OF THESE FOODS LIKE RICE OR FULL-FAT DAIRY TO SEE HOW YOUR BODY TOLERATES 'EM.

"PALEO" IS REALLY JUST SHORTHAND FOR EATING REAL, NOURISHING FOODS THAT DON'T WRECK OUR METABOLIC, DIGESTIVE, AND IMMUNE SYSTEMS.

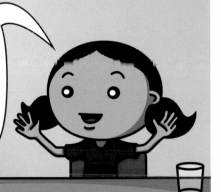

I FEEL GREAT EATING THIS WAY. I'M HEALTHIER AND STRONGER, TOO!

BESIDES, FRESH, SEASONAL, WHOLE INGREDIENTS ARE INSANELY DELICIOUS!

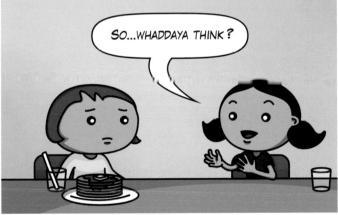

SO...WHADDAYA THINK?

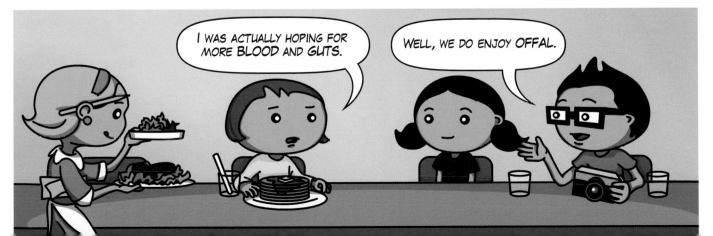

I WAS ACTUALLY HOPING FOR MORE BLOOD AND GUTS.

WELL, WE DO ENJOY OFFAL.

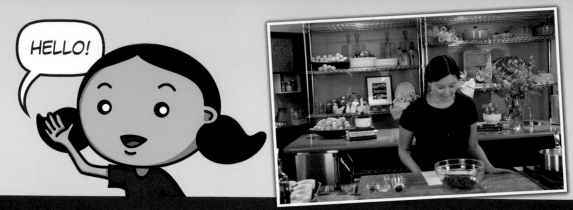

HELLO!

MY NAME IS MICHELLE, AND I'M A FOODAHOLIC.

My waking thoughts are preoccupied with food: finding it, cooking it, savoring it. Perhaps it's genetic: my family has always shared my obsession with all things gustatory. In Cantonese—my parents' native tongue—my mother, father, sister, and I can all be described as *wai sek*: we live to eat.

In fact, I like to think that my parents chose to settle in Northern California in part because of the region's collective enthusiasm for fresh ingredients and flavors. (Reality: they moved here from Hong Kong to be closer to relatives.) Regardless of how they ended up in the San Francisco Bay Area, my sister and I benefitted from growing up in the very heart of the slow food movement. Even as children, we knew in our bones that food is much, much more than fuel; it's one of the singular pleasures of life.

My love for food started with the tastes, sights, and aromas of my mother's kitchen. My mom was (and is) an excellent cook, and as a child, I was her little shadow as she prepared supper each night. It didn't take long for me to master the art of lingering next to her cutting board until she'd hand me a scrap of succulent roast duck or barbecued pork.

My mom's kitchen skills were enhanced by her uncanny ability to identify individual ingredients by taste and reverse-engineer recipes. "I can make that," she'd say after trying a dish at a restaurant. I'd scoff, but she was always right. Through years of close observation, I managed to learn a thing or two from my mother—and in particular, how to create splendid meals from pantry items: savory pan-fried chow mein, steaming bowls of soup noodles, and juicy dumplings with spicy dipping sauces.

My mom was the first of my many food idols, and from her, I gained a deep and abiding love for magically transforming simple ingredients into mouth-watering family feasts. And yes, I'm using the word "feast" for good reason. Here's what a typical weekend dinner looked like at our house:

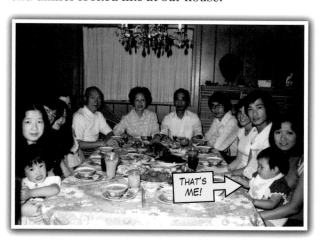

THAT'S ME!

In keeping with Chinese tradition, our cramped little house was a multigenerational one. We lived under one roof with my grandparents, and my aunts and uncles regularly gathered around our dining room table for cozy, family-style suppers. And night after night, my mom somehow managed to create multiple dishes by herself *from scratch*.

Here's the mathematical formula my mother used to calculate the number of courses she'd prepare:

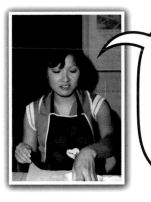

TAKE THE NUMBER OF DINNER GUESTS, AND SUBTRACT ONE. TONIGHT, THERE'LL BE 13 OF US AROUND THE SUPPER TABLE, SO I'M GOING TO MAKE 12 DIFFERENT DISHES.

OH, AND SOUP, TOO.

I often catch myself wishing that I'd inherited my mom's culinary chops. (My older sister certainly did.) There is, however, one thing my mom most certainly passed down to me: an infatuation with food and flavor.

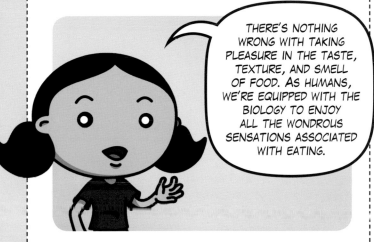

THERE'S NOTHING WRONG WITH TAKING PLEASURE IN THE TASTE, TEXTURE, AND SMELL OF FOOD. AS HUMANS, WE'RE EQUIPPED WITH THE BIOLOGY TO ENJOY ALL THE WONDROUS SENSATIONS ASSOCIATED WITH EATING.

But as I was growing up, so was the industrial food complex. I was a child of the 1970s and 1980s—the same decades that saw an explosion in the global manufacture of factory-processed foods. Flavor scientists were ushering in a brave new world of chemically enhanced food products, and Madison Avenue was pushing these concoctions through television screens right into our living rooms.

Forget home-cooked meals; you can now start your day with rainbow-colored cereals and end it with a trip to the fast food drive-thru window. Who needs fresh produce when you can pick up some fruit-flavored gummy snacks and a bag of chips? And who wants to slave over a hot stove when you can just nuke a plastic tray of macaroni and fake cheese that's been expertly engineered to massage all the pleasure centers in your brain?

A good chunk of my childhood was spent planted in front of the television, so not surprisingly, I had a long and torrid affair with some of the unhealthi-est, most highly processed concoctions pitched over the airwaves. The more flavor-enhancing chemical additives, the better. Want examples?

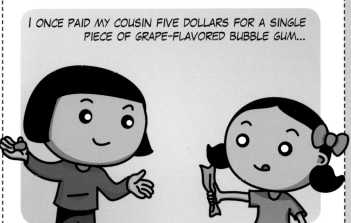

I ONCE PAID MY COUSIN FIVE DOLLARS FOR A SINGLE PIECE OF GRAPE-FLAVORED BUBBLE GUM...

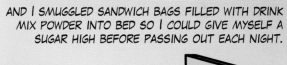

AND I SMUGGLED SANDWICH BAGS FILLED WITH DRINK MIX POWDER INTO BED SO I COULD GIVE MYSELF A SUGAR HIGH BEFORE PASSING OUT EACH NIGHT.

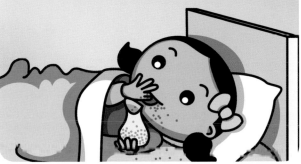

Needless to say, I loved sweets. When I was 15, I landed an after-school job at the frozen yogurt joint down the street, which meant I could slurp up all the sugary, artificially flavored froyo I wanted. (Hey—the stuff's non-fat, so it must be healthy, right?) I used my tip money from the yogurt shop to purchase my school lunches from the vending machines. My meal of choice: two bags of chips, chased down with a can of soda.

If it weren't for the fact that my mom continued to whip up dinner from scratch every night, I'm sure I would've turned fluorescent from all the food dyes I was ingesting.

It wasn't until I moved to Berkeley for college that I realized that it was much cooler to be "health con-scious." Those scrawny young hippies on Telegraph

Avenue were all about salads and whole grains, so I decided to do my part to fit in with all the patchouli-oiled, sandal-wearing masses. I chomped on whole-grain loaves and lugged around a gigantic box of gravel-like grain clusters, shoveling handfuls of it into my mouth at every opportunity. Shockingly, I failed to detect any improvement in my health.

But I wasn't ready to give up on processed foods. Better living through chemistry, right? I decided to major in Nutrition and Food Science so I could become a flavor scientist and create Frankenfoods.

I'm not joking. At the time, I idolized a friend's mother, who held the patent on a chemical spray that made microwaved meals turn golden brown, thereby mimicking the effects of oven-cooked food.

Somehow, through it all, my love for food and flavors remained, and even blossomed. I met a boy in school (who later became my partner-in-crime and husband), and together, Henry and I made excursions around the San Francisco Bay Area to the best restaurants we could afford on our student budgets.

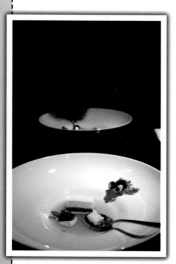

After Henry and I got student jobs on campus, we blew entire paychecks on lavish meals at places like the iconic Chez Panisse—but we also loved cheap eats. Berkeley's Cheeseboard Pizza was one of our haunts, and we sought out the area's best ethnic grub whenever possible, from freshly sliced sashimi and fiery North Indian chaat to overstuffed burritos and rib-sticking Eritrean stews served with injera bread. Every Thursday night, a small group of us would venture across the bay to explore yet another hole-in-the-wall eatery in San Francisco.

I was in food heaven.

Over the course of many great meals made with fresh, local ingredients, I came to fully appreciate the importance of food quality. Sure, I still subscribed to conventional wisdom about the benefits of low-fat eating, but I started making regular visits to farmer's markets and seeking out organically grown whole foods. I was lucky enough to enjoy some of the freshest, most flavorful ingredients in the Bay Area, and the scales were finally falling from

my eyes. I no longer dreamed of a career developing flavor compounds for food conglomerates.

Instead, when I graduated from college, I decided to use my foundation in biochemistry to become…

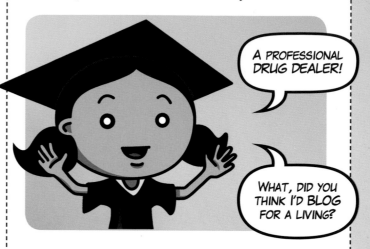

A PROFESSIONAL DRUG DEALER!

WHAT, DID YOU THINK I'D BLOG FOR A LIVING?

I moved to San Francisco to earn a doctorate in clinical pharmacy just as the Bay Area food scene exploded. My big sister moved back from southern California, too, and started her career as a chef, working in some of the most acclaimed kitchens in San Francisco.

Like my mom, Fiona is a culinary genius, with a talent for cobbling together shockingly good flavor combinations. With my sister cooking with some of the best chefs around, I finally had an "in." I eagerly followed the openings and closings of local foodie hotspots. And when I'd fly back east to visit Henry (who was attending law school), we descended like vultures on restaurants in New York City. Forget seeing the sights; I was there to eat.

Fittingly, after Henry moved back to the Bay Area, he proposed to me in the middle of a lavish ten-course meal. It's the only tasting menu I don't recall eating. I was too busy hyperventilating.

After our wedding, we settled in San Francisco, where Henry toiled as a litigator in a downtown law firm, and I got a job working as a night shift hospital pharmacist. We almost never cooked at home. With two incomes and no kids, we continued to eat our way through the city. When we weren't breaking bread at restaurants with friends, we were chowing on take-out. And I'm not just talking about pizza and Chinese; in our food-crazed city, every conceivable cuisine was available to us, from Burmese to Moroccan and everything in between. I didn't hold back. Any money I didn't put in the bank was frittered away on food experiences and cookbooks. (I didn't cook from any of them, mind you; they were strictly for pleasure reading.)

Admittedly, it got a little nuts. For a while, my goal in life was to visit a particular sushi joint until I scored an invitation to sit at the VIP counter. And I didn't hesitate to book flights to faraway cities when I wanted to dine at Alinea in Chicago or taste the pies at Pizzeria Bianco in Phoenix. We'd grab our passports and head off to Italy or Japan just so I could sample the *bollito misto* in Florence or experience a *shojin-ryori* meal in Kyoto. Exercise was reserved for the weekend, when we'd run or bike through the city—straight to our favorite bakery to gorge on pizza, muffins, scones, and cheese rolls.

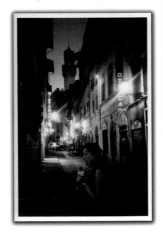

It wasn't until after we had children and moved to the suburbs that I took notice of the muffin-top that was emerging from my waistband. Once our two boys were born, I was determined to get rid of the loose flesh—and get stronger, too. Carrying small, wriggly toddlers had left me with a bad case of Mommy Thumb, an inflammation of the tendons below my thumb, and I didn't want to live life with a brace permanently wrapped around my wrist.

So I did what any crazy-busy working mom would do: I subscribed to fitness magazines and ordered a bunch of home exercise DVDs. For well over a year, I did heart-pounding cardio moves in the garage by myself every night. I counted calories. I strapped a high-tech monitor around my sweaty arm and tracked my caloric expenditure. I lost weight.

But I was also starving and miserable and tired and cranky. I wasn't any stronger, and I was achy all the time. My gut felt terrible every time I worked night shifts. Worst of all, my muffin-top didn't go away.

In the meantime, my husband had embarked on a mission of his own to improve his health and fitness. After the birth of our second kid, Henry could no longer disappear to the neighborhood gym, so he bought a set of weights and began exercising in our garage. He logged his workouts online, and started digging into the various approaches to better health that he came across on the Internet.

And that's how we first stumbled upon Paleo eating.

When Henry first learned about the Paleo approach to nutrition, he and I shared a good laugh about it. No heart-healthy whole grains? No beans? *Ha!*

But the more my husband looked into this real-food approach, the more he became convinced of its benefits. He soon transitioned to eating Paleo, while I sat back and scoffed. I figured that Henry's dalliance with this "caveman" thing wouldn't last long. After all, I'm the one with a nutrition degree, and the Paleo framework went against everything I'd learned. I was certain that all that protein and fat was going to send Henry to an early grave.

So naturally, I did my best to sabotage his diet.

I knew of my husband's weakness for pizza, so I made a point of regularly baking his favorite thin-crust pies. And if that didn't work, well…I guess I could take out a bigger life insurance policy on him.

But my husband can be stubborn. Henry stuck to his guns, and to my surprise, he didn't just survive eating Paleo—he *thrived*. Here I was, suffering through hour-long cardio workouts and obsessively recording my calories each night, and I didn't feel any healthier. Sure, my bathroom scale told me I'd shed some pounds, but my food cravings were off the charts.

Meanwhile, my husband had joined a local Cross-Fit gym, where he did high-intensity workouts just three times a week. He ate according to a Paleo template, and was in better shape than when he was in college. His blood work and body composition were excellent, and he was happily gobbling up all the stuff I secretly wanted to eat.

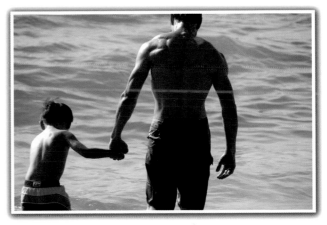

I had to give this Paleo thing a try.

In 2010, while on a family trip to Alaska, I made the decision to go Paleo. Despite being on a cruise ship, I immediately cut out all grains, legumes, sugar, and processed food from my diet. (Seeing other passengers dragging their oxygen tanks to the buffet lines was more than a little motivating.)

When I got home, I went online and read everything I could about the science behind the Paleo framework. I vacuumed up every morsel of information from books and blogs. I quit doing all the crazy cardio and started going to CrossFit classes. I was all-in. I had joined the cult of Paleo.

And now, I'm the healthiest I've ever been.

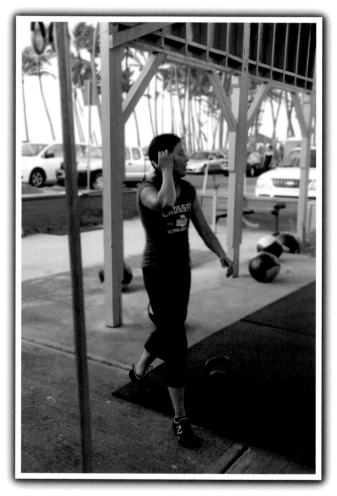

I'd been mentally and physically lagging after a decade of working graveyard shifts, but once I changed my diet, my energy levels shot up, and my digestive problems disappeared entirely.

My moods were sunnier, too. I was a much nicer mommy. Paleo managed to both whittle down my midsection and fuel me with enough spunk to wrangle two small boys, hold down a full-time night shift job as a hospital pharmacist, cook for a houseful of hungry cavepeople, lift heavy(ish) stuff at the gym, develop a bestselling app, and maintain a blog.

Oh, right—the blog. I suppose I should say a few words about my little corner of the Internet.

Nom Nom Paleo started on a whim. For years, I'd been a voracious consumer of food blogs. I was entranced by bloggers who posted tantalizing recipes and gorgeous photographs of their meals. Each site was unique and inspiring in its own way, but all of them made me want to cook. But having switched to a Paleo lifestyle, I found myself craving a food blog that reflected my new approach to eating.

One day, as I gazed at the food porn on my laptop screen, I mused: "I want to start a Paleo food blog."

Henry glanced over at me. "Really? What would you call it?" he asked.

"Nom Nom Paleo."

"Huh? What's a 'Nom Nom'?"

"You know—the noise you make when you're eating something incredibly mind-blowing, and you're just scarfing it down. Like this!"

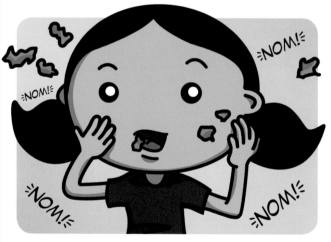

That night, my husband unveiled a blog he'd created for me called—you guessed it—Nom Nom Paleo. Henry knew I was much too lazy to launch a site on my own. "Jump right in," he prodded. "Don't overthink it. Just put up content that you'd find useful if you were a reader." He's such an enabler.

So I started blogging. I shot photographs of my meals and documented my culinary adventures. I discussed my Paleo (and Paleo-ish) meals around town. I offered kitchen shortcuts and reviewed my favorite cooking tools. I posted recipes, and did my best to make Paleo easy and accessible for obsessive gastrophiles and rookie cooks alike.

And I haven't looked back since.

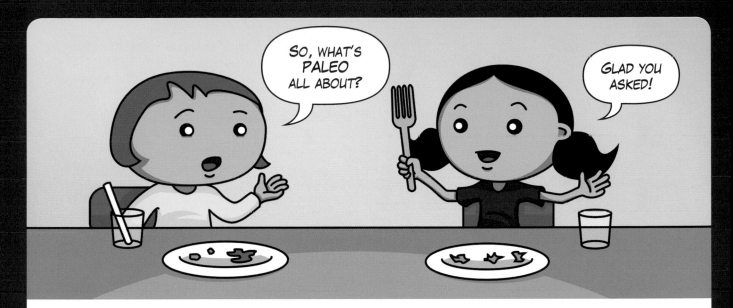

FOR OPTIMAL HEALTH, WE SHOULD EAT MORE LIKE OUR HUNTER-GATHERER ANCESTORS. IN OTHER WORDS, WE SHOULD GET BACK TO EATING REAL, NATURALLY OCCURRING INGREDIENTS.

The "caveman" label makes this sound like a weird fad diet, but trust me: it isn't. Over the past 200,000 years, humans have biologically adapted best to whole foods: plants, meat, seafood—all of them packed with the nutrients our bodies evolved to thrive on.

Agriculture came on the scene a mere 10,000 years ago—a tiny fraction of our evolutionary history. There simply hasn't been enough time and evolutionary pressure for humans to completely adapt to eating modern foods like wheat, sugar, chemically processed vegetable and seed oils, and other "Neolithic" foods. It's not a coincidence that many modern diseases of civilization—including autoimmune disorders, cardiovascular disease, type 2 diabetes, and rampant obesity—have accompanied the global spread of industrialized food. That's why the Paleo approach emphasizes returning to a more ancestral approach to eating.

But here's the thing to keep in mind: we're not trying to precisely replicate cavemen diets. Yes, a few Paleo die-hards may approach their diets this way, but there isn't just one definitive, monolithic, one-size-fits-all "Paleo diet." Some Paleo eaters choose to go super-low-carb, while others of us are happy to munch on a baked potato or a bowl of white rice every now and then. There are Paleo eaters who can't imagine life without dairy, and more orthodox folks who refuse to touch even a pat of butter with a ten-foot pole. The Paleo tent is big enough to fit a host of different approaches, but the core tenets of ancestral eating remain the same:

---

1. PRIORITIZE WHOLE, UNPROCESSED, NUTRIENT-RICH, NOURISHING FOODS. Eat vegetables, grass-fed and pastured meats and eggs, wild-caught seafood, and some fruit, nuts, and seeds.

2. AVOID FOODS THAT ARE LIKELY TO BE MORE HARMFUL THAN HEALTHFUL. Especially when regularly consumed, certain foods can trigger inflammation, cause digestive problems, or derail our natural metabolic processes, such as grains, legumes, sugar, and processed seed and vegetable oils.

Once a baseline of health is established, we can slowly reintroduce some of these foods (like dairy, white potatoes and rice—not processed junk foods) to see where each of us sits on the spectrum of food tolerance.

Transitioning to a Paleo lifestyle can seem like a daunting task, but remember: it's not about deprivation. Go Paleo, and you won't have to stress out about counting calories, balancing macronutrients, or starving yourself. Paleo isn't specifically intended to be a low-carb or weight-loss diet, but by eliminating processed foods, added sugar, and grains, and by consuming deliciously nourishing foods like vegetables, meat, and healthy fats, you can eat until you're full—and still improve your body composition and overall health.

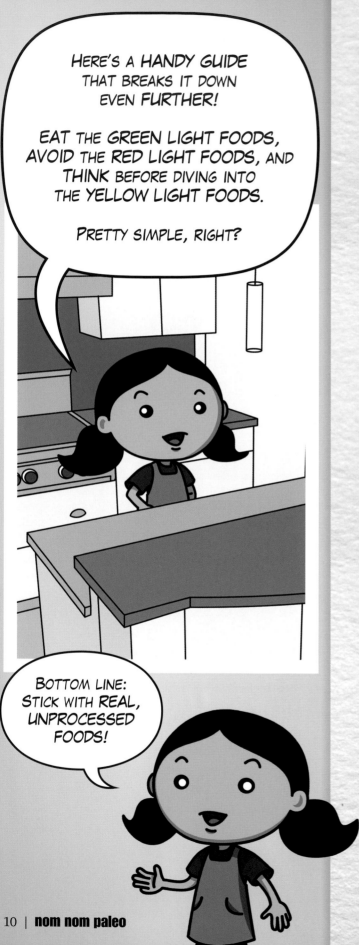

HERE'S A HANDY GUIDE THAT BREAKS IT DOWN EVEN FURTHER!

EAT THE GREEN LIGHT FOODS, AVOID THE RED LIGHT FOODS, AND THINK BEFORE DIVING INTO THE YELLOW LIGHT FOODS.

PRETTY SIMPLE, RIGHT?

BOTTOM LINE: STICK WITH REAL, UNPROCESSED FOODS!

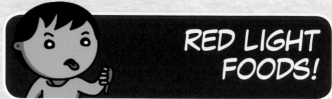

RED LIGHT FOODS!

PROCESSED FOODS:

Processed foods are almost always made with cheap, unpronounceable, terrible-for-you additives like artificial dyes, trans fats (a.k.a. hydrogenated oils), chemical preservatives, and high-fructose corn syrup. Stay away.

SUGAR + ARTIFICIAL SWEETENERS:

I'm guessing you already know that foods with added sugar or artificial sweeteners aren't good for you, right?

GRAINS:

Grains are cheap, but they're nutrient-poor relative to fruits and vegetables, and contain proteins like gluten that can cause gut permeability and inflammation. Some people are more intolerant to grains than others, but even if you don't have celiac disease, regular consumption of large amounts of grains can be harmful. For instance, oats may be gluten-free, but they contain a compound called avenin that can similarly compromise your body's digestive and immune systems. Boo.

LEGUMES:

Like grains, legumes—which include beans, peas, and even peanuts (which aren't nuts at all)—aren't your healthiest option. Sure, beans are plentiful and full of minerals, but their nutrients aren't readily bioavailable to our bodies due to the phytates in legumes. And while it's possible to make legumes less harmful by taking the time to soak, sprout, cook, and ferment them, there are many more nutrient-rich (and far less time-consuming) options available to you. Soy, in particular, should not be part of your regular diet; commercially available soy is typically genetically modified, and contains isoflavones that may disrupt normal endocrine function.

PROCESSED VEGETABLE + SEED OILS:

Vegetable and seed oils are processed with chemical solvents like hexane in order to remove offending odors and flavors—but that's not all. These oils are also high in omega-6 polyunsaturated fatty acids, and highly susceptible to oxidation and rancidity. Yuck.

ALCOHOL:

Face it: booze isn't great for your liver or your judgment.

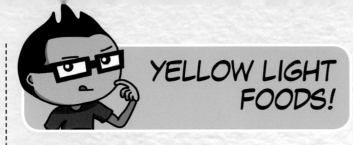

YELLOW LIGHT FOODS!

GREEN LIGHT FOODS!

FRUIT:

Don't get me wrong: fruit is awesome. But don't eat it in place of vegetables, which are generally more rich in vitamins and nutrients (and lower in sugar). It's particularly easy to overconsume dried fruits, so don't spike your sugar levels by gorging on an entire bag of raisins.

NUTS + SEEDS:

In order to properly prepare nuts and seeds for human consumption, you have to soak, sprout, and dehydrate them, which is a lot of work for something that nature didn't intend for us to eat in large quantities. It's fine to use nuts and seeds to add texture and flavor to your dishes, but don't go nuts with nuts.

STARCHES:

If you're trying to lose body fat, starches aren't your best bet. But if you're lean, active, and looking to replenish your muscle glycogen after a hard workout, eat some starchy foods like chestnuts, plantains, beets, taro, peeled white or sweet potatoes, or other tubers.

DAIRY:

Full-fat dairy from pastured, grass-fed ruminants can be a fantastically nutrient-rich source of protein, calcium, conjugated linoleic acid, and fat-soluble vitamins A, D, and K_2. However, in some people, dairy can also trigger a host of health issues, from histamine responses to acne. If you're worried you might have a sensitivity to dairy, try removing it from your diet for 30 days; then, slowly reintroduce it to see how it affects you.

By the way, with the exception of ghee (a traditional Indian preparation of clarified butter which removes any potentially problematic milk solids), all but one of the recipes in this book are dairy-free. (But personally, I do eat small amounts of high-quality dairy in the form of grass-fed butter and raw heavy cream in my coffee.)

NATURAL SWEETENERS:

If you're treating yourself to a sweet treat on a special occasion, try to stick with those that are sweetened with a bit of maple syrup or raw honey—and not agave nectar, which (despite its "all-natural" reputation) is actually a highly processed, high-fructose product.

ANIMAL PROTEIN:

The most sustainable, healthful, and flavorful animal protein comes from healthy beasts that chow on whatever nature intended them to eat. So prioritize grass-fed (and grass-finished) beef, lamb, and goat, as well as wild game. (Eat the odd bits, too!) These animals offer meat that's full of anti-inflammatory omega-3 polyunsaturated fatty acids, antioxidants, and other nutrients.

By the way, you won't find any grass-fed pigs because they're omnivores. Instead, look for fully pastured pork. It's your best bet if you love swine. Choose pastured chicken and eggs, too—not just for health reasons, but also for ethical and environmental ones.

Wild-caught sustainable seafood is another excellent source of protein packed with vitamins, minerals, and beneficial long-chain omega-3 fatty acids. Consult the Monterey Bay Aquarium Seafood Watch for the latest recommendations, and then go get some.

VEGETABLES:

Everything your mom told you about the health benefits of vegetables is true (except the stuff about how spinach instantly quadruples the size of your biceps so you can pummel your bearded romantic rival). Buy in-season, pesticide-free produce at your local farmer's market, and supplement with frozen organic veggies.

HEALTHY COOKING FATS:

Don't make the mistake of demonizing all dietary fats simply because some aren't good for you. Instead, head over to page 29 to read my top picks for cooking fats.

FERMENTED FOODS:

One of the best things you can do for your health is to eat fermented foods like sauerkraut, kimchi, kombucha, and coconut kefir. There's a reason why most traditional diets include probiotics: fermentation increases the good bacteria, vitamins, and enzymes in foods, and makes nutrients more available for absorption by our bodies. Plus, fermented foods are tasty.

SPICES:

Spices make life worth living. That is all.

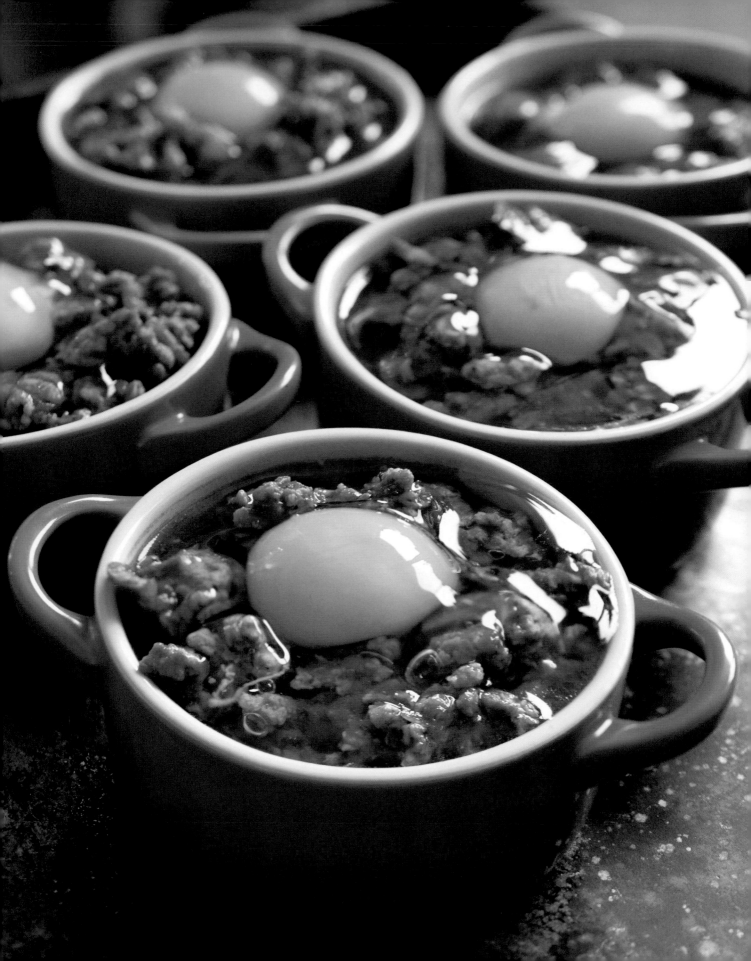

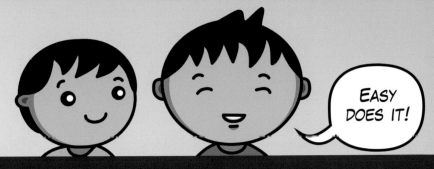

EASY DOES IT!

IT'S ALL ABOUT SIMPLE FEASTS FOR MODERN BEASTS.

Paleo eating can seem daunting and mysterious, but my goal is to help translate the "rules of the road" into delicious, easy-to-prepare meals for you and your family. In this book, you'll find recipes that reflect the way I eat on an everyday basis—and I'm the queen of lazy, so if I can do this, you can, too.

Overall, my diet is fairly "clean." I cook entirely gluten- and soy-free, and steer clear of legumes and processed seed and vegetable oils. I rarely make "Paleo-fied" treats like pancakes or cookies, but I'm not "Paleo perfect." Sometimes, a bit of sugar will creep into my diet (in the form of super-dark chocolate), and I've been known to cook with butter. But that's me. Your approach to Paleo doesn't have to mirror mine—it just needs to work for *you*.

Certainly, if you're on a weight-loss journey, suffering from an immunological disorder, or committing to a month-long dietary reset, a strict approach to Paleo may be the ticket. But remember: this is not about slavishly and mindlessly mimicking the diets of our Paleolithic ancestors. This template simply gives us a starting point from which to decide how to feed ourselves in the modern world. I make my own choices by considering the health risks and consequences of the foods I eat—and I also weigh the gustatory experience, too. Here's my approach:

STICK TO THE PALEO ROADMAP.

Yes, there may be an occasional detour, and every now and then, some gastronomic off-roading can be fun and well worth the indulgence. But we need to keep picking ourselves up and moving in the right direction, which means avoiding dietary potholes like gluten, soy, added sugar, processed junk, and other inflammatory foods as much as possible.

SIMPLE AND QUICK DOES THE TRICK.

Cooking becomes an overwhelming chore when we get too wrapped up in frustratingly complicated, time-consuming recipes. To be practical and sustainable, ancestral eating has to be easy. I have my hands full as a night shift worker and a busy mom, so I'm always on the lookout for shortcuts in the kitchen. But despite my emphasis on convenience…

IT BETTER BE CRAZY DELICIOUS.

I've heard it before: "I could never go Paleo—there's nothing to eat."

What these skeptics mean is that they can't conceive of Paleo fare being anywhere near as scrumptious as their meals at the diner down the street, or as satisfying as the crinkly bag of half-eaten fluorescent cheese poofs next to them on the couch. To get people to maintain a Paleo lifestyle, it's important to show how food can be healthy *and* insanely good.

The recipes in this book were created with these three guiding principles in mind. Sure, you might quibble with a couple of my strategies and ingredients; I'll concede right now that cavemen didn't use pressure cookers or make ghee. But everything was designed with an eye toward practicality, sustainability, and deliciousness. My recipes feature a depth and complexity of flavor that will keep you coming back for seconds and thirds.

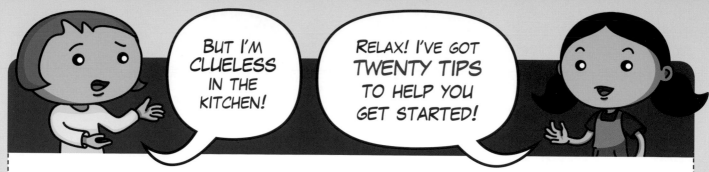
1. READ THE RECIPE FIRST.

Have you ever realized halfway through cooking a new recipe that you're missing a key ingredient? It's a gut punch, so take a minute or two to read—and understand—all the instructions from start to finish before you dive in. And if you're planning a multi-dish meal, be sure to pick recipes that can be prepared at the same time. It's kind of impossible to simultaneously oven-roast three dishes at three different temperatures if you have only one oven.

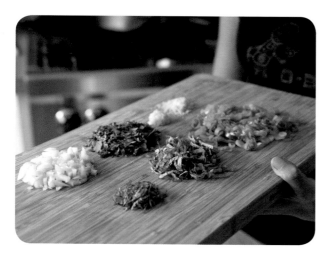

2. SET YOUR MISE EN PLACE.

In French, *mise en place* means "set in place," and refers to a key kitchen practice: preparing ingredients in advance. Before you start cooking, measure out your dry and wet ingredients, take out your kitchen gadgets and equipment, and do your chopping, mincing, slicing, and dicing. Setting your *mise en place* will enable you to cook without distraction.

3. GET A HEAD START ON AROMATICS.

Professional chefs often keep tubs of *mirepoix* (chopped carrots, onions, and celery) or *soffritto* (chopped onions, garlic, and celery) handy so they can quickly add an aromatic foundation to everything from soups and stews to braises and sauces. This isn't mandatory, but it can't hurt—especially if you find yourself routinely cooking for a crowd.

4. CLEAN AS YOU GO.

No one wants to tackle a gigantic pile of dirty pots and pans at the end of the night. Besides, it doesn't take much to clean up as you cook. Just keep a towel handy, and toss all your kitchen scraps into a large bowl as you go along. (I'll admit it: I stole this marvelous "garbage bowl" idea from Rachael Ray.)

5. "MEAT" YOUR DEFROST BOWL.

There's nothing magical about my defrost bowl: it's just a big container in my fridge that I use to thaw frozen meat. Every few days, I transfer some meat from my freezer to my trusty defrost bowl. Then, when it's time to cook, I grab whatever's no longer icy. My defrost bowl serves another purpose, too: it forces me to cook my meat before it spoils, which keeps me from stuffing my face with take-out.

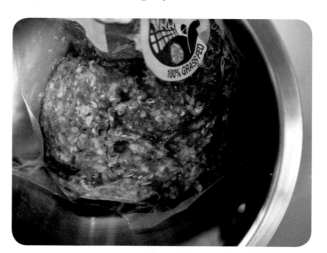

6. QUICK-THAW MEAT.

Need a faster way to thaw your frozen foods? Soak 'em in a hot water bath. It takes just minutes to thaw small to medium cuts of meat. As food guru Harold McGee points out, all you have to do is submerge the packaged meat in hot tap water for 15 to 30 minutes or until thawed, and you'll be good to go. (The ex-germophobe in me was highly skeptical of this process, but don't be alarmed; studies show that this is perfectly safe.)

7. DIVERSIFY YOUR COOKING METHODS.

One-pot meals can be a life-saver, but don't narrow your focus to a single method of cooking at the expense of learning others. By deploying a variety of different approaches to food prep, you can have a roast in the oven and still whip up a number of sides using your stove, steamer, slow cooker, pressure cooker, or backyard grill. Not only will you become a more efficient kitchen ninja, but you'll also enjoy a wider range of flavors and textures.

8. MAKE SURE YOUR OVEN'S READY.

Oven thermometers are cheap, so invest in one and make sure your oven's properly calibrated. Hot spots can also be a problem, so if you know that a certain corner of your oven runs hotter, do your best to avoid it, or rotate your food to make sure it cooks evenly. Obviously, if the dish you're making requires the use of an oven, preheat it in advance, and make sure the racks are placed at the appropriate levels. Then, while the temperature's rising, you can leisurely prep your ingredients. Make your oven wait for you, and not the other way around.

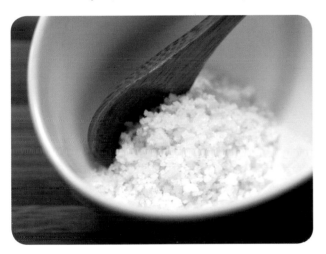

9. KNOW YOUR SALT.

Salt is a healthy, essential seasoning for just about any dish, but selecting the right kind to use can be baffling. Personally, I prefer kosher salt and sea salt to regular table salt, which is highly processed and often contains chemical additives like dextrose and ferric ferrocyanide. Most of my recipes in this book call for kosher salt—and by "kosher salt," I mean Diamond Crystal brand, and not the denser crystals made by Morton's. Remember: not all salts are created equal. If you're using Morton's kosher salt or fine sea salt (or have only table salt on hand), use roughly half the amount specified in my recipes.

10. SALT MEATS EARLY.

I typically try to season my meats with salt at least a few hours (and up to a couple of days) before cooking. At first, the salt draws moisture from the meat, but once the protein fibers loosen up, they'll reabsorb the savory juices, resulting in a more tender and succulent dish. When salting meat, here's a good rule of thumb from Chef Judy Rodgers of San Francisco's Zuni Café: for every 4 pounds of meat, season with 1 tablespoon of kosher salt.

11. BLOT BEFORE YOU SEAR.

If you want to develop a nice char on your steaks and roasts (and who doesn't?), use a paper towel to thoroughly dry your meat before applying high heat. Otherwise, the moist surface will yield steam instead of tasty brown bits. Alternatively, let your salted meat rest uncovered in the fridge for a day or two before cooking.

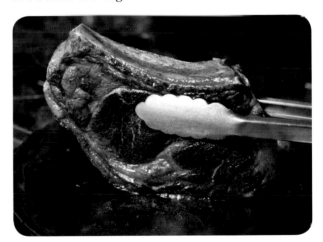

12. MAKE SURE YOUR PAN IS HOT.

If you're searing your proteins, be sure to start with a hot pan that's spacious enough to accommodate the contents with room to spare. Otherwise, your food won't develop the delicious sear you're after. Test your skillet for heat by adding a bit of cooking fat; once it shimmers, you'll know the pan's ready for action. Also, don't keep moving the meat around the pan. Be patient; the meat should remain in contact with the bottom of the skillet until the browned edges naturally release.

13. HAVE A TASTE OR TWO (OR SEVEN).

Only you know what your palate likes best, so don't be afraid to taste your food during each (edible) step of the cooking process, and adjust the seasoning accordingly.

14. THE BROILER IS YOUR FRIEND.

Don't be afraid of your oven's broiler setting. I'm convinced that more folks would use their broilers if only they knew of the versatility of this tool. There's a reason why salamander broilers are a mainstay in virtually every professional kitchen: broilers can be used to quickly cook everything from thin stalks of asparagus to herb-stuffed whole fish. Just make sure your food is 4 to 6 inches away from the heating element, and watch it like a hawk to prevent scorching or burning. After all, there are better ways to test the smoke alarms in your house.

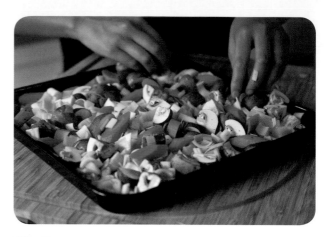

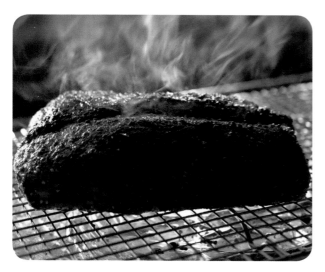

15. REST YOUR MEAT.

Even after a hunk of meat is removed from the heat source, it'll continue to cook. The bigger the piece of meat, the greater the rise in internal temperature. If you slice into the meat right away, the compression of the muscle fibers caused by the cooking process will push the meat's juices out all over your cutting board. But once the meat has cooled slightly (5 to 10 minutes), its muscle fibers will relax and widen, enabling it to retain more of its innate juiciness. So give it a rest, people.

16. GO AGAINST THE GRAIN.

By cutting meat against the grain, you're actually tenderizing it before your teeth get in on the action. A piece of meat is made of muscle fibers and connective tissues, and while our pearly choppers are usually up to the job of gnawing and mashing them up, slicing meat against the grain (perpendicular to the direction of the muscle fibers) makes it easier for your teeth and jaws to do their thing. To find the grain, gently pull at the meat in opposite directions at the same time, and all will be revealed.

17. ROAST OFF YOUR VEGETABLES.

Don't let your vegetables rot in the fridge. Before stocking up on fresh produce, take all the uneaten veggies out of the crisper, and slice them up. Toss the pieces in a baking tray with some fresh herbs, kosher salt, pepper, and your favorite cooking fat. Roast it all in the oven at 425°F for 30 to 45 minutes or until the vegetables are toasty on the outside and tender on the inside. Eat 'em with everything.

18. ONE WORD: BRINNER.

You can't go wrong with breakfast for dinner, or dinner for breakfast. After all, there's no rule that says that your first meal of the day must pop out of a toaster or waffle iron. Likewise, there's nothing stopping you from dishing up sunny-side-up eggs and a rasher of bacon for dinner (with a big side of vegetables, of course).

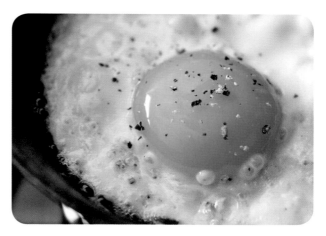

19. ALWAYS MAKE EXTRA.

There's no such thing as too many leftovers. Even if you're cooking only for yourself, a fridge packed with fully cooked emergency protein and vegetables can be a life-saver when you're pressed for time.

20. Ooh, Mommy: Use Umami!

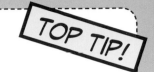

Last but not least, here's my favorite tip of all: stock up on ingredients that boost umami, like fish sauce, mushrooms, and tomatoes. My obsession with deliciousness is matched only by my laziness—and simply adding umami-rich ingredients allows me to maximize flavor with minimal effort.

But what exactly *is* umami?

Until the late 1800s, the conventional wisdom was that humans can detect only four fundamental tastes: sweet, salty, sour, and bitter.

But then along came Auguste Escoffier, the author of *Le Guide Culinaire*, and one of the greatest chefs of the late nineteenth century. Escoffier began serving up dishes that tasted like nothing anyone had experienced before, like *tournedos Rossini*, a filet mignon served with foie gras and black truffles. The chef's secret ingredient, however, was a special reduction made of veal stock. Foods cooked with Escoffier's veal stock tasted more robust, complex, and satisfying—even though the stock itself wasn't sweet, salty, sour, or bitter.

Escoffier had stumbled upon the fifth taste: *umami*.

In Japanese, "umami" means "deliciousness," and describes a robust, savory, mouth-filling quality to food. How did Japan get the naming rights even though Escoffier was wowing rich European diners with his umami-packed dishes in France? Because no one could put their finger on this fifth taste until a University of Tokyo chemist named Kikunae Ikeda did some detective work in 1907.

For generations, Japanese cooks had used a seaweed stock called *dashi* to imbue their food with a unique richness. Intrigued by this effect, Ikeda did some digging, and finally uncovered the essence of this flavor: a chemical compound called glutamate and ribonucleotides like inosinate and guanylate.

WHEN SOMETHING TASTES INSANELY AWESOME IN A WAY THAT'S NOT SWEET, SALTY, SOUR, OR BITTER, GUESS WHAT? YOU'RE EXPERIENCING UMAMI!

And here's the best thing about umami-rich foods: when you combine them, the sum tastes even better than the parts. That's right: you can exponentially kick up the flavor dimensions of a dish simply by adding the right mix of components.

That's why Big-O Bacon Burgers (page 226) are so nomtastic. They combine beef, bacon, and mushrooms—all of which are high in umami. And with just a handful of rich, savory ingredients, Slow Cooker Kalua Pig (page 234) has a flavor-to-effort ratio that's off the charts.

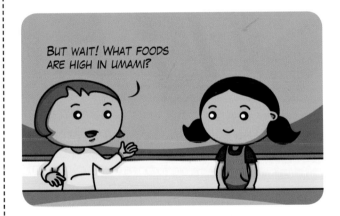

BUT WAIT! WHAT FOODS ARE HIGH IN UMAMI?

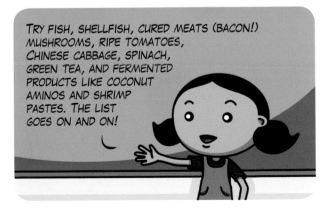

TRY FISH, SHELLFISH, CURED MEATS (BACON!) MUSHROOMS, RIPE TOMATOES, CHINESE CABBAGE, SPINACH, GREEN TEA, AND FERMENTED PRODUCTS LIKE COCONUT AMINOS AND SHRIMP PASTES. THE LIST GOES ON AND ON!

Even if you don't have these ingredients on hand, you can instantly amp up your dishes with just a splash of fish sauce or a pinch of Magic Mushroom Powder (page 35). You're welcome!

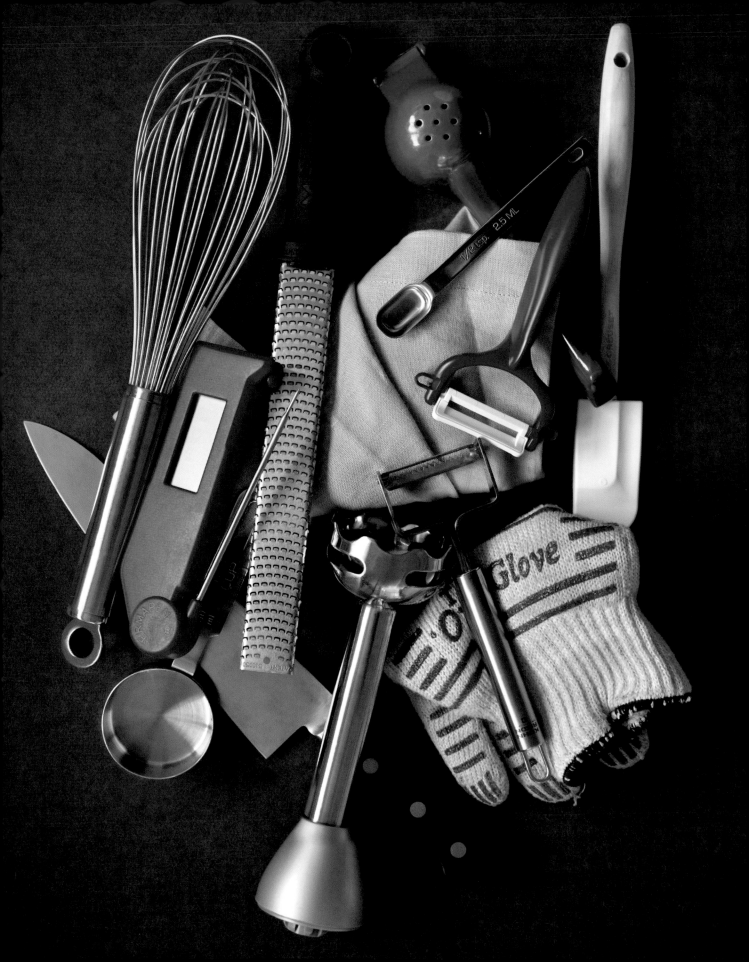

TOOL TIME!

I'll admit it: I'm a gadget queen. I spend hardly any money on clothes or shoes, and jewelry ain't my thing. But drop me off at a kitchen supply store, and you'll need to return with a truck to help me haul my purchases home. I'm always on the lookout for quality equipment that'll streamline and enhance the cooking experience. Plus, they're just plain fun.

But does everyone need fancy doodads to cook like a champ? Not at all. Just because I compulsively hoard cooking tools doesn't mean you need to spend a fortune to outfit your kitchen. You can throw together insanely delicious meals with nothing more than a few versatile basics. Remember: with an unlimited budget (and infinite storage space), anyone can assemble a dream kitchen with every tricked-out piece of equipment imaginable—but it won't guarantee culinary success. Kitchen tools are helpful, but it's the quality of the ingredients and what you actually do with your equipment that counts.

CHEF'S KNIFE

Have you ever noticed how professional chefs carry their knives around with them? It's not just because pointy blades are handy in a street fight. Knives are a chef's most valuable and versatile tool; even when there's no heat source in sight, a good cook with a sharp knife can create something wonderful.

Get yourself a sturdy, well-balanced chef's knife made of carbon or stainless steel—its broad, tapered blade makes for a great all-purpose kitchen knife. You'll be spending a lot of time with this indispensable tool, so get yourself a good one. Look for high-quality full-tang or forged knives. Hand-wash and hand-dry your blades, and keep them sharp. Treat your chef's knife with care, and it'll be your best friend in the kitchen for years to come.

PARING KNIFE

A small, short-bladed paring knife is useful in situations where a bigger blade is too cumbersome. You don't have to splurge on an expensive paring knife, though; even a cheap one—if it's kept sharp—can help make quick work of small, detailed tasks on the cutting board.

CUTTING BOARD

Choosing a cutting board can present a baffling dilemma: Should you get a wooden or plastic one? If you get a wooden one, should you choose an end-grain or edge-grain board? How big should it be? What about food safety concerns? Here's my take: you should invest in an end-grain wooden cutting board. The latest research suggests that contrary to popular belief, plastic cutting boards are more prone to contamination. Of course, your personal preferences (and budget) will ultimately dictate your selection, but whatever you do, choose a durable, heavy board that offers plenty of cutting space and a satiny, knife-gripping surface. You're going to be doing a lot of slicing and chopping on this baby, so invest in a quality board.

KITCHEN SHEARS

A sharp pair of scissors can help handle a host of tasks in the kitchen, from trimming herbs to butterflying chicken. Choose well-balanced, high-carbon stainless steel shears with micro-serrations on the blades to help firmly grip the slippery foods you'll be cutting. And for easy cleaning, make sure the blades can be fully separated.

Knife Sharpener

Think sharp knives are more dangerous than dull ones? Think again. Always keep your blades honed for maximum precision, efficiency, and safety.

Peelers

I keep three vegetable peelers in the kitchen: one with a regular blade, one with a serrated edge for grabbing on to smooth-skinned vegetables and fruit, and one that makes quick work of julienning zucchini into "spaghetti." Always keep in mind that peelers aren't just for peeling—they can also make fine edible shavings of vegetables for garnishes, pickles, and salads.

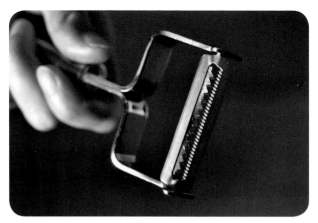

Rasp Grater

If you're serious about cooking, you need a rasp grater. Originally designed for use by woodworkers, rasp graters have since been adopted by home cooks and culinary pros who use them to finely zest citrus and grate ginger. This grater's tiny, sharp teeth slice food into delicate ribbons, thereby increasing the surface area of the food and intensifying the flavors that hit your tongue.

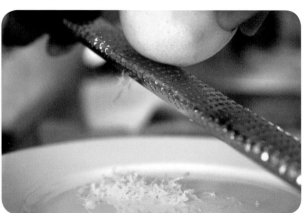

Spatulas

Are you tired of your cheap plastic spatulas melting into misshapen lumps of goo? Get some spatulas with silicone heads. They're heat-resistant, non-stick, and food-safe. Pick spatulas with flat heads; that way, you can scrape food against the rim of a bowl or slip it cleanly under the edge of a fried egg.

Tongs

No need to buy anything fancy here; just get a basic pair of locking tongs with wide-scalloped pincers.

Pepper Mill

If you don't have one, get one. I'm serious. Just about every single one of my recipes demands ground black pepper. Besides, freshly cracked peppercorns taste a bazillion times more intense and flavorful than the stuff that comes out of a shaker.

Measuring Cups + Spoons

When buying liquid measuring cups, avoid plastic ones. Go with glass, which will withstand the heat of the steaming broths and sizzling oils you're going to pour into them. And when selecting measuring spoons, choose the narrow, flat-bottomed ones; not only will they actually fit inside the mouths of your spice containers, but you can rest them on your kitchen counter without fear of spills.

Instant-Read Thermometer

Want to prepare perfectly cooked slow-roasted meats? Get yourself an instant-read probe thermometer with a display that sits outside the oven. It's not expensive, so don't be penny-wise and pound-foolish: invest in a good thermometer so you don't screw up your pricy meat.

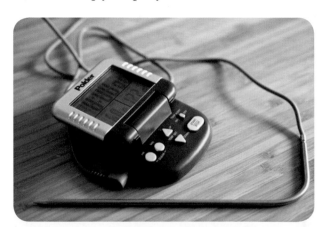

Oven Mitts / Gloves

Got an oven? Then you'll need oven mitts (unless, of course, you happen to be a robot). Yes, towels work fine, too, but I prefer to slip on a pair of super-heat-resistant Kevlar or Nomex gloves with five fingers for maximum dexterity.

Wire Racks

You can never have too many wire racks. Besides, they don't take up much storage space. Use them to keep your roasted meats from sitting in a puddle of grease in the oven or to make sure your crispy chicken nuggets don't go limp and soggy.

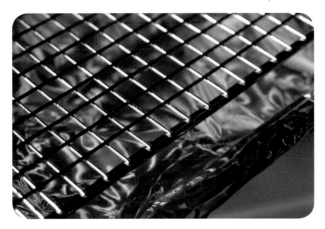

Rimmed Baking Sheets

Cookie sheets can be used for much more than just baking cookies. Use 'em to roast meats and veggies or to crisp up batches of kale chips.

Skillets (8-inch + 12-inch)

For just a fraction of the cost of copper or clad metal cookware, cast-iron skillets offer super-efficient heat conduction and retention. Once properly seasoned, cast iron develops a natural nonstick finish, and doesn't react to or absorb the flavors of the food you're cooking. To maintain these skillets, scrub them clean with hot water (but no soap or detergent), and then wipe them dry before rubbing a bit of melted fat onto all surfaces. If you're cooking acidic foods, however, use enameled cast-iron or stainless steel pans with copper or aluminum cores.

Saucepan

A saucepan is essentially a high-sided pan. This little pot is super-versatile: use a saucepan for everything from boiling eggs to heating leftovers.

Dutch Oven

A Dutch oven is a heavy, enamel-coated, high-sided pot made of cast iron. With excellent heat retention and tight-fitting lids, these pots help ensure even cooking and are perfect for soups, braises, and stews. Sear meat in a Dutch oven on the stove, and then pop it into the oven to finish cooking. Dutch ovens can be expensive, so if you're still saving up for one, use a heavy-gauge pot with a lid for now.

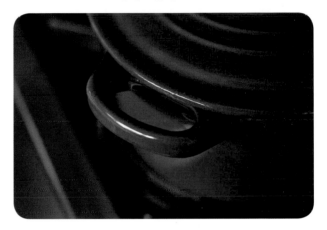

Stockpot

You probably have room for just one stockpot, so get one that's big enough to handle a multitude of tasks, from simmering broths to boiling crabs.

Food Processor

Food processors can be expensive, but focus on value rather than cost. Think about it: Would you rather be hanging out with your family and friends, or weeping over a cutting board piled high with raw onions and wishing you'd bought a food processor?

Blender

Immersion blenders (also known as stick blenders) aren't expensive, and they're perfect for quickly puréeing soups, sauces, marinades, and mashes—as well as for whipping up condiments like Paleo Mayonnaise (page 40). A full-sized blender can accomplish the same thing (I'm awfully fond of my high-powered Vitamix), but an immersion blender is often the best choice for lazy home cooks like me who don't want to wash a bunch of extra stuff.

Pressure Cooker + Slow Cooker

Ready to read my love letters to these time-saving appliances? Turn the page!

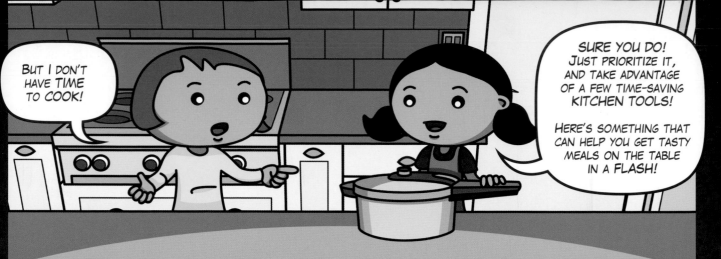

COOK UNDER PRESSURE!

Pressure cooking is a game-changer—especially for home cooks with hectic schedules like me. When I'm pressed for time but craving foods that usually take forever to prepare (like bone broth, tough cuts of meat, or braised winter vegetables), I turn to one of my pressure cookers. Dinner will be on the table in minutes instead of hours.

But what *is* a pressure cooker?

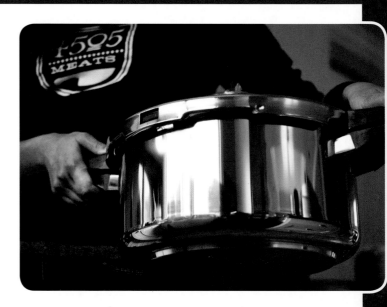

A pressure cooker is a specialized pot with a locking, airtight lid and a valve system that regulates the internal temperature. These pots can raise the temperature of boiling water under pressure, thereby cooking food faster. When a sealed pot is heated, the pressure from the steam raises the temperature up to 250°F, forcing the steam—a fantastically efficient heat conductor—through foods, thus shortening the cooking time by as much as two-thirds. What's more, with all the liquids kept in the pot, the contents are guaranteed to be tender and concentrated with intense flavors. Pressure-cooked foods also retain all the nutrients that ordinarily get lost in the cooking process.

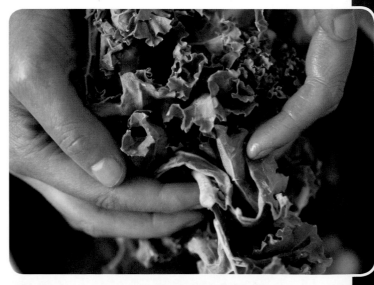

Although pressure cookers are popular in many parts of the world, many home cooks in Western societies have never used one. If you're among the uninitiated, don't be afraid to try it. Pressure cookers have been around for 300 years, and modern versions are packed to the gills with safety features and back-up safety valves, so accidents are exceedingly rare. Like riding a bicycle, pressure cooking can seem tricky and daunting at first, but with just a little practice, you'll soon revel in the freedom it affords you. Whee!

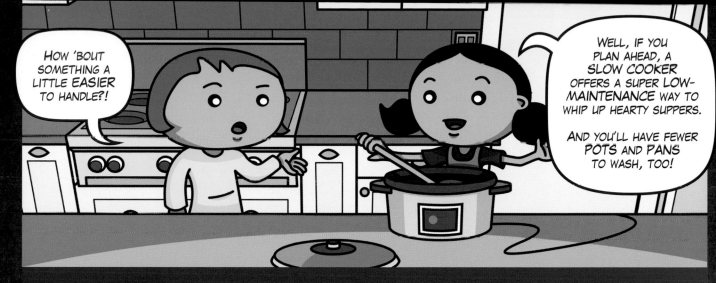

SET IT AND FORGET IT!

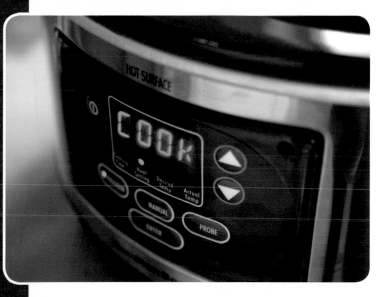

Cover your ears, Paleo people. I'm about to let you in on a deep, dark secret about slow cookers: when it first came to market in the early 1970s, the beloved appliance that we routinely use to simmer savory, meaty stews was originally intended for cooking beans.

Luckily, slow cookers have proved much more versatile. This cheap, no-frills countertop appliance offers an easy way for us to cook food at a low, steady temperature for hours. There's no need to babysit the pot—just set it and forget about it. After working a long night shift, I like to chuck the components of a hearty stew into my slow cooker before conking out; eight hours later, I wake to the intoxicating aroma of a delicious, ready-made meal. My family gets a home-cooked supper, and I get to sleep in. Win-win.

Best of all, the slow cooker's low temperature and prolonged simmering helps to break down the collagen in meat; as a result, even tough cuts end up perfectly tenderized. But remember:

1. Unless you're a fan of overcooked food, don't use the "high" setting; it's much too hot for low, slow cooking.

2. Resist the temptation to add more liquid to the pot than the recipe specifies. Your ingredients will release (and cook in) their own juices, and the slow cooker will trap all the liquid, so there shouldn't be any need to add extra moisture to the dish. For example, my Slow Cooker Kalua Pig (page 234) is prepared with no additional liquid at all.

STOCKING YOUR PALEO KITCHEN

Okay—you've tossed out all your dried pasta and beans. Your vegetable oil's been relegated to the trash bin of history, and that unopened tub of peanut butter's in the garbage, next to all your boxes of crackers and sugary cereal. Now what?

Simple: fill your kitchen with the good stuff that's going into your family's belly.

Your kitchen should be well-stocked with real, whole, nourishing grub: grass-fed and pastured meats, fresh vegetables and fruit, healthy cooking fats, seasonings, spices, and condiments.

Here are some key ingredients to help you get started:

LEAFY GREENS

Pick your favorite greens, and keep plenty of them on hand. Butter lettuce is great for wraps, spinach and kale are wonderful in salads, and cabbage is terrific in stews. Choose fresh, bright, in-season greens, and find ways to incorporate them into your main dishes or sides. Or if you're super-lazy (like I can be), buy a few bags of pre-washed greens—it's better than not eating your veggies.

CRUCIFEROUS VEGETABLES

Cauliflower, broccoli, cabbage, bok choy, and other cruciferous vegetables (a.k.a. "brassicas") are incredibly versatile: roast them in fat, stir-fry them, throw them in stews and braises, or steam and mash them.

AVOCADOS

I always stock up on bags of avocados at our neighborhood warehouse store. Once they're ripe, I put them in the fridge where they'll keep for at least a week. Avocados are a great source of monounsaturated fats, and they're just plain yummy. We keep them on hand to quickly make guacamole (see page 51) and to top lettuce-wrapped tacos or scrambled eggs.

MUSHROOMS

Mushrooms—both fresh and dried—are rich in glutamate, making them a first-rate flavor enhancer. Toss them in your savory dishes for a blast of umami. (By the way, you should always store fresh mushrooms in a paper bag in the refrigerator. No one likes slimy mushrooms.)

ASPARAGUS

I know spring has sprung when I spy these perky green spears at the local farmer's market. Asparagus is easy to prepare: lop off the woody ends, coat them with ghee, season with salt and pepper, and broil for a few minutes. Drizzle with lemon juice or balsamic vinegar, and you'll have an instant side dish.

NIGHTSHADES

Nightshades like tomatoes, eggplants, and peppers add deep, rich flavors to cooked dishes, but they're also high in alkaloids, which can cause problems for some folks. I've never felt any ill effects from eating these foods, so I incorporate them in many of my cooked dishes—but if you find that you're particularly sensitive to alkaloids, avoid them.

GOURDS + SQUASHES

No matter the season, squashes play a big role in my cooking. In the summertime, cucumbers and zucchini take center stage, and when it starts getting chilly, I turn to the warm, comforting flavors of butternut squash, pumpkins, and kabocha squash.

ROOTS + TUBERS

Need to feed your glycogen-starved muscles after a hard workout? Forget the sports drinks; grab some root vegetables instead. I prefer sweet potatoes, but you can also go for taro, carrots, beets, turnips, or whatever your heart desires. Bake 'em or roast 'em or nuke 'em or boil 'em or steam 'em, and you'll have a handy and tasty source of post-workout carbs. Frankly, I eat them even when I'm not exercising. They add sweetness and depth to all sorts of dishes, from braises and stews to purées and salads.

GINGER

Always keep fresh ginger root in your freezer. When you're ready to use it, just break off a knob, peel off some skin, and slice it into coins or finely grate it.

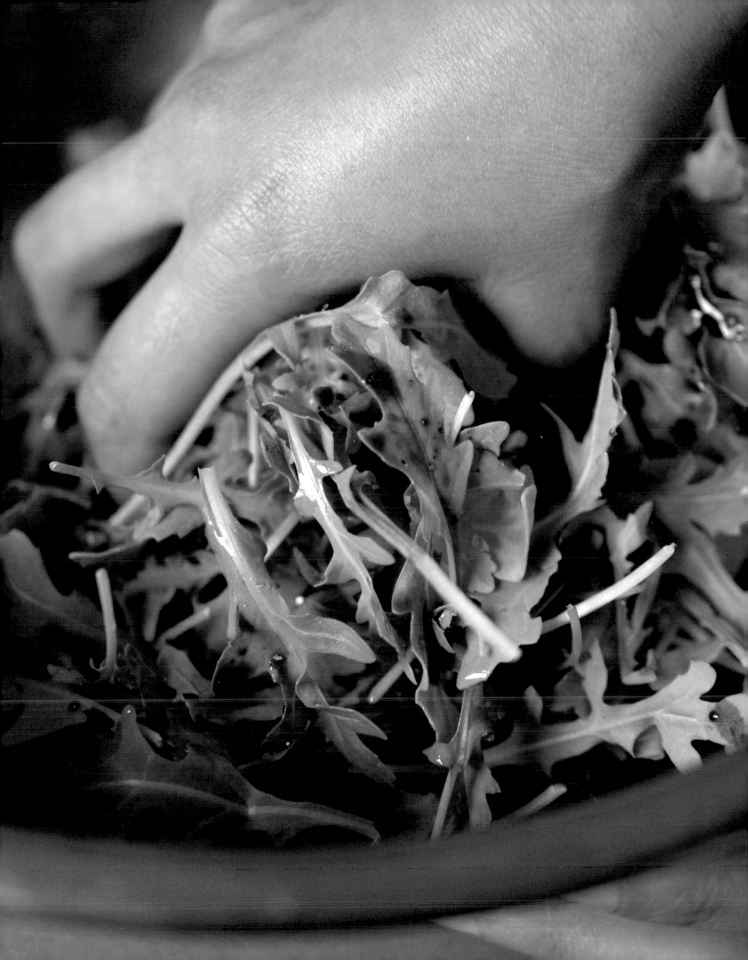

FRESH HERBS

Fresh herbs add brightness and flavor to your meals, so make sure you have plenty on hand. At the market, pick herbs with a clean, fresh aroma and vibrantly colored leaves. Better yet, grow your own herb garden. Make sure you always keep some fresh Italian parsley, cilantro, thyme, basil, and mint in your kitchen. I store my herbs wrapped in paper towels and sealed in an airtight bag. Kept this way, most herbs will last for up to a week in the fridge.

ALLIUMS

The word "allium" is derived from the Greek for garlic, and refers to the family of aromatic vegetables at the heart of my favorite savory dishes. Onions, garlic, shallots, leeks, and chives all belong to the allium family of plants, and I can't imagine life without them.

ASSORTED FROZEN VEGETABLES

Sometimes, you just need vegetables *stat*. That's why I keep bags of broccoli, spinach, carrots, winter squash, and green beans (yes, green beans are Paleo-compliant) in my freezer. It's easy to add them to stews, soups, and other dishes to round out my meals.

FERMENTED VEGETABLES

Containers of sauerkraut, kimchi, and pickles are always in my refrigerator. I love the tangy crunch these condiments add to my dishes. Plus, these lacto-fermented vegetables help promote the growth of healthy bacteria in your gut.

FRESH FRUIT + BERRIES

I don't often eat fruit as a snack—I don't crave the sugar, and there are plenty of other ways I can get my fill of fiber and phytonutrients. But that's not to say that we don't enjoy fruit. Fresh, organic strawberries and blueberries are wonderful in the summertime, as are apples in the fall. If you're looking to shed body fat, I suggest limiting your fruit intake, but otherwise, ripe, seasonal fruits can add a bright note of sweetness to your diet.

FROZEN FRUIT

Once upon a time, our family subsisted on "healthy" smoothies. Our freezer was packed with packages of frozen fruit, and it seemed like our blender was always whirring away on the counter. These days, we make smoothies only as an occasional treat, but I still keep a few bags of frozen berries in the fridge for those occasions when we need a burst of sweetness in a recipe or an icy treat like Summer Berry Soup (page 254) or Strawberry Banana Ice Cream (page 260).

ACIDS

Acids are a key component in cooking, and one of the most valuable flavor enhancers in your pantry. A splash of acid often adds much-needed tartness and brightness to your finished dishes. Plus, acids are responsible for tenderizing your proteins, keeping your sliced apples from turning brown, and making vinaigrettes possible. Use acidic ingredients such as vinegar or citrus as a counterpoint to the sweet, salty, or bitter notes in your cooking.

Vinegar lends a delicious acidity to your foods. Stock up on a variety of vinegars: apple cider vinegar, aged balsamic vinegar, sherry vinegar, red wine vinegar, and white vinegar, to name just a few. Each has distinct notes that can wake up your dishes in unique ways. For example, apple cider vinegar can lend your food a fruity sweetness, while aged balsamic vinegar offers a deep, dark, tangy-sweet intensity.

Similarly, a fresh squirt of citrus can nicely balance out the flavors in your recipes. That's why I keep a big bag of limes in my refrigerator (and "borrow" lemons from my neighbor's tree).

Remember: salt isn't the only ingredient at your disposal to adjust the flavors of a dish; acids can be an equally powerful seasoning.

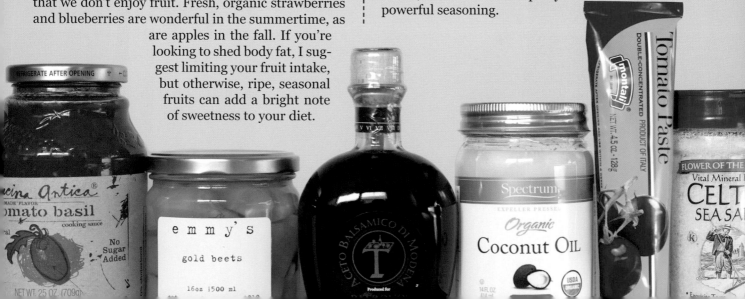

SALT

Some Paleo eaters avoid salt entirely, but I use kosher salt (the airy, flaky Diamond Crystal brand) in most of my savory dishes. I like its coarseness, which makes it easy to pinch and sprinkle. (This may explain why it's the standard cooking salt used by most chefs.) Plus, unlike table salt, kosher salt is free of additives, and it's not highly refined or processed. For a few recipes that call for a finer grain of salt or more complex flavor profiles, I opt for sea salt or flavored salts rather than processed table salt. Note, however, that kosher salt and sea salt have virtually no iodine content, so make sure you're getting enough iodine from other sources like seafood.

SPICES + SEASONINGS

Think Paleo food is bland? Nothing could be further from the truth. To be sustainable, Paleo eating has to be tasty, and spices go a long way toward perking up our palates. Seek out your local spice purveyor and follow your nose. Stock up on curry powder, red chile pepper flakes, Chinese five spice, cumin, cinnamon—whatever floats your boat. And don't be afraid to use them in your dishes. In our kitchen, we have two spice drawers, and they're overflowing with fragrant seasonings and blends.

FISH SAUCE

Fish sauce (called *nước mắm* in Vietnamese) is a staple ingredient in a number of Southeast Asian cultures. Anchovies and salt are fermented in wooden barrels and then slowly pressed to produce the intense, savory liquid. Yes, it smells a little gross, but don't judge a condiment by its nose. Just a splash of the stuff can lend a deep umami quality to all your dishes.

Sadly, most of the fish sauce in supermarkets and Asian grocery stores are full of additives: hydrolyzed wheat protein, sugar, MSG, chemical preservatives—you name it. Luckily, new Paleo-friendly fish sauces are becoming more widely available. Red Boat Fish Sauce—made with just anchovies and salt—is my favorite brand. Make sure you always have a bottle of this magical liquid at the ready.

ANCHOVIES

Keep a few tins of anchovies packed in olive oil in your pantry. If you don't have fish sauce, use some minced anchovy to subtly deepen the umami in your dishes.

CAPERS

I used to abhor capers and pick them out of my food, but over the years, I've come to develop a fondness for these bright and tart bursts of flavor. Stock a jar in your pantry in case of flavor emergencies.

COCONUT AMINOS

This dark, salty, aged coconut tree sap tastes remarkably similar to soy sauce, but without gluten or soy.

THAI CURRY PASTES

Raid your local Asian grocery for Paleo-friendly curry pastes. You'll be thankful for them when you realize you have guests coming over for dinner and no clue what to serve.

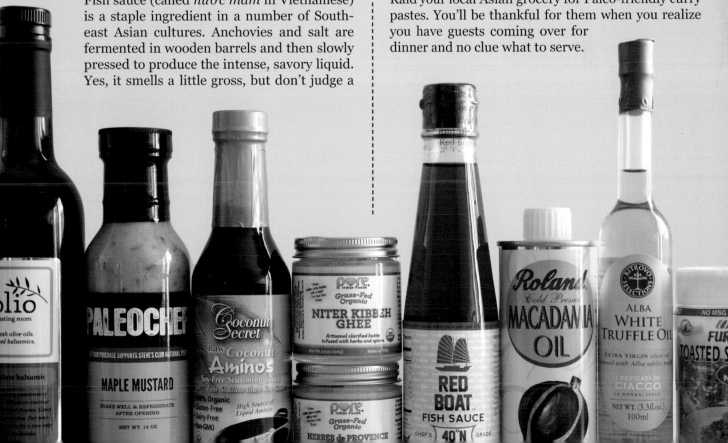

MUSTARD

The sharp, vinegary tang of Dijon-style mustard goes well with more than just sausages and roast beef. It acts as a tasty emulsifier in marinades, mayonnaise, and vinaigrettes, too.

PREPARED SAUCES + DRESSINGS

It's always better to make your own sauces and dressings from scratch, but to stay sane, I keep a few bottles of marinara sauce and various salad dressings in the pantry. All feature Paleo-friendly ingredients, and enable me to quickly throw together a meal.

TOMATO PASTE

Just one spoonful will add depth and umami to your stews and braises.

COCONUT MILK

When choosing coconut milk, always pick the shelf-stable, full-fat, sulfite-free variety in BPA-free cans.

COCONUT FLOUR + ALMOND FLOUR

I use these gluten-free flours sparingly, but once in a while, I'll grab some coconut flour or almond flour to whip up baked goods or to add a crunchy crust to savory dishes.

ARROWROOT POWDER + TAPIOCA FLOUR

Pure arrowroot powder is a gluten-free starch made from the pulp of arrowroot tubers. Tapioca flour is a similar starch, but it's derived from cassava root. A light dusting of either starch on the outside of your favorite protein yields a thin, crunchy coating on deep-fried items. Also, both can be used interchangeably as Paleo-friendly thickeners for sauces, puddings, and other foods. Note, however, that both arrowroot powder and tapioca flour lose their thickening power at high temperatures, so take your dish off the heat as soon as it's ready.

ANIMAL PROTEINS

Read about how to stock your fridge and freezer with healthy and sustainable meats, poultry, seafood, and eggs on pages 11 and 209.

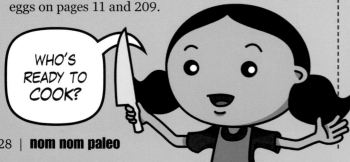

WHO'S READY TO COOK?

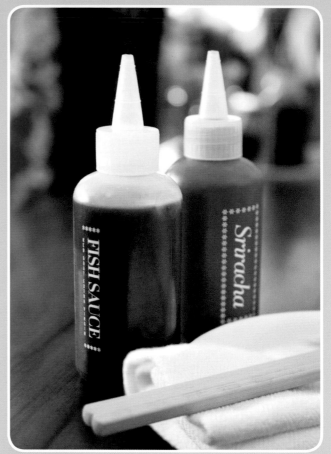

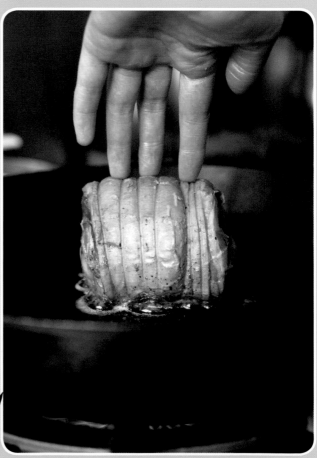

BUT WHAT ABOUT COOKING FATS?

Think that vegetable and seed oils are made by taking a bunch of garden-fresh veggies like kale and cabbage and squeezing 'em really, really hard until they release a stream of golden ooze? Nope. The vast majority of vegetable and seed oils found on supermarket shelves are highly processed with chemical solvents and full of omega-6 polyunsaturated fatty acids. These oils are so unstable that even when stored at room temperature, they oxidize and turn rancid to some degree. Heat accelerates this oxidation, and the formation of free radicals will assault the healthy cells in your body.

Instead, choose healthy saturated fats that remain stable when exposed to heat. And don't be afraid of the word "saturated." Most people assume it means that the fat is super-duper artery clogging, when it actually refers to the fact that there are no double-bonds between the individual carbon atoms of the fatty acid chain. In other words, the chain of carbon atoms is fully "saturated" with hydrogen atoms, making it more chemically stable.

Still skeptical? A meta-analysis of more than twenty studies covering a third of a million people over twenty-three years of age found that "[t]here is no significant evidence for concluding that dietary saturated fat is associated with an increased risk of coronary heart disease, stroke, or cardiovascular disease."[1]

GHEE

Ghee—a traditional Indian preparation of clarified butter—is infused with the rich flavor of butter, but without the potentially problematic milk solids. It's incredibly versatile, and over the years, ghee has become my favorite high-temperature cooking fat. My recipe for ghee is on page 36. (Of course, if you're okay with high-quality butter from grass-fed cows, more power to you. I happen to love cooking with it, too.)

RENDERED ANIMAL FATS

Lard, tallow, bacon drippings, and duck fat are wonderful cooking fats that infuse your foods with incredible flavor. But just to be clear, I'm talking about fats from grass-fed or pastured meats—not the pro-inflammatory animal fats from Concentrated Animal Feeding Operation (CAFO) beasties.

COCONUT OIL

At long last, scientists are finally recognizing the virtues of coconut oil and lauding this highly stable saturated fat for its antioxidant, antimicrobial, antibacterial, and antifungal properties. Coconut oil can also help with insulin control and protect against liver damage.

MACADAMIA NUT OIL

With its mild flavor, macadamia nut oil is a wonderful alternative to coconut oil—especially for those who can't stand even the faintest taste of coconut.

EXTRA-VIRGIN OLIVE OIL

Extra-virgin olive oil is best used uncooked or for low to medium-temperature cooking. I love drizzling the stuff on roasted vegetables and mixing it with acids to make flavorful salad dressings.

[1]Siri-Tarino P., Sun Q., Hu F. B., & Krauss R. M., "Meta-analysis of prospective cohort studies evaluating the association of saturated fat with cardiovascular disease," *Am J Clin Nutr.* 2010 March; 91(3): 535–546.

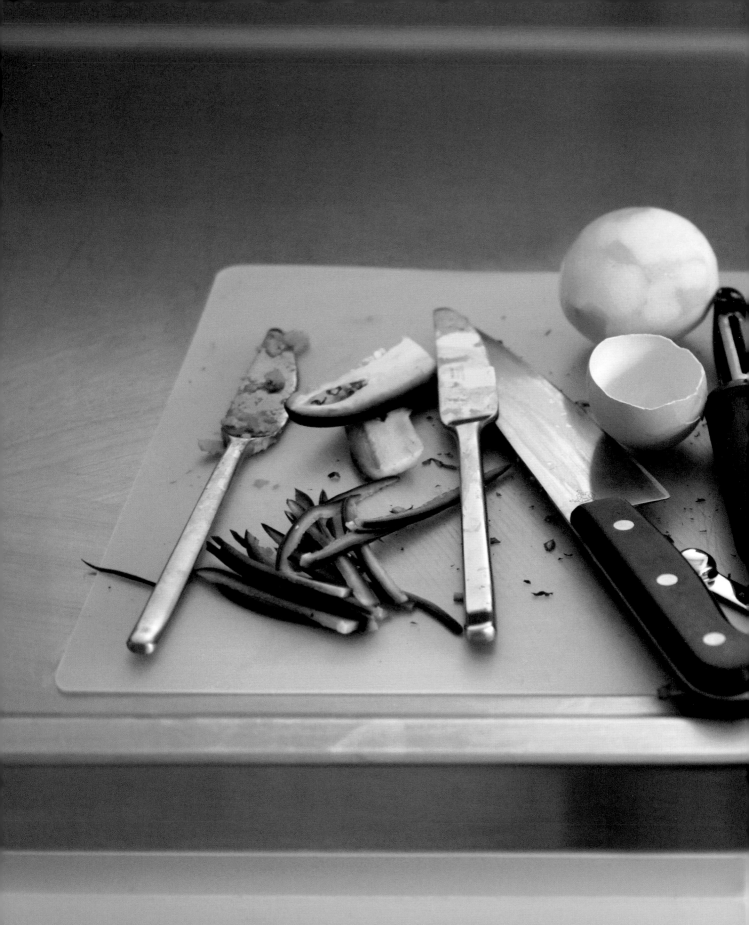

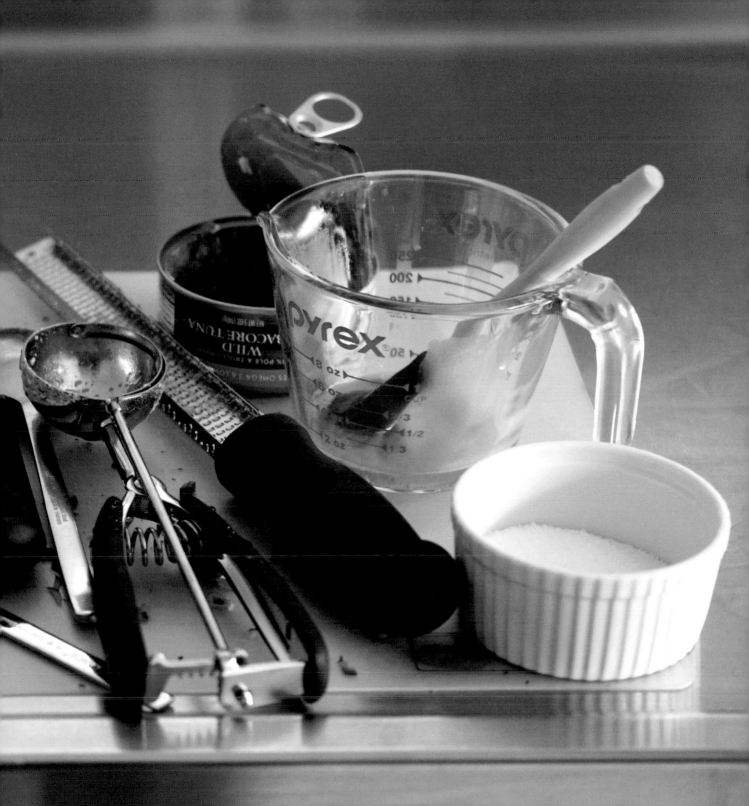

RECIPES:
FOOD FOR HUMANS

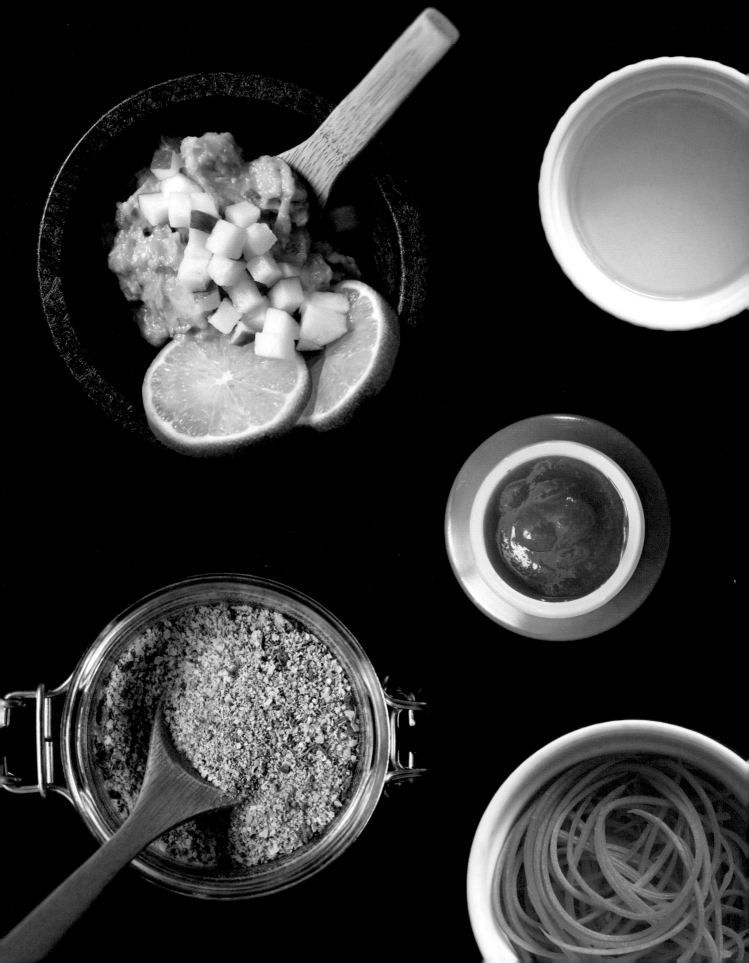

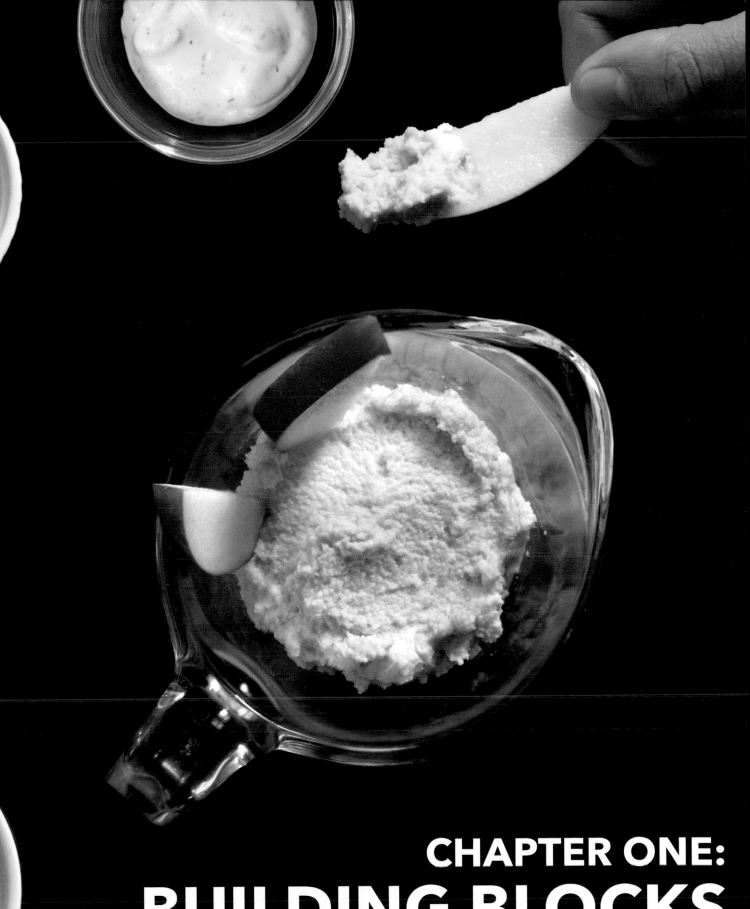

CHAPTER ONE:
BUILDING BLOCKS

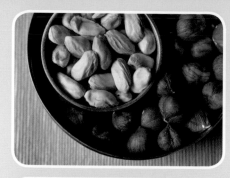
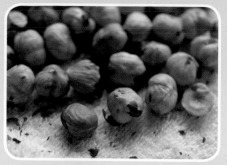
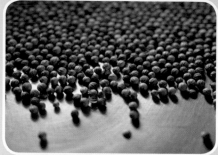
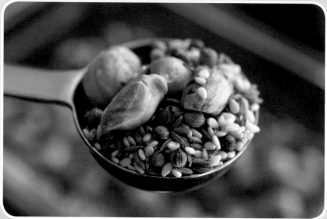
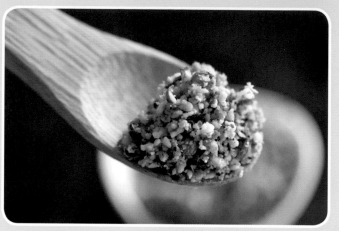

DUKKAH

Dukkah (pronounced *doo-kah*) is an ancient Egyptian spice blend traditionally served alongside olive oil as a "dip" for bread. But as an unrepentant bread-abstainer, I've found an even *better* use for this crumbly nut and spice blend: I sprinkle it on all sorts of meats and vegetables before roasting or grilling 'em. With dukkah's smoky, nutty flavors and inviting crunch, it's long been one of my go-to seasonings.

Makes 1½ cups
Hands-on time: 20 minutes
Total time: 20 minutes

⅓ cup raw **hazelnuts**
¼ cup **coriander seeds**
2 tablespoons **cumin seeds**
⅓ cup raw **sesame seeds**
¼ cup shelled roasted **pistachio nuts**

DO THIS:

1. Preheat the oven to 350°F with the rack in the middle position. Spread the hazelnuts on a foil-lined baking sheet and roast them in the oven for 10 to 15 minutes or until golden and fragrant. Transfer the hazelnuts to a clean kitchen towel and cool them for about 5 minutes. Use the towel to rub off the papery hazelnut skins.

2. Toast the coriander seeds in a skillet over medium-low heat for 1 minute or until fragrant. Shake the pan constantly to keep the seeds from scorching. Transfer the seeds to a bowl. Using the same method, toast the cumin seeds, and then add them to the same bowl. Lightly brown the sesame seeds in the same manner, and transfer all but 1 tablespoon to the bowl.

3. Add the cooled hazelnuts and pistachio nuts to the bowl of toasted seeds. Cool the mixture slightly. Then, in small batches, coarsely grind the ingredients in a clean spice grinder.

4. Mix in the reserved whole sesame seeds, and you're done. Dukkah will keep in a covered container in the refrigerator for a few months, so make extra and save some for a rainy day.

  ~ ADD TEXTURE TO YOUR CARROT + CARDAMOM SOUP (PAGE 115) WITH A SPRINKLE OF DUKKAH!

MAGIC MUSHROOM POWDER

This spice blend is truly magical—and one of my most highly sought-after secrets. If fish sauce is liquid umami in a bottle, this stuff is powdered umami in a jar, and an indispensable tool in your kitchen arsenal. Despairing about not having enough time to prepare a meal? Just sprinkle some of this flavorful dust on anything you cook, and bask in the admiring gazes of your dinner guests.

By the way, I know this goes without saying, but don't skimp out and use some cheapo blend of dried mushrooms. Dried porcini mushrooms have an intense flavor and aroma that you won't want to dilute.

Makes 1¼ cups
Hands-on time: 5 minutes
Total time: 5 minutes

1   ounce dried **porcini mushrooms**
⅔   cup **kosher salt**
1   tablespoon **red pepper flakes**
2   teaspoons dried **thyme**
1   teaspoon freshly ground **black pepper**

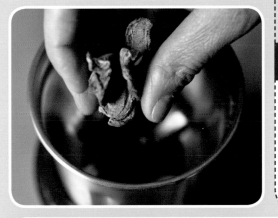

DO THIS:

1. Pulse the dried mushrooms in a clean spice grinder until they're finely ground. Transfer the mushroom powder to a bowl, and add the salt, red pepper flakes, thyme, and pepper. Mix thoroughly to incorporate.

2. Store the powder in an airtight container. It'll keep for several months, but I bet you'll run out well before then.

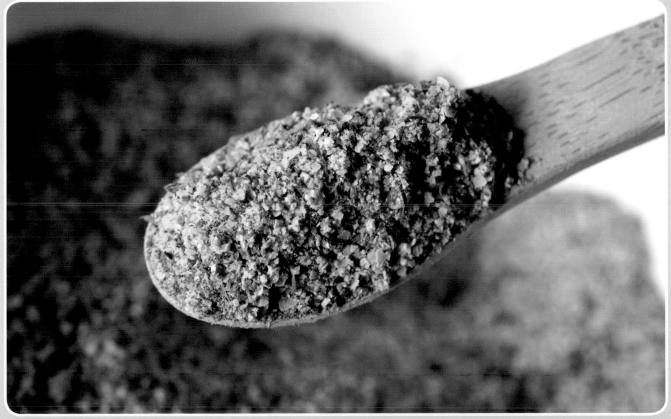

USE THIS POWDER IN PLACE OF SALT, AND REMEMBER: A LITTLE GOES A LONG WAY.

GHEE (CLARIFIED BUTTER)

Makes ¾ cup | Hands-on time: 15 minutes | Total time: 15 minutes

Got some high-quality butter from grass-fed cows sitting in your fridge? Excellent. Remove the dairy solids by rendering a pot of ghee, a traditional Indian preparation of clarified butter. The process is simple and quick, and you'll end up with a lactose- and casein-free cooking fat that's deliciously nutty and shelf-stable for months. Plus, ghee has an incredibly high smoke point—close to 500°F!—making it a fantastic choice for high-heat cooking.

I love ghee for its subtle flavor and versatility. Toss a tray of autumn root vegetables with melted ghee prior to oven-roasting, or sear off a beautiful flank steak in a red-hot cast-iron skillet slicked with shimmering ghee. You'll see what I mean.

GET:

1   cup (2 sticks) **unsalted butter**

BUT IF AT ALL POSSIBLE, USE BUTTER FROM GRASS-FED COWS. YOU'RE PUTTING THIS IN YOUR BODY, SO GET THE GOOD STUFF!

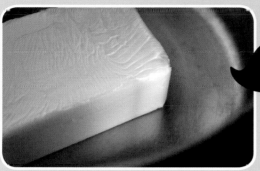

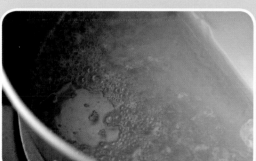

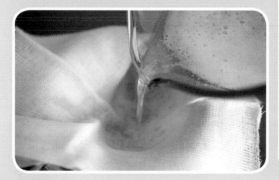

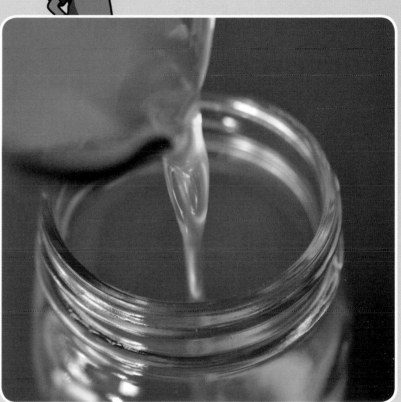

DO THIS:

1. Melt the butter in a saucepan over low heat. As it melts, the clear fat will separate from the milk solids. Continue simmering gently, and keep a close eye on the melted butter. Bubbles will form and then gradually get smaller, until the surface of the butter resembles a foam.

2. Soon, you'll see the milk solids brown, and some of the solids will clump together. Remove the pan from the heat when the milk solids turn a deep golden brown and start falling to the bottom, about 8 to 10 minutes after the melted butter starts bubbling.

3. Place a fine-mesh strainer on top of a heat-safe bowl or cup, and tuck a triple layer of cheesecloth into the strainer. Carefully strain the butter through the cheesecloth, and discard the milk solids.

4. Store the ghee in a sealed container. After the milk solids have been removed, the ghee no longer requires refrigeration—but if you keep your homemade stash in the fridge, it'll last up to a year.

BONUS RECIPE! → TO MAKE NITER KIBBEH, AN ETHIOPIAN SPICE-INFUSED GHEE, JUST ADD TWO MINCED GARLIC CLOVES, HALF A CHOPPED YELLOW ONION, HALF A CINNAMON STICK, A TEASPOON OF FINELY GRATED GINGER, AND A QUARTER TEASPOON OF TURMERIC WHEN YOU SIMMER THE BUTTER. IT'LL KEEP IN THE FRIDGE FOR UP TO A FULL YEAR!

SLOW-ROASTED TOMATOES

Got extra tomatoes sitting around? A nice long stint in the oven will concentrate their flavors and make each bite candy-sweet. Slow-roasted tomatoes can rescue almost any dish with a blast of toothsome umami.

Makes 4 servings
Hands-on time: 5 minutes
Total time: 2 hours

 ~ THEY'LL KEEP FOR UP TO A WEEK IN A SEALED CONTAINER IN THE FRIDGE!

20 **plum tomatoes**
Kosher salt
Freshly ground **black pepper**
2 tablespoons dried **herbs** of choice (I like basil or thyme)
¼ cup **avocado oil** or fat of choice

DO THIS:

1. Preheat the oven to 300°F with the rack in the middle position, and line a rimmed baking sheet with heavy-duty aluminum foil.

2. Cut each tomato in half lengthwise. Arrange them in a single layer, cut-side up, on the baking sheet. Season with salt, pepper, and herbs. Drizzle the oil on the tomatoes.

3. Roast in the oven for 2 hours or until the edges are lightly browned, rotating the baking sheet occasionally.

CARAMELIZED ONIONS

You know how some recipes call for cooking onions "8 to 10 minutes until caramelized"? Total lie. It takes a *looong* time to properly caramelize onions, folks. But once you have some on hand, you can toss 'em on just about anything for a transformative burst of smoky sweetness. They're well worth the time and effort.

Makes ½ cup
Hands-on time: 50 minutes
Total time: 50 minutes

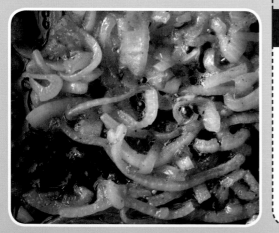

2 tablespoons **ghee** or fat of choice
3 medium **yellow onions**, thinly sliced
Kosher salt

DO THIS:

1. Heat the ghee in a skillet over medium heat. Add the sliced onions, and let them cook undisturbed for 1 to 2 minutes.

2. Season liberally with salt, and gently turn over the pile of onions every 3 or 4 minutes to ensure even cooking. Once the onions have softened and significantly reduced in volume, about 15 minutes, turn the heat to medium-low.

3. Continue cooking, turning over the onion pile every 10 minutes or so, for 30 minutes or until golden brown.

 ~ THE CARAMELIZED ONIONS WILL KEEP FOR UP TO A WEEK IN A COVERED CONTAINER IN THE REFRIGERATOR.

ROASTED BELL PEPPERS

Raid my refrigerator, and you'll almost always find a stash of roasted bell peppers. These sweetly piquant vegetables are incredibly versatile: you can snack on these vibrant, smoky peppers straight out of the icebox, toss them on some leftover protein as a flavorful topping, or dress them to make a quick and colorful salad. Plus, they're easy to make, and keep for up to a week (covered, of course) in the fridge. What's not to like?

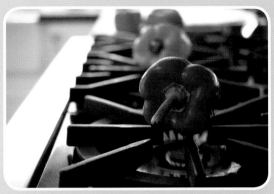

Makes 1 cup
Hands-on time: 15 minutes
Total time: 30 minutes

3   medium **bell peppers**
     Balsamic vinegar (optional)
     Extra-virgin olive oil
     (optional)

DO THIS:

1. Position the bell peppers directly on the burners of a gas range, and crank the heat to high.

2. Char the peppers for about 5 minutes, rotating every so often with a pair of tongs. Blacken the entire surface of the peppers—it'll be easier to remove the skin later.

3. Once the peppers are nicely blackened, toss them into a large bowl and cover tightly with plastic wrap or a lid. Leave them in there for at least 15 minutes, and up to a few hours. Let 'em sweat.

4. When you're ready, peel the peppers with your fingers. The papery skins should come right off.

5. Remove the stems, tops, and seeds. Use a sharp knife to trim off the soft ribs, and slice the peppers into strips. Drizzle with balsamic vinegar and olive oil, if desired.

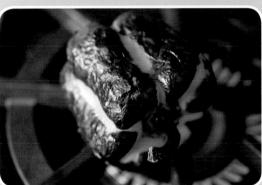

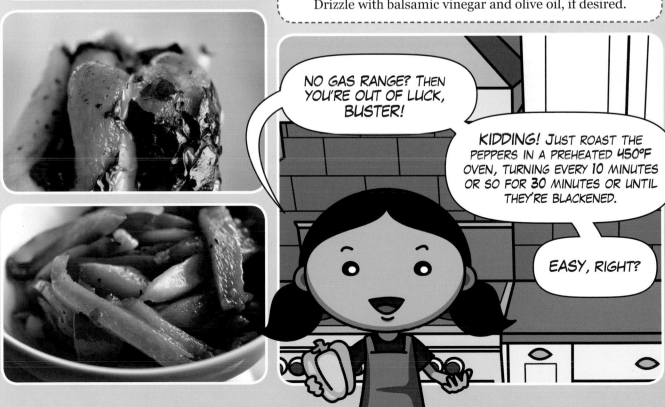

PALEO MAYONNAISE

I know what you're thinking: *Why on earth should I make my own mayonnaise? I can just buy it!*

Well, for starters, homemade Paleo-friendly mayonnaise is nothing like the jar of hyper-processed yellowing goo that's sitting in your fridge. This stuff's made with real, whole ingredients and good-for-you oils. Besides, this creamy flavor booster is more flavorful than any store-bought mayo, and a breeze to make. It's versatile, too; use it as a condiment or as a base for everything from deviled eggs and tuna wraps to chicken salads and spicy party dips.

Convinced? Good, 'cause I want you to try two of my favorite ways to make mayo. Roll up your sleeves!

Makes ¾ cup
Hands-on time: 20 minutes
Total time: 20 minutes

GET:

1	large **egg yolk**
¼	teaspoon **kosher salt**
¼	teaspoon **Dijon-style mustard**
1½	teaspoons fresh **lemon juice**
1	teaspoon distilled **white vinegar**
¾	cup **macadamia nut** or **avocado oil**

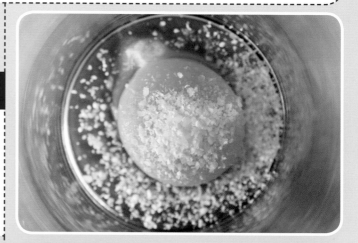

MAKE MAYO WITH A HAND WHISK:

No fancy kitchen gadgets required—all you need is a whisk and some elbow grease!

1. In a medium-sized bowl, whisk together the yolk, salt, mustard, lemon juice, and vinegar for about 30 seconds, or until the yolk thickens and the color brightens.

2. Pour about one-third of the oil in a slow, steady stream into the bowl while whisking the mixture vigorously for about 1 minute to create an emulsion. (A measuring cup works fine, but I like to drizzle my oil from a squeeze bottle; it helps me maintain a light, steady stream.)

3. After the oil is incorporated, slowly add half of the remaining oil and continue to whisk rapidly. Once it's emulsified, repeat with the rest of the oil. You'll soon have a mayonnaise that's thick enough to hold its own shape.

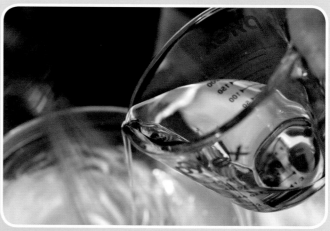

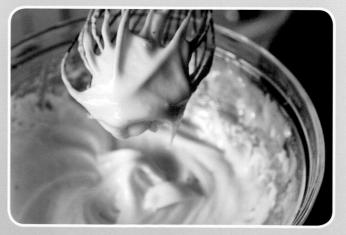

BONUS: THIS MAKES FOR A TERRIFIC WORKOUT, TOO!

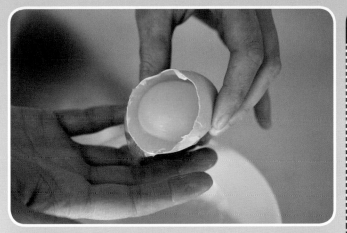

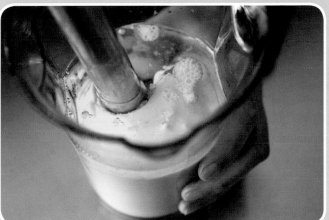

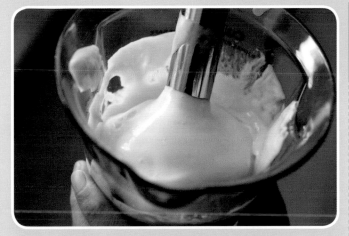

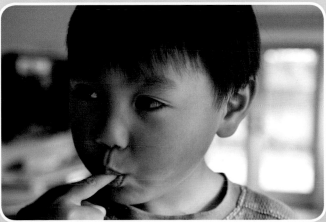

WHAT'S GOING ON?

Like a vinaigrette or butter, mayo's an *emulsion*—a combination of two types of liquids that don't normally mix, like oil and water. But by slowly adding one liquid to the other while mixing super-rapidly, a suspension of tiny droplets is formed.

It also helps to use an *emulsifier*, like mustard or egg yolk. Emulsifiers contain molecules that bind fats and water together, keeping your mayo from looking like the contents of your mom's lava lamp.

Makes 1 cup
Hands-on time: 5 minutes
Total time: 5 minutes

GET:

1	large **egg yolk**
1	tablespoon fresh **lemon juice**
1	tablespoon **water**
1	teaspoon **Dijon-style mustard**
1	cup **macadamia nut** or **avocado oil**
	Kosher salt

MAKE MAYO WITH AN IMMERSION BLENDER:

I learned about this game-changing mayo-making method from J. Kenji López-Alt of Serious Eats. It requires an immersion blender, but it's fast, stress-free, and foolproof. You must try this.

1. Throw the egg yolk, lemon juice, water, and mustard into an immersion blender cup. Add the oil to the contents in the cup.

2. Place the head of an immersion blender at the bottom of the cup, and pulse away. As the emulsion forms, carefully lift and tilt the head of the immersion blender so that the mayonnaise forms evenly.

3. Season with salt to taste. If you're not using the mayo right away, cover and store it in the fridge. It should keep for up to a week or two. (Or, as Michael Ruhlman sagely tweeted, "until it tastes bad.")

 I KNOW IT'S TEMPTING, BUT NEVER LICK THE HEAD OF YOUR STICK BLENDER. DUH!

PALEO SRIRACHA

Makes 2¼ cups | Hands-on time: 20 minutes | Total time: 20 minutes

Question: Who doesn't love sriracha?

Answer: People who haven't tried it yet.

But I know you. You're a sriracha connoisseur. The first time you spied it on the table at your favorite Vietnamese joint and squirted some onto a spoonful of *phở*, you were hooked. You squealed when you spotted little squeeze packets of sriracha at the food truck near your office. You sought out the rooster-emblazoned bottle with the green top at Asian supermarkets. You stockpiled the stuff in your pantry and ate the spicy, umami-packed condiment with, well, everything.

And why not? Sriracha's been anointed as The World's Greatest Condiment and The Most Amazing Condiment on the Planet. Matthew Inman of The Oatmeal calls it "a delicious blessing flavored with the incandescent glow of a thousand dying suns"—and you know that's no exaggeration. Sriracha is *magic*.

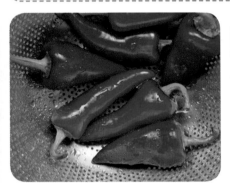 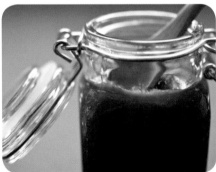 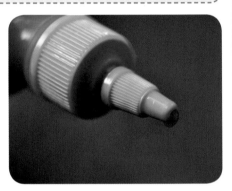

But then you made the switch to Paleo. And for the first time, you read the ingredients on your store-bought squeeze bottle of sriracha. You saw that it contains stuff you don't recognize, like potassium sorbate, sodium bisulfite, and xantham gum. It felt like someone let all the air out of your hot-sauce-loving balloon.

You couldn't bear to toss out your sriracha. But you ate it less frequently. And when you did, you felt a gnawing guilt about ingesting all those chemical preservatives. Every time you passed by your pantry, you eyed that bright crimson-orange bottle with longing—until the little voice in your head whispered: "*Faileo.*"

Finally, after weeks of sriracha withdrawal, you decided to take matters into your own hands. Furiously searching the Internet, you found a recipe for do-it-yourself sriracha—but it called for a week of fermentation and daily stirring. And patience isn't one of your virtues. You want sriracha *today*. Sad face.

But what if I were to tell you that there is a recipe for a quick, Paleo-friendly version of the world-famous "Rooster Sauce"? Would you pledge to me your undying love?

LOOKS LIKE YOU'RE JUST GONNA HAVE TO LOVE ME FOREVER!

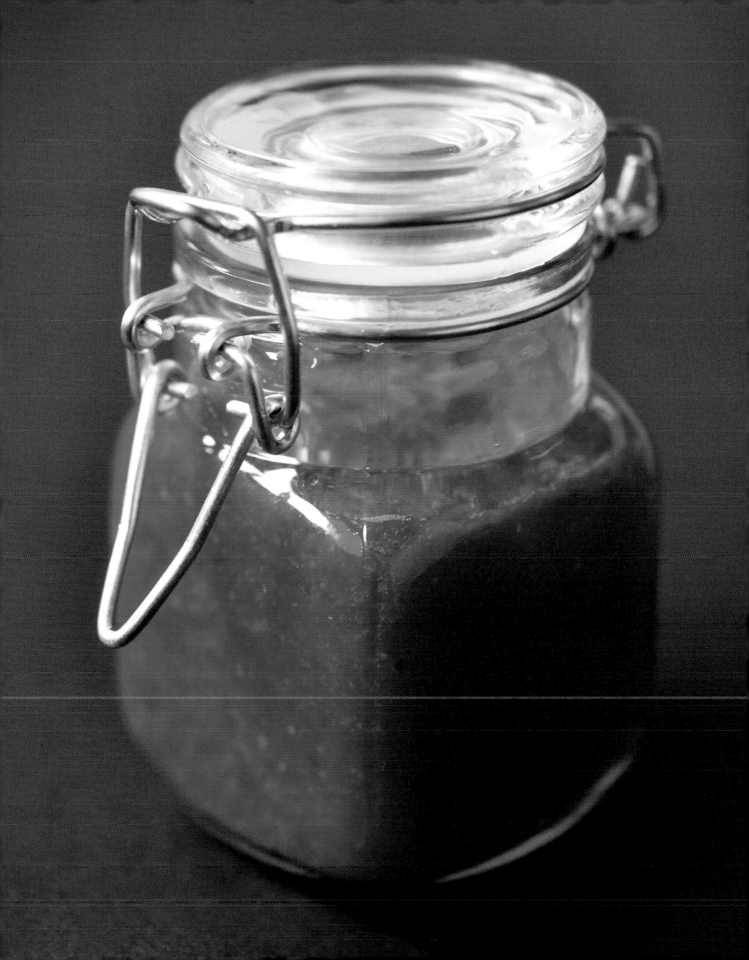

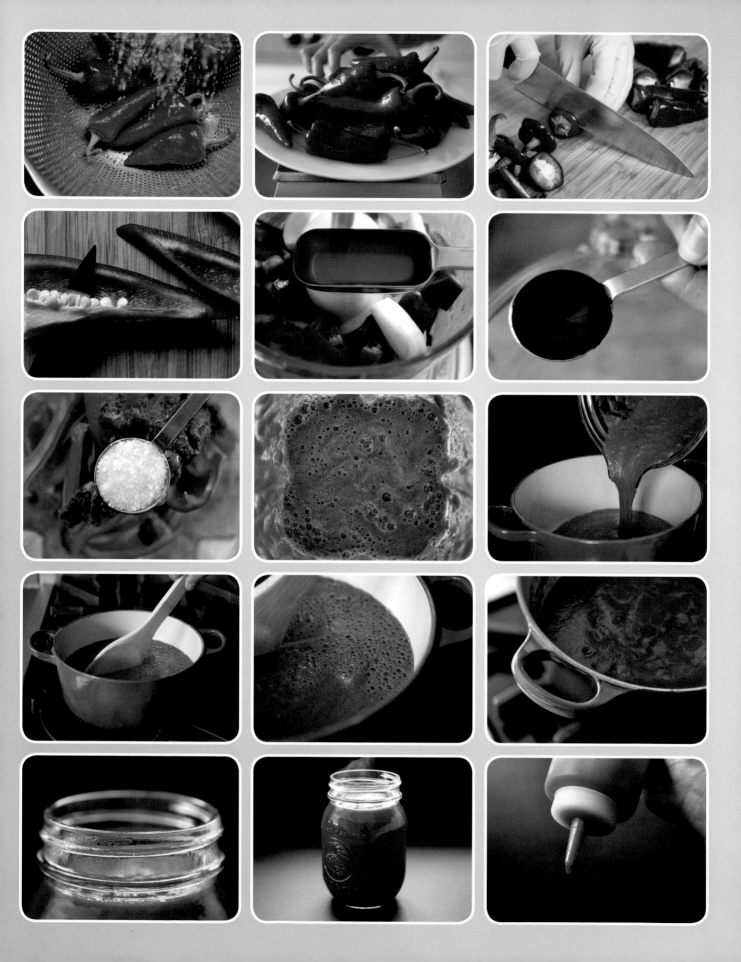

This sriracha ain't just Paleo-friendly—it's also super-fast. Most sriracha recipes require prolonged fermentation to boost the umami in the fiery red sauce, but I've found a way around the interminable waiting period. The secret? You can just add the umami yourself, in the form of tomato paste and fish sauce.

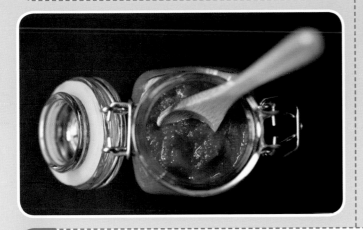

GET:

1½	pounds fresh **red jalapeño peppers**, stemmed, seeded, and roughly chopped
8	**garlic cloves**, smashed and peeled
⅓	cup **apple cider vinegar**
3	tablespoons **tomato paste**
3	tablespoons **honey** (see note below)
2	tablespoons Paleo-friendly **fish sauce**
1½	teaspoons **kosher salt**

DO THIS:

1. Throw the peppers, garlic, vinegar, tomato paste, honey, fish sauce, and salt into a high-speed blender. Purée until smooth.

2. Pour the purée into a saucepan and bring it to a boil over high heat. Don't worry about the froth on top—it'll cook off.

3. As soon as the sauce boils, turn down the heat to low and maintain a simmer for 5 to 10 minutes, stirring occasionally. Once the foam subsides, the sauce should be a vibrant red color, and you shouldn't be able to detect any raw vegetable smell. Taste and adjust for salt if necessary.

4. Transfer the sriracha to a jar (or three) and cool it. You can keep it in the fridge, covered, for up to a week. Behold: Paleo Sriracha!

PRO TIPS:

BURNING HANDS AND STINGING EYES NOT YOUR IDEA OF FUN? THEN BE SMART: USE GLOVES WHEN HANDLING THE PEPPERS.

ALSO, IF YOU PREFER EXTRA-FIERY SRIRACHA, LEAVE IN SOME OF THE JALAPEÑOS' RIBS AND SEEDS, AND/OR USE HOTTER PEPPERS (LIKE SERRANOS OR EVEN SUPER-SPICY LUMBRE PEPPERS).

SRIRACHA MAYONNAISE

BONUS RECIPE!

Makes ½ cup
Hands-on time: 1 minute
Total time: 1 minute

6	tablespoons **Paleo Mayonnaise** (page 40)
2	tablespoons **Paleo Sriracha** (above)

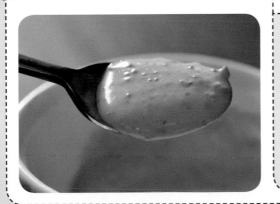

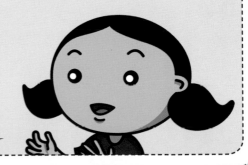

MIX THE MAYONNAISE AND THE SRIRACHA TOGETHER IN A BOWL. THE END.

MACADAMIA NUT "RICOTTA"

Makes 1 1/2 cups | Hands-on time: 5 minutes | Total time: 5 minutes
Raise your hand if you miss cheese!

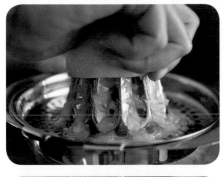
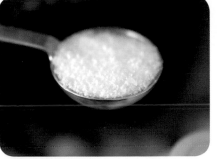
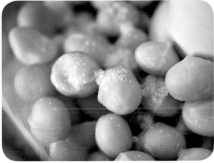
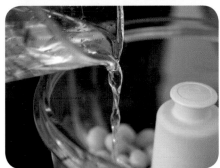
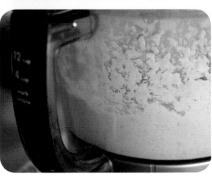
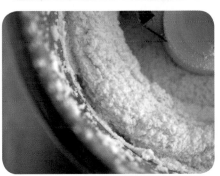

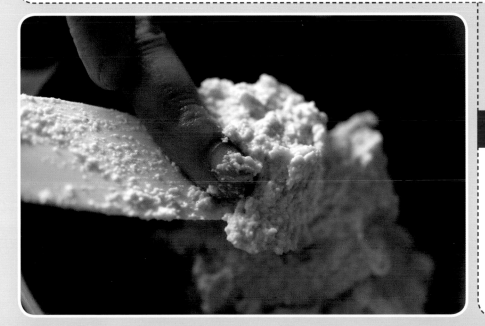

2   cups raw **macadamia nuts**
1   teaspoon **kosher salt**
    Juice from ½ medium
    lemon (about 1 tablespoon)
½   cup **water**

DO THIS:

In a food processor or a high-powered blender, purée the ingredients together until smooth.

If necessary, scrape down the sides with a spatula and/or add a bit more water. The resulting texture should resemble—you guessed it!—ricotta cheese.

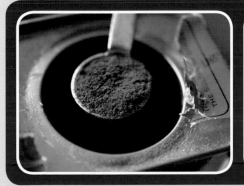

KA-POW!

Amplify the color and flavor by mixing in ¼ teaspoon of smoked paprika. Or add minced sundried tomatoes and fresh basil.

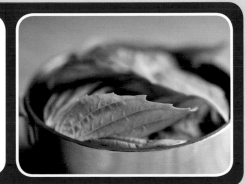

 ~ THIS "RICOTTA" WILL KEEP FOR UP TO A WEEK IN AN AIRTIGHT CONTAINER IN THE FRIDGE.

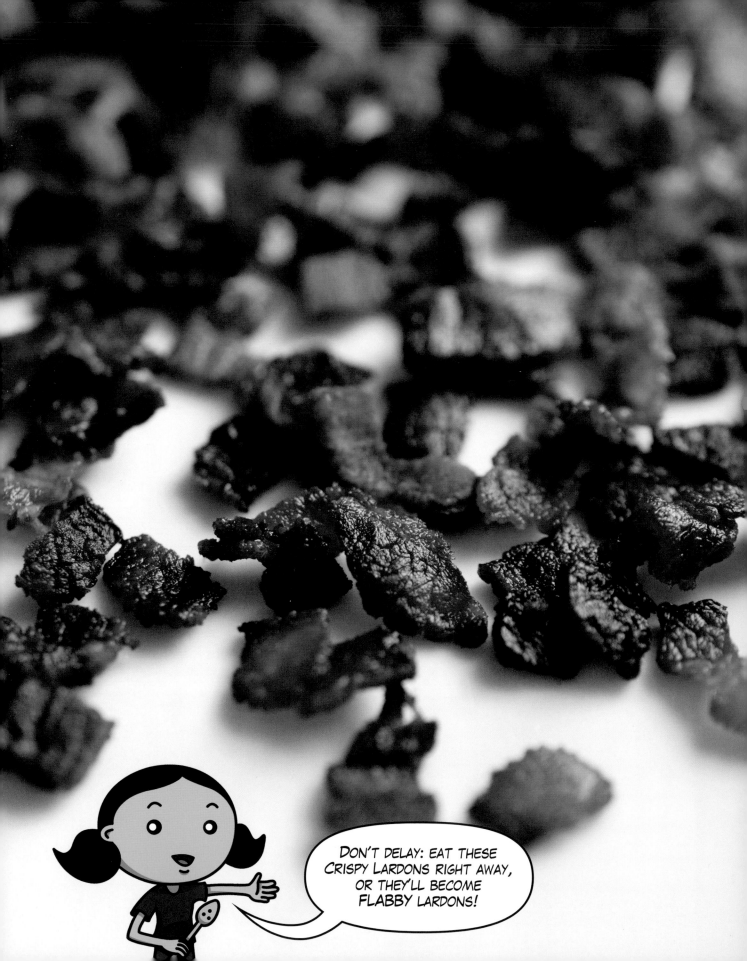

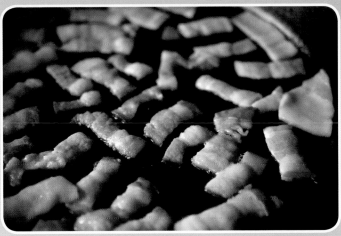
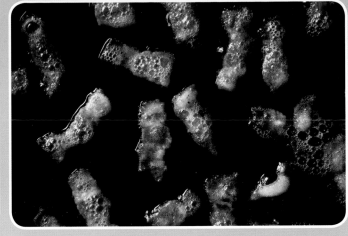
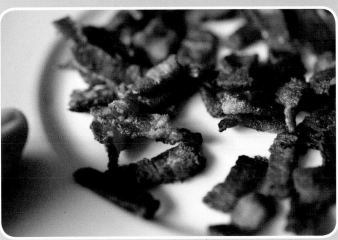
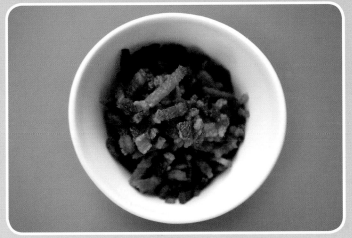

CRISPY LARDONS

Admit it: swine makes it fine. No one's saying that bacon should be your primary source of protein or fat, but it certainly lends a full-bodied, smoky crunch to whatever you're eating. So if you have some extra bacon sitting in your fridge, why not fry some lardons and punch up your meals with some savory, porky love?

Makes ½ cup
Hands-on time: 25 minutes
Total time: 25 minutes

6 slices **bacon**

DO THIS:

1. Slice the bacon crosswise into ¼-inch pieces. (Slicing bacon can be a slippery, messy exercise in frustration. Make it easier on yourself by putting it in the freezer for 20 minutes before you try to cut it up. Or just keep your bacon in the freezer in 3-slice portions, and it'll be ready for the cutting board at a moment's notice.)

2. Toss the bacon into a large skillet and cook it over medium heat. By heating the skillet and bacon together, you'll lower the chances of scorching the bacon in a too-hot pan.

3. Slowly render the bacon until the drippings are released and the bits get crunchy (approximately 15 minutes). Use a slotted spoon to transfer the bacon bits to a paper towel–lined plate. And don't forget to reserve the liquid bacon fat to make Five-Minute Bacon Aïoli (page 60)!

⌐ REPEAT AFTER ME: TURKEY BACON IS FAKIN' BACON!

QUICK-PICKLED CARROT STRINGS

Need a little something to perk up your meals? The tang of pickled carrot strings adds a fresh crispness to any dish. Here's a simple recipe that takes just half an hour to make, featuring a sweet brine made with apple juice instead of sugar. So grab a bunch of carrots and your trusty julienne peeler, and let's get to work!

Makes 3 cups
Hands-on time: 5 minutes
Total time: 30 minutes

GET:

- ¼ cup **apple juice**
- ½ cup **apple cider vinegar**
- ½ teaspoon **kosher salt**
- 3 large **carrots**, julienned

DO THIS:

Combine the apple juice, vinegar, and salt in a bowl and mix well. Drop in the carrot strings (I shred mine with a julienne peeler), making sure to completely submerge them in the brine. Cover the container and refrigerate for at least 30 minutes—they'll keep for up to a week.

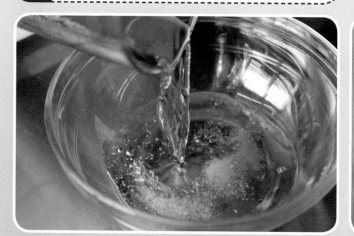

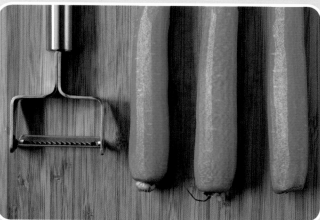

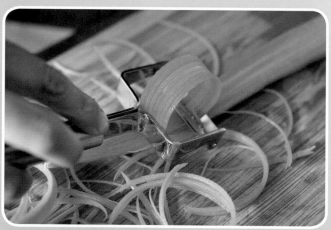

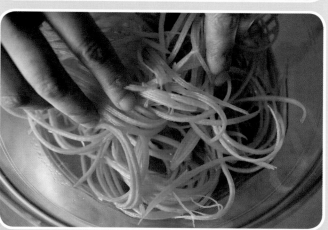

CRAZY FOR PICKLES? TRY THESE MODIFICATIONS!

The method above will work with any number of different vegetables, so don't limit yourself to carrots. Try pickling paper-thin slices of red onion and cucumber, or julienned daikon and radishes. And while you're at it, add a little heat to your apple juice brine with a pinch of red pepper flakes. After all, a garnish of tart, colorful pickles is often all that's needed to perk up a ho-hum weeknight meal.

THE TERM "PICKLE" IS DERIVED FROM "PEKEL," A DUTCH WORD THAT REFERS TO A SALTY BRINE ORIGINALLY USED TO PRESERVE MEATS!

HOLY 'MOLY (EASY GUACAMOLE)

Holy moly—I love guacamole. I routinely put my husband in charge of whipping up this green goodness because his version is my favorite by far: it's the perfect mix of chunky and creamy, savory and spicy. Henry uses just a few ingredients, so it's always a breeze to make a batch to accompany our meats and vegetables.

By the way, if you're looking for a quick and healthy finger food to accompany your homemade guacamole, try raw jicama. Popular in Asia, South and Central America, and the Caribbean, this taproot vegetable has a refreshingly apple-crisp texture. Dip your jicama sticks in guacamole, and you'll never crave chips again.

Makes 4 servings
Hands-on time: 15 minutes
Total time: 15 minutes

1   small **shallot**, minced
    Juice from 1 small **lime**
½   teaspoon **kosher salt**
3   medium **Hass avocados**, halved, pitted, and peeled
    Freshly ground **black pepper**
    Chile powder (optional)

DO THIS:

1. In a small bowl, combine the shallot, lime juice, and salt. Leave the mixture alone for about 10 minutes so the acid can take some of the bite off the shallot.

2. Mash half of the avocado flesh in a bowl with a fork. Add the shallot mixture to the mashed avocado and stir to combine.

3. Cube the remaining half of the avocado into ¾-inch pieces and add it to the mixture in the bowl. Gently incorporate the mashed avocado and the cubed avocado.

4. As a finishing touch, add pepper (and, if desired, some chile powder) to taste. Eat immediately.

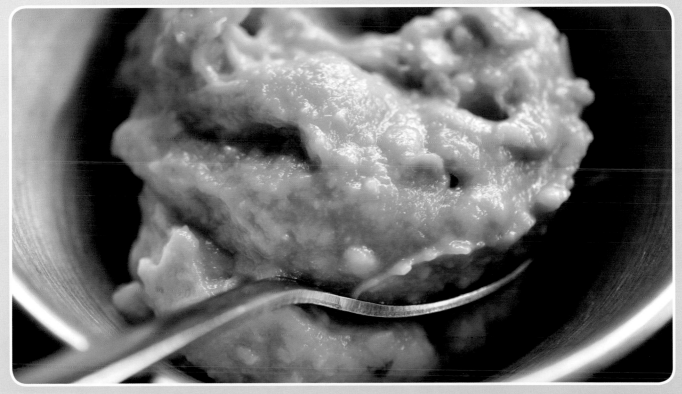

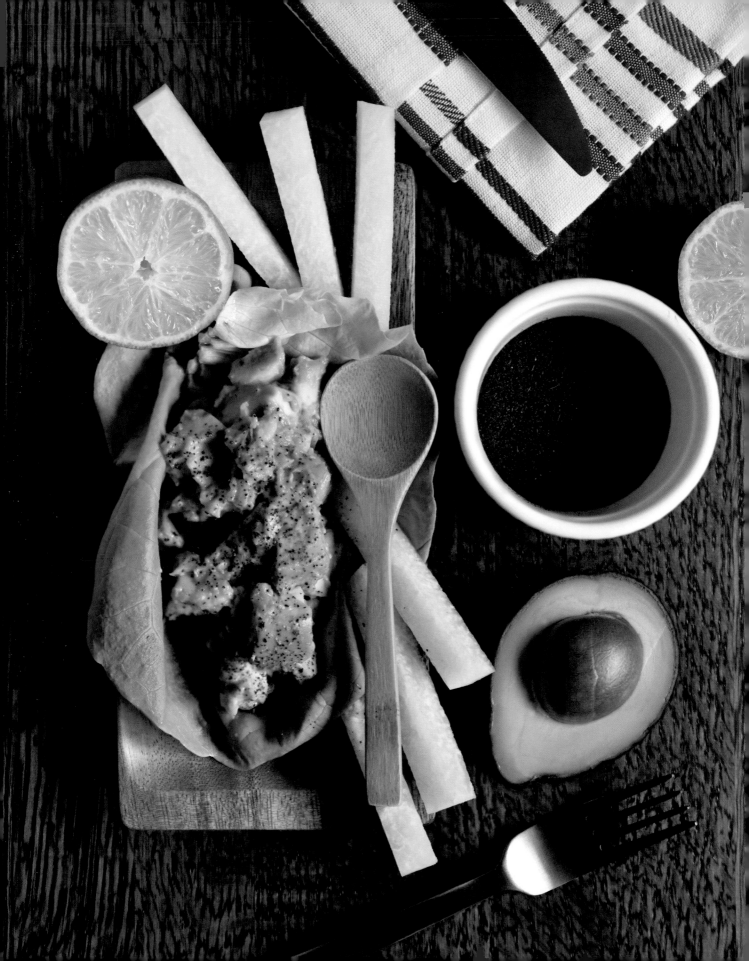

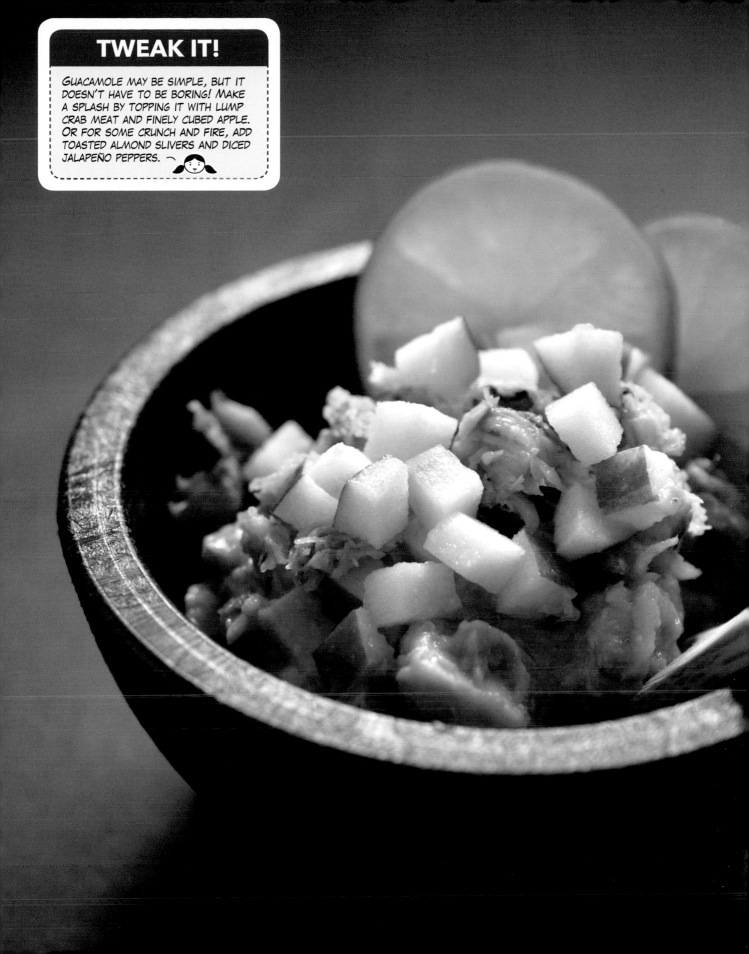

TWEAK IT!

GUACAMOLE MAY BE SIMPLE, BUT IT DOESN'T HAVE TO BE BORING! MAKE A SPLASH BY TOPPING IT WITH LUMP CRAB MEAT AND FINELY CUBED APPLE. OR FOR SOME CRUNCH AND FIRE, ADD TOASTED ALMOND SLIVERS AND DICED JALAPEÑO PEPPERS.

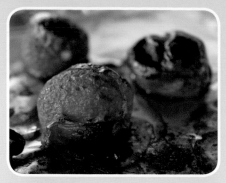
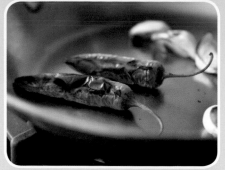
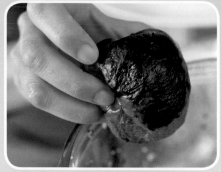
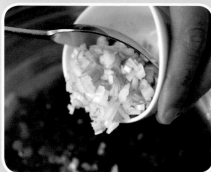
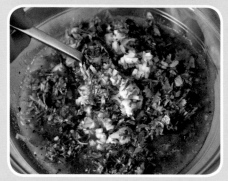
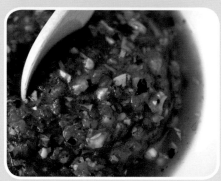

SALSA ROJA ASADA

Want to add some heat to your meals? Use this lip-tingling fire-roasted salsa to punch your food in the face!

Makes 2 cups
Hands-on time: 20 minutes
Total time: 20 minutes

- **1** pound plum **tomatoes**
- **2** medium **serrano** or **jalapeño peppers**
- **4** **garlic cloves**, unpeeled
- **½** teaspoon **kosher salt**
- Juice from ½ small **lime**
- **1** large **shallot**, finely minced
- **¼** cup chopped fresh **cilantro**

DO THIS:

1. Position an oven rack about 4 to 6 inches from the heating element, and preheat the broiler. Place the tomatoes on a foil-lined baking sheet and roast under the broiler for 5 minutes or until the skins are blistered and blackened on top. Flip the tomatoes over, and roast for another 5 minutes.

2. Meanwhile, roast the chile peppers and garlic in an ungreased skillet, turning occasionally, for about 15 minutes or until the garlic is softened and charred and the peppers are nicely blistered. (Watch them carefully; the peppers will probably be done first.)

3. When the garlic and peppers are cool enough to handle, peel the garlic and remove the stems from the peppers. (Want a milder salsa? Use jalapeño peppers, and remove the seeds and ribs.)

4. In a food processor, grind up the peppers, garlic, and salt. Be careful when removing the lid—the spicy contents will make your eyes water.

5. Add the tomatoes to the food processor and pulse until a thick purée develops. Transfer the salsa to a bowl and stir in the lime juice, shallot, and cilantro. Taste and adjust for seasoning.

STORE THE SALSA IN A COVERED CONTAINER IN THE REFRIGERATOR FOR UP TO 4 DAYS. AND BY THE WAY: IF YOU'VE NEVER TRIED ADDING SALSA TO YOUR SCRAMBLED EGGS, WHAT ARE YOU WAITING FOR?

SPICY PINEAPPLE SALSA

You'll love the sweet, tangy bursts of flavor that this tropical salsa lends to everything from salads to steaks.

Makes 2 cups
Hands-on time: 10 minutes
Total time: 10 minutes

1½ cups finely diced fresh **pineapple**
1   **Persian cucumber**, peeled and cut into ¼ inch dice
1   **jalapeño pepper**, cut into ¼-inch dice (with ribs and seeds removed if you can't stand the heat)
¼   cup finely chopped **red onion**
¼   cup minced fresh **cilantro**
2   tablespoons **extra-virgin olive oil**
     Juice from 1 small **lime**
     Kosher salt
     Freshly ground **black pepper**

DO THIS:

Combine everything in a bowl and season to taste with salt and pepper. The salsa will keep in an airtight container in the fridge for up to 4 days.

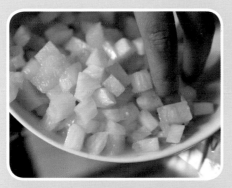
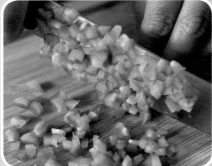
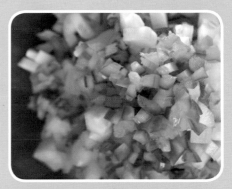
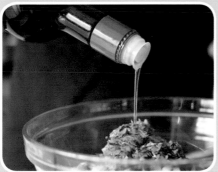
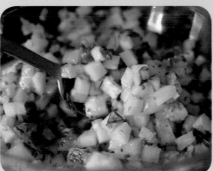
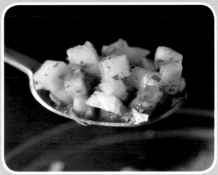

SPICY MANGO SALSA

BONUS RECIPE!

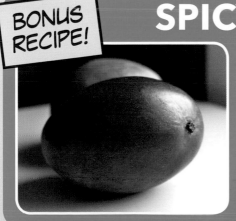

NOT IN A PINEAPPLE KIND OF MOOD? NOT A PROBLEM. IN ITS PLACE, SIMPLY SUBSTITUTE A MEDIUM-SIZE MANGO, PITTED, PEELED, AND DICED SMALL. TRUST ME: MANGO ADDS A WONDERFULLY CRUNCHY BRIGHTNESS TO YOUR DISHES.

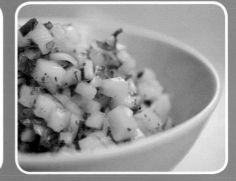

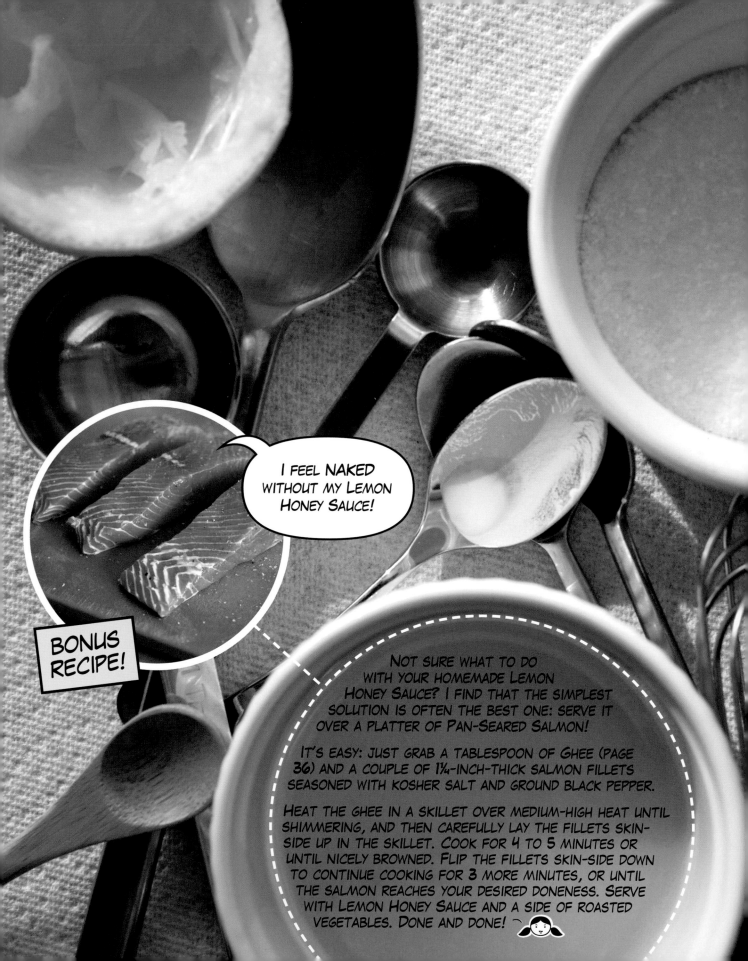

I FEEL NAKED WITHOUT MY LEMON HONEY SAUCE!

BONUS RECIPE!

NOT SURE WHAT TO DO WITH YOUR HOMEMADE LEMON HONEY SAUCE? I FIND THAT THE SIMPLEST SOLUTION IS OFTEN THE BEST ONE: SERVE IT OVER A PLATTER OF PAN-SEARED SALMON!

IT'S EASY: JUST GRAB A TABLESPOON OF GHEE (PAGE 36) AND A COUPLE OF 1¼-INCH-THICK SALMON FILLETS SEASONED WITH KOSHER SALT AND GROUND BLACK PEPPER.

HEAT THE GHEE IN A SKILLET OVER MEDIUM-HIGH HEAT UNTIL SHIMMERING, AND THEN CAREFULLY LAY THE FILLETS SKIN-SIDE UP IN THE SKILLET. COOK FOR 4 TO 5 MINUTES OR UNTIL NICELY BROWNED. FLIP THE FILLETS SKIN-SIDE DOWN TO CONTINUE COOKING FOR 3 MORE MINUTES, OR UNTIL THE SALMON REACHES YOUR DESIRED DONENESS. SERVE WITH LEMON HONEY SAUCE AND A SIDE OF ROASTED VEGETABLES. DONE AND DONE!

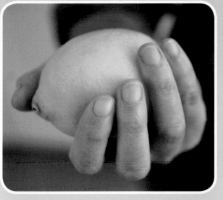
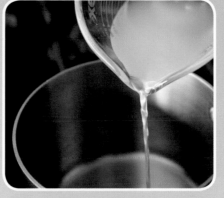
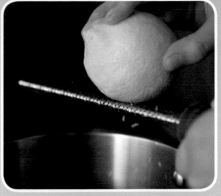
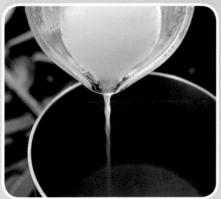
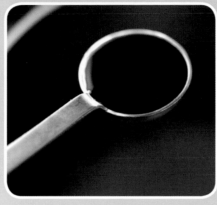
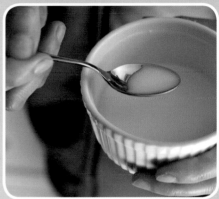

LEMON HONEY SAUCE

I know the feeling. Sometimes, you just want to pour sauce all over your food. This sweetly tart sauce should do the trick: it's lip-smackingly delicious, a cinch to make, and a perfect partner for seafood or poultry.

Makes 1 cup
Hands-on time: 10 minutes
Total time: 10 minutes

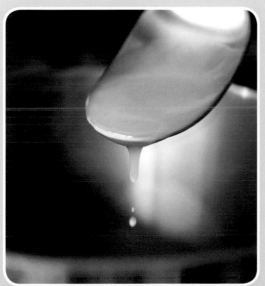

½ cup **chicken broth**
Finely grated zest from 1 small **lemon**
⅓ cup fresh **lemon juice** (from about 2 small lemons)
2½ tablespoons **honey**
1 teaspoon **coconut aminos**
½ teaspoon grated fresh **ginger**
1 tablespoon **arrowroot powder**, dissolved in about 1½ tablespoons water

DO THIS:

1. In a small saucepan, combine the broth, zest, juice, honey, coconut aminos, and grated ginger, and bring to a boil. Take the pot off the burner and cool the sauce for a few minutes.

2. Stir the dissolved arrowroot powder into the sauce while it's still hot, but not boiling. Cool slightly before serving. It'll keep for 3 days in a covered container in the fridge.

 DRIZZLE SOME LEMON HONEY SAUCE ON YOUR ROASTED VEGETABLES FOR A PUNCH OF INSTANT FLAVOR!

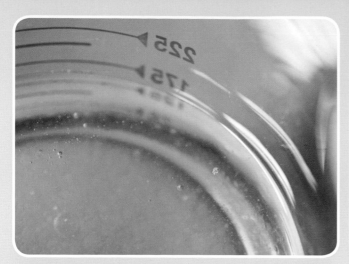
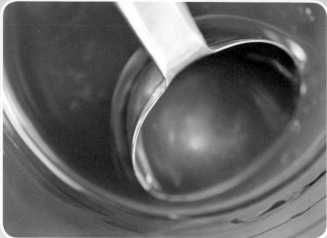
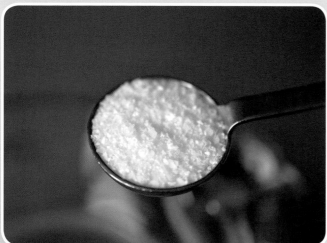
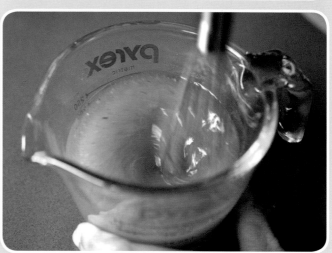

HONEY MUSTARD DRESSING

With just a few pantry ingredients and a few minutes, anyone can whip up this zippy dressing. Even you!

Makes ½ cup
Hands-on time: 5 minutes
Total time: 5 minutes

3 tablespoons **apple cider vinegar**
2 tablespoons **extra-virgin olive oil**
2 tablespoons **honey**
2 teaspoons **Dijon-style mustard**
¼ teaspoon **kosher salt**
Freshly ground **black pepper**

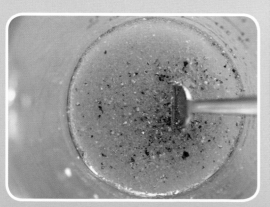

DO THIS:

In a small bowl, thoroughly whisk the vinegar, olive oil, honey, mustard, and salt until combined. Season to taste with pepper. Use the dressing immediately, or refrigerate in a sealed jar for up to 3 days. (Just remember to shake well before serving.)

MAKE A SIMPLE FRUIT SALAD POP BY TOSSING IT WITH HONEY MUSTARD DRESSING!

CITRUS VINAIGRETTE

If you're tired of tossing salads with nothing but oil and vinegar, give this tangy dressing a whirl. Don't leave out the mustard—just a bit helps bind the olive oil and juice together and gives this vinaigrette a nice bite.

Makes ¾ cup
Hands-on time: 5 minutes
Total time: 5 minutes

½ cup **extra-virgin olive oil**
2 tablespoons fresh **lemon juice**
2 tablespoons fresh **orange juice**
1 teaspoon **Dijon-style mustard**
1 teaspoon **kosher salt**
Freshly ground **black pepper**

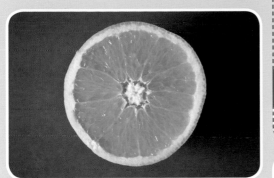

DO THIS:

Whisk together the oil, juices, mustard, salt, and pepper to taste.

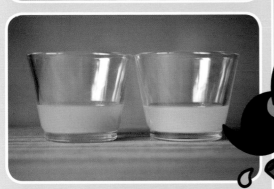

A VINAIGRETTE'S AN EMULSION: A COMBINATION OF TWO LIQUIDS THAT NORMALLY DON'T MIX, LIKE AN OIL AND AN ACID.

THEY'RE OFTEN BOUND TOGETHER BY AN EMULSIFIER, LIKE EGG YOLK.

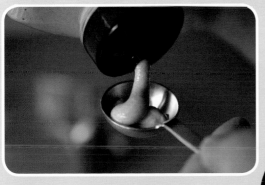

BUT MY FAVORITE EMULSIFIER IS MUSTARD, WHICH STABILIZES DRESSINGS WHILE ADDING A SUBTLE BOOST OF FLAVOR!

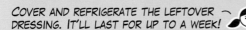

COVER AND REFRIGERATE THE LEFTOVER DRESSING. IT'LL LAST FOR UP TO A WEEK!

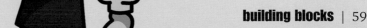

FIVE-MINUTE BACON AÏOLI

Makes 1 cup
Hands-on time: 5 minutes
Total time: 5 minutes

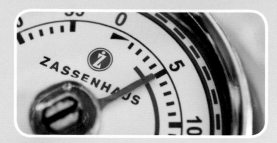

Yes, that's exactly what I said. Bacon aïoli. In just five minutes.

½ cup **macadamia nut oil**
½ cup liquid, room temperature **bacon drippings**
1 large **egg yolk**
2 **garlic cloves**, finely minced
1 tablespoon **sherry vinegar**
1 tablespoon **Dijon-style mustard**
Kosher salt
Freshly ground **black pepper**

DO THIS:

1. In a liquid measuring cup, combine the macadamia nut oil and bacon drippings.

2. In an immersion blender cup, toss the egg yolk, garlic, sherry vinegar, and mustard, and season with salt and pepper to taste. Mix with an immersion blender for about 30 seconds, or until the ingredients are well combined.

3. Add the oil and bacon drippings, and place the head of the immersion blender in the bottom of the cup. Pulse away. As the aïoli forms, carefully lift and tilt the head of the blender so that the thick, bacon-infused emulsion forms evenly. This rich, smoky dressing will keep in a covered container for up to 3 days in the refrigerator.

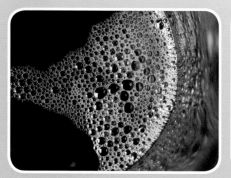
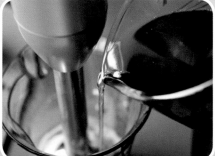
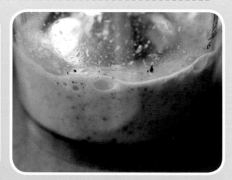

WHAT'S AÏOLI, YOU ASK? AÏOLI'S A GARLICKY PROVENÇAL MAYONNAISE. THINK OF IT AS A QUICK AND EASY FLAVOR ENHANCER FOR EVERYTHING FROM SEARED TUNA AND SUMMERY SALADS TO CRUDITÉS AND HARD-BOILED EGGS.

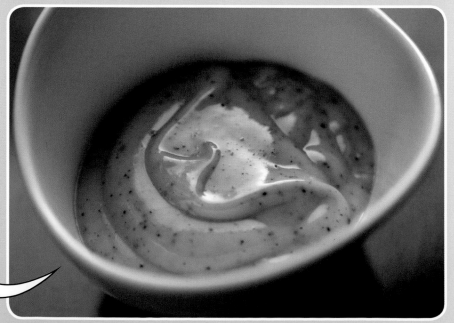

I HOPE YOU SAVED SOME BACON DRIPPINGS WHEN YOU MADE CRISPY LARDONS (PAGE 49)!

AVOCADO + BASIL DRESSING

Sick of vinaigrettes? Wistful for creamy salad dressings? You know—the ones that you can't eat anymore because they're loaded with high-fructose corn syrup, soybean oil, and Yellow Number 5? Believe it or not, with a few pantry staples, you can whip up a fresh, thick dressing in minutes. Here's one of my favorites.

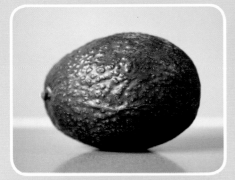

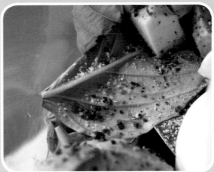

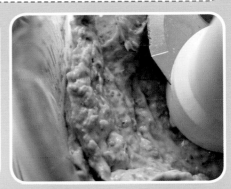

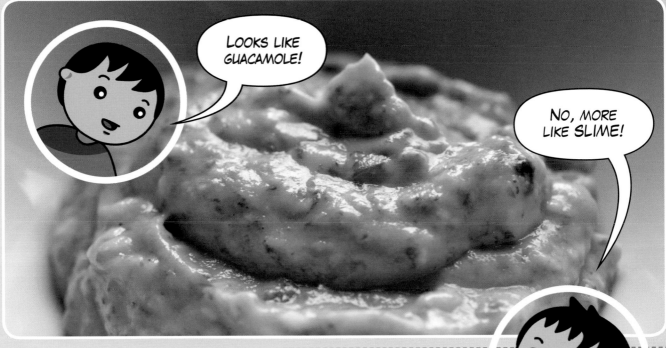

Makes 1 cup
Hands-on time: 10 minutes
Total time: 10 minutes

DO THIS:

1. Add all the ingredients to the work bowl of a food processor, and blitz until well combined.

2. The dressing should be thick and chunky, but if it's too dense for your taste, add a bit of water to thin it out to your desired consistency.

1 medium **Hass avocado** pitted, peeled, and cubed
1 cup packed fresh **basil**
1 **garlic clove**
Juice from 1 large **lime**
¼ cup **extra-virgin olive oil**
Kosher salt
Freshly ground **black pepper**
½ teaspoon **Aleppo pepper** or **red pepper flakes**

PALEO RANCH DRESSING

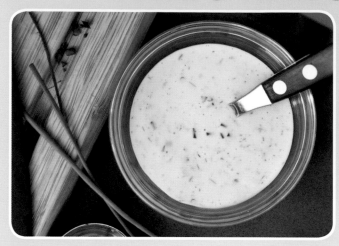

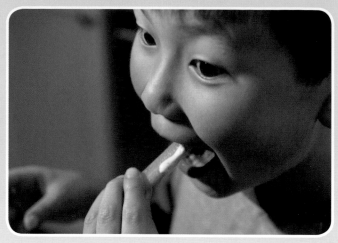

Pop quiz, hotshot: What's the best-selling salad dressing in the United States?

Why, it's ranch dressing, of course! (If you guessed wrong, you really ought to pay closer attention to the title of the recipe on this page.)

Invented by the owners of Santa Barbara's Hidden Valley Ranch in the mid-1950s, this creamy condiment long ago overtook Italian dressing in the hearts and minds of salad-tossing Americans. These days, supermarket shelves are brimming with ranch-flavored products, from snack chips to marinades—but store-bought ranch dressing isn't considered a health food for good reason. The stuff's made with hyper-processed canola-heavy mayonnaise and a multitude of chemical additives. *No bueno.*

Knowing this, I avoided ranch dressing for years, but Owen kept asking for it. "Carrot sticks just don't taste the same if I can't dip them in ranch dressing," my son reasoned. True enough.

"Want ranch dressing?" I asked. "Then we're going to have to come up with a recipe together." We did, and this creamy, herby dressing turned out to be one of the easiest condiments I've ever Paleo-fied.

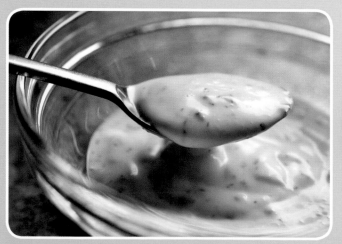

Makes 1 cup
Hands-on time: 10 minutes
Total time: 10 minutes

½ cup **Paleo Mayonnaise** (page 40)
⅓ cup full-fat **coconut milk**
1 tablespoon fresh **lemon juice**
1 tablespoon minced fresh **Italian parsley**
1 tablespoon minced fresh **chives**
1 teaspoon **onion powder**
½ teaspoon dried **dill**, or 1 teaspoon fresh dill
1 teaspoon **kosher salt**
½ small **garlic clove**, minced

DO THIS:

Stir the ingredients together in a bowl until smooth. If desired, cover and refrigerate to thicken slightly before serving. This ranch dressing will keep for up to a week in the refrigerator.

MY KIDS HAPPILY EAT THEIR VEGGIES WHEN I INCLUDE A LITTLE
CONTAINER OF RANCH DRESSING IN THEIR PACKED LUNCHES!

LOUISIANA RÉMOULADE

Although rémoulade was invented in France, it's the Creole version that makes me swoon. The addition of paprika lends a ruddy complexion and piquant flair to this classic condiment. Rémoulade is often served with seafood—it's fantastic with Fried Salmon Patties (page 180) or Spicy Coconut Shrimp (page 176)—but don't underestimate the versatility of this creamy dressing. You'll love it on everything from Chicken Nuggets (page 195) to Perfect Hard-Boiled Eggs (page 120). Or just slather it on some homemade Roast Beast (page 229). After all, rémoulade was originally made to accompany meat.

Makes 1 cup
Hands-on time: 10 minutes
Total time: 10 minutes

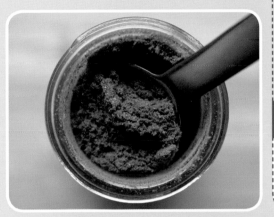

1	cup **Paleo Mayonnaise** (page 40)
2	tablespoons **Dijon-style mustard**
2	teaspoons **capers**, minced
1½	teaspoons fresh **lemon juice**
1	teaspoon **garlic powder**
1	teaspoon **onion powder**
1	teaspoon **paprika**
½	teaspoon **ancho chile powder**

DO THIS:

Stir together all the ingredients in a bowl until smooth and thoroughly combined. Refrigerate the rémoulade in a covered container, and it'll keep for up to a week.

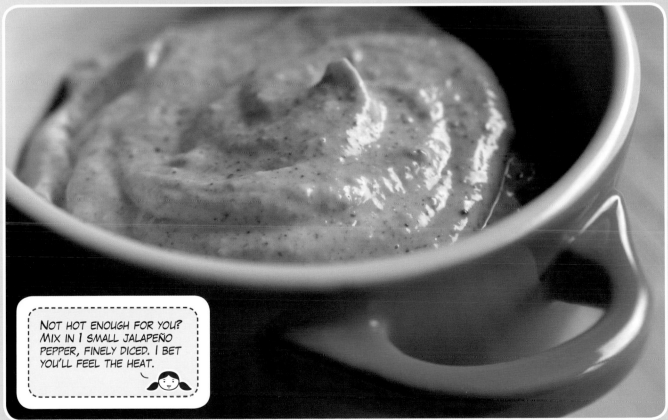

NOT HOT ENOUGH FOR YOU? MIX IN 1 SMALL JALAPEÑO PEPPER, FINELY DICED. I BET YOU'LL FEEL THE HEAT.

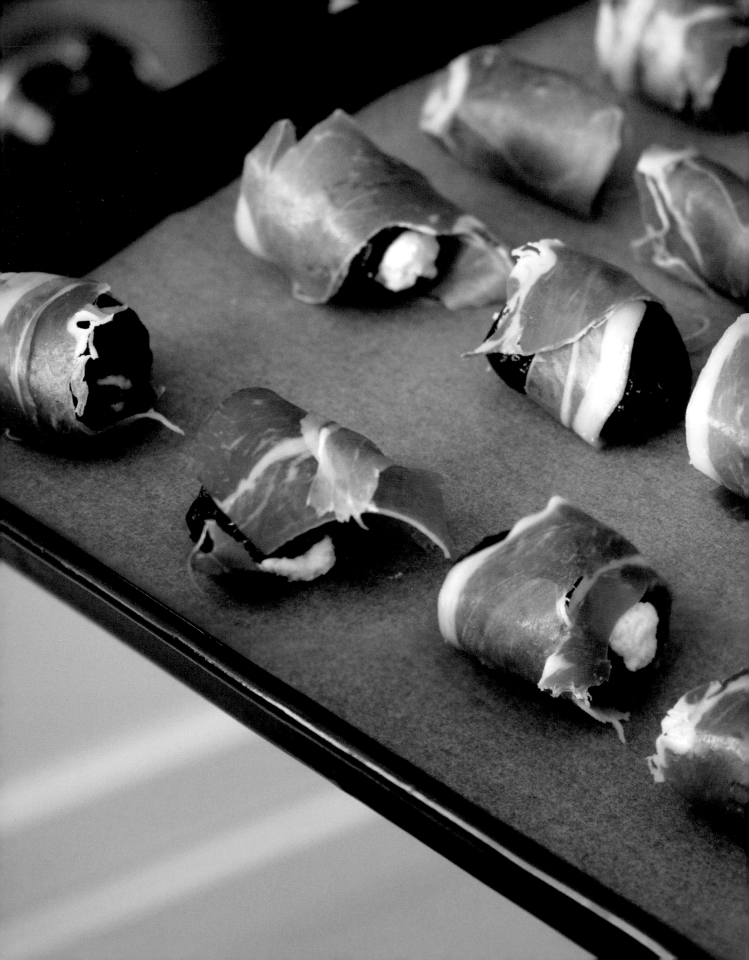

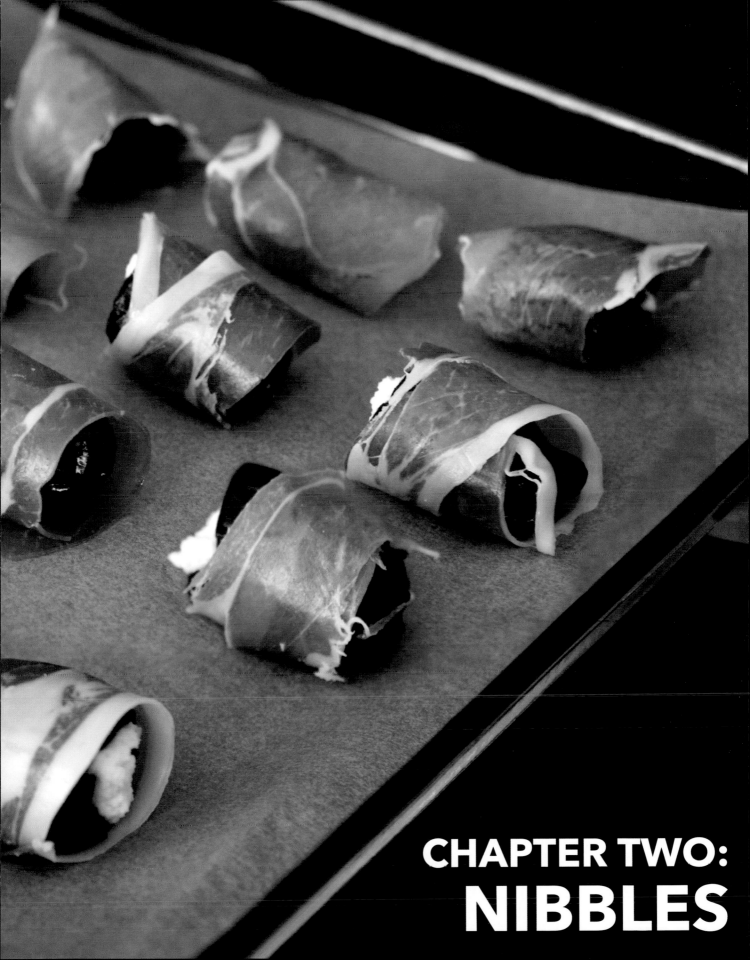

CHAPTER TWO:
NIBBLES

ROASTED ROSEMARY ALMONDS

Those tiny bags of roasted, spiced almonds from gourmet markets are delicious, but they're not exactly wallet-friendly. Plus, store-bought nuts are typically cooked in decidedly non-Paleo fats, like highly processed seed oils. The solution? Roast your own almonds. I've done this successfully with a number of different spices, but rosemary's my hands-down favorite; the woody herb lends a warm, piney aroma to the nuts. A note of warning, though: roasted almonds are dangerously addictive. Proceed with caution.

Makes 2 cups
Hands-on time: 5 minutes
Total time: 20 minutes

1	tablespoon **ghee** or fat of choice
2	cups whole, raw, skin-on **almonds**
2	tablespoons dried **rosemary**
2	teaspoons **kosher salt**
¼	teaspoon freshly ground **black pepper**

DO THIS:

1. Melt the ghee in a large skillet over medium-low heat.

2. Throw in the nuts, making sure they're in a single layer. Stir until the almonds are coated in the ghee, and then add the rosemary, salt, and pepper. Taste and adjust the seasoning.

3. Toast the almonds, stirring often, until slightly darkened and aromatic, about 8 to 12 minutes. Transfer the nuts to a plate and cool to room temperature before serving. You can also store them in an airtight container for up to a week—though I think they taste best on the first day.

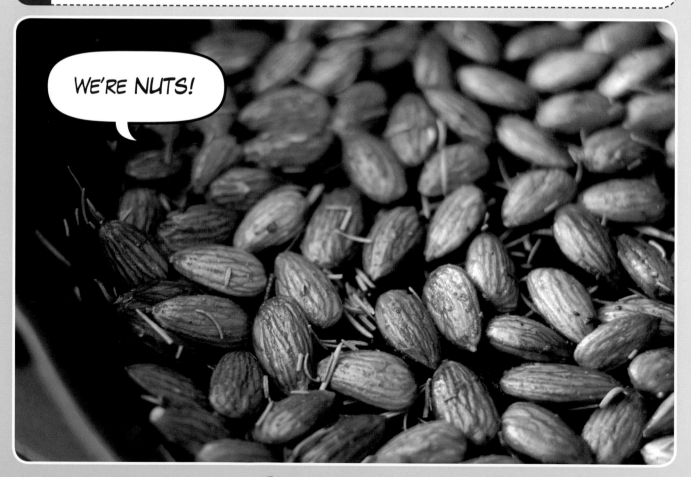

WE'RE NUTS!

THESE NUTS ARE HEAVENLY WHEN SERVED WITH APRICOTS OR GRAPES!

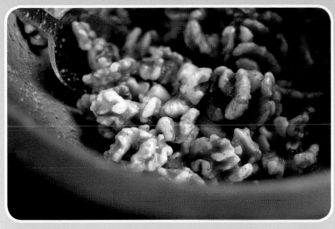
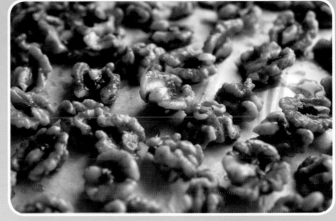
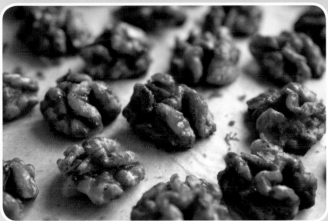
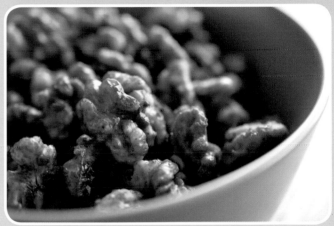

MAPLE-SPICED WALNUTS

These glazed walnuts add a bright, crunchy sweetness to your dishes—and they're dead simple to make.

Makes ¾ cup
Hands-on time: 20 minutes
Total time: 20 minutes

6	ounces raw **walnuts**
2	tablespoons **maple syrup**
1	tablespoon melted **ghee** or **coconut oil**
½	teaspoon **kosher salt**
¼	teaspoon **cayenne pepper**

DO THIS:

1. Preheat the oven to 350°F with the rack in the middle position.

2. Add the walnuts, maple syrup, melted ghee, salt, and cayenne to a bowl, and stir to combine the ingredients. Make sure the nuts are well coated, and then spread them in a single layer on a parchment-lined baking sheet.

3. Bake the nuts for 15 minutes or until fragrant, stirring often to ensure even cooking. Keep a close eye on the walnuts—particularly in the last few minutes—to prevent scorching.

4. Take the walnuts out of the oven, and give them one final toss. They'll still be sticky, but the coating will harden once the nuts cool down.

 THESE CANDIED NUTS CAN HELP BALANCE THE FLAVORS AND TEXTURES OF A SALAD OF SPICY OR BITTER GREENS!

AH, CHIPS. (OR, IF YOU'RE A BRIT, CRISPS.)

LEGEND HAS IT THAT POTATO CHIPS WERE INVENTED A DECADE BEFORE THE CIVIL WAR BY GEORGE CRUM, AN AFRICAN AMERICAN CHEF AT THE MOON LAKE LODGE IN SARATOGA SPRINGS, NEW YORK. AS THE STORY GOES, CRUM'S INVENTION WAS TRIGGERED BY A FLASH OF ANGER AT A CUSTOMER WHO HAD SENT BACK HIS ORDER OF FRENCH FRIES, COMPLAINING THAT THEY WERE TOO THICK AND SOGGY. IN A FIT OF SPITE, CRUM CUT UP ANOTHER POTATO INTO PAPER-THIN SLICES. DEEP-FRIED AND TOSSED IN A SHOWER OF SALT, THESE "FRIES" WERE MEANT AS A SARCASTIC RETORT TO THE CUSTOMER'S COMPLAINT, BUT TO CRUM'S SURPRISE, HIS "SARATOGA CHIPS" BECAME A HUGE HIT.

CRUM'S TALE IS LIKELY APOCRYPHAL, BUT CRUNCHY, SALTY CHIPS WERE HERE TO STAY. BY THE START OF THE TWENTIETH CENTURY, CHIPS HAD ALREADY BECOME AMERICA'S SNACK FOOD OF CHOICE.

TODAY, MASS-MANUFACTURED POTATO AND CORN CHIPS (NOT TO MENTION ALL SORTS OF CHEESY, POOFY THINGS) ARE EVERYWHERE. EVERY YEAR, AMERICANS CONSUME OVER 1.2 BILLION POUNDS OF HYPER-PROCESSED, ARTIFICIALLY COLORED, CHEMICALLY ENHANCED CHIPS. THAT'S A TON OF HYDROGENATED OILS, ACRYLAMIDE, AND MSG, PEOPLE.

WHAT DO YOU SAY WE MAKE SOMETHING TASTIER AND HEALTHIER, BUT JUST AS CRUNCHY AND SAVORY?

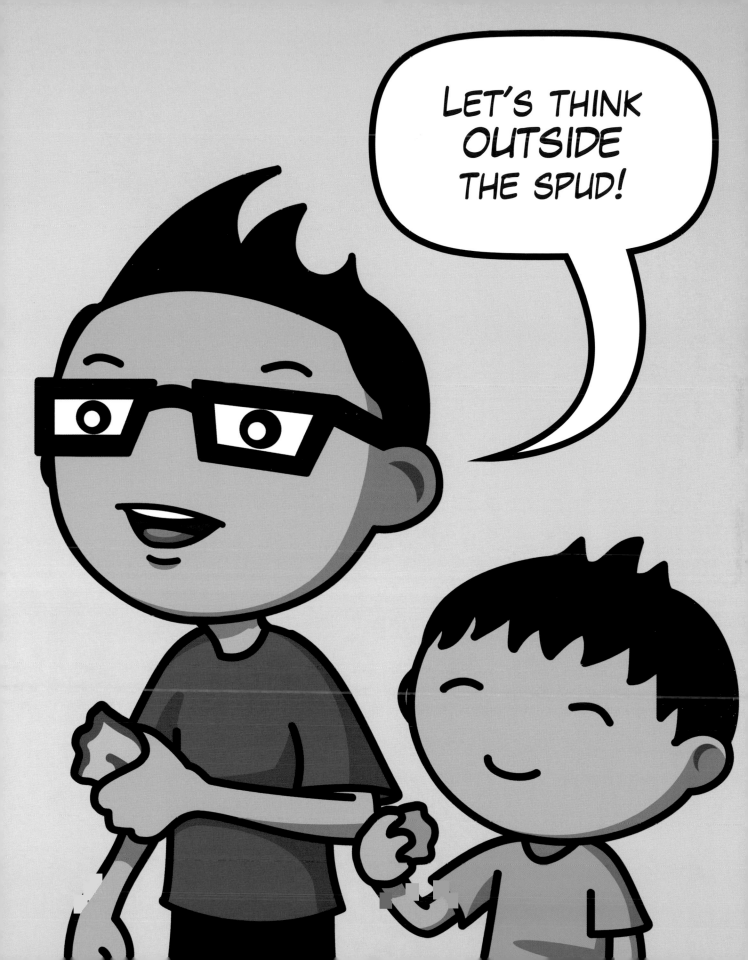

BRUSSELS SPROUTS CHIPS

The next time you trim Brussels sprouts in preparation for roasting, don't chuck the outer leaves into the trash. Instead, bake them into salty, crunchy, irresistible Brussels sprouts chips. Waste not, want not, right?

Makes 2 cups
Hands-on time: 10 minutes
Total time: 30 minutes

2 cups **Brussels sprouts leaves** (the outer leaves trimmed from about 2 pounds of sprouts)
2 tablespoons melted **ghee** or fat of choice
Kosher salt
Finely grated zest from 1 small **lemon** (optional)

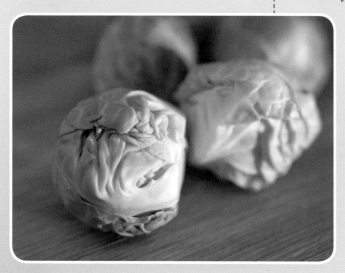 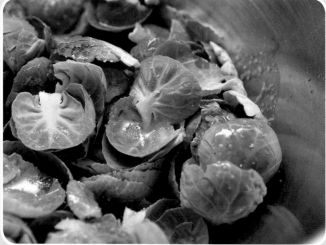

DO THIS:

1. Preheat the oven to 350°F, and line two rimmed baking sheets with parchment paper.

2. In a large bowl, mix the leaves and melted ghee. Season with salt to taste.

3. Arrange the leaves in a single layer on the baking sheets, and bake each tray for 8 to 10 minutes or until crispy and brown around the edges.

4. If desired, grate some lemon zest over the crispy Brussels sprouts leaves, and serve immediately.

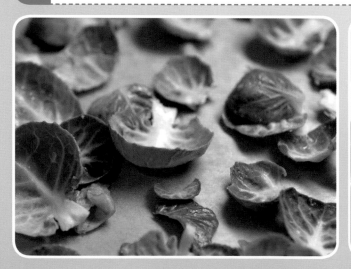 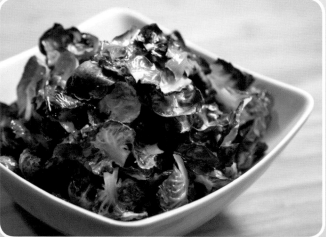

YOU CAN ALSO DEEP-FRY 'EM, BUT ONLY IF YOU DON'T MIND THE SPLATTER AND CLEAN-UP!

APPLE CHIPS

For us, apple chips are a family affair. Every autumn, when my husband's uncle distributes boxes of apples from his trees, I know that my mother-in-law will soon appear on our doorstep with bags of freshly baked apple chips. Using a mandoline slicer, she thinly cuts Fuji apples before dusting them with cinnamon and slowly baking them until they're crisp. Each bag of these light, crunchy chips takes her several hours to make, but we've been known to polish 'em off in a matter of minutes. Yes, they're *that* good.

Makes 8 servings
Hands-on time: 10 minutes
Total time: 3 hours

5   large Granny Smith or Fuji **apples**, cored and cut crosswise with a mandoline into uniform ⅛-inch-thick slices

2   teaspoons ground **cinnamon** (optional)

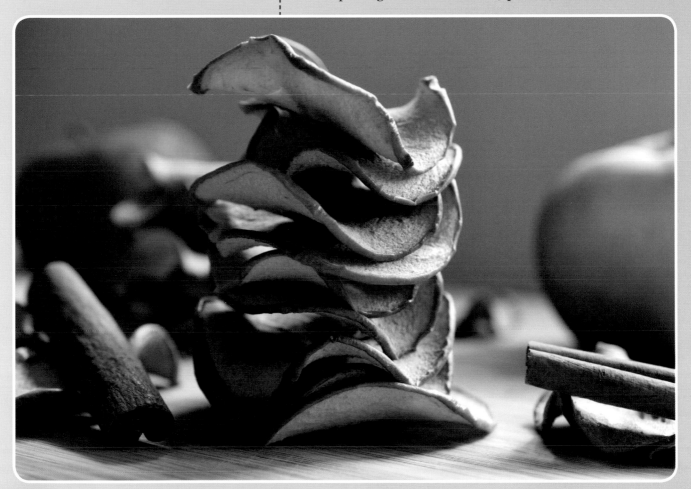

DO THIS:

1. Adjust the racks in the oven so that they're evenly spaced, and preheat the oven to 225°F on the convection bake setting. (Alternatively, you can use the regular bake setting, but without the circulating hot air, you'll have to bake the apple slices one tray at a time on the middle rack.)

2. Arrange the apple slices on several parchment-lined baking sheets, and if desired, dust with cinnamon. Bake for 1½ hours on convection bake (or 2 hours on regular bake), flipping the chips over midway through the cooking time. Turn off the oven, leaving the chips inside to fully dehydrate. Once they're cool, serve or store the chips in a sealed container for up to 3 days.

 EVER TRY SLOW COOKER KALUA PIG (PAGE 234) ON AN APPLE CHIP? IT'S NOT WEIRD. IT'S GOOD.

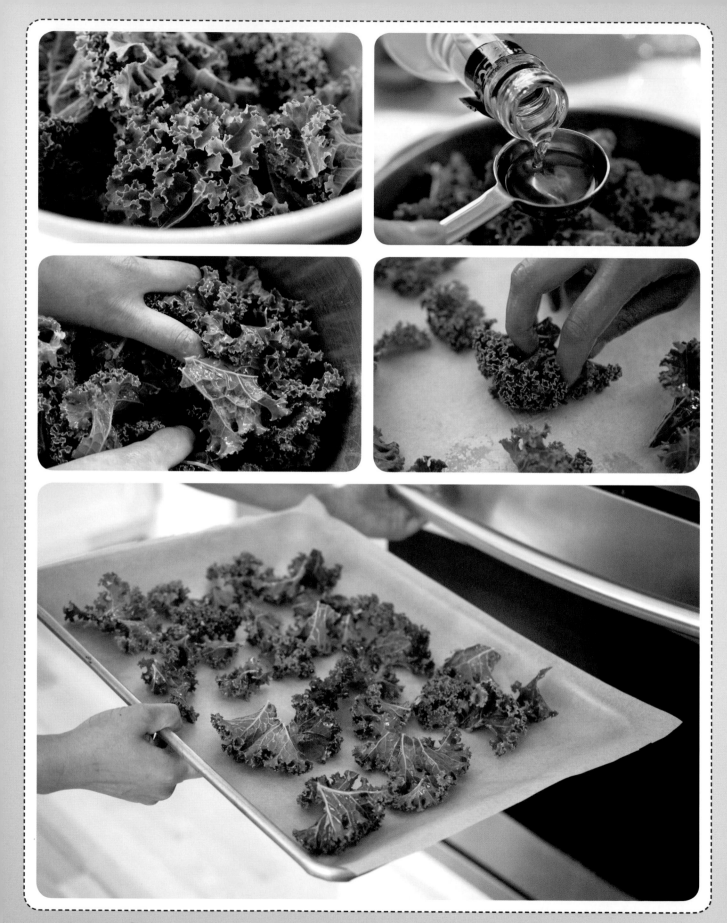

KALE CHIPS

Kale chips are the most addictive superfood known to mankind. Combining the salty crunch of potato chips and the nutrient load of a bottle of vitamins, these crisps will disappear before you can bake up a second batch. Even your vegan pals will give you an enthusiastic round of high-fives after they sample your chips.

Makes 3 cups
Hands-on time: 10 minutes
Total time: 25 minutes

1 pound **kale** (about 2 large bunches), washed, stemmed, and thoroughly dried
2 tablespoons **macadamia nut oil** or fat of choice
Fleur de sel, **Magic Mushroom Powder** (page 35), or seasoning salt of choice
Finely grated zest from 1 small **lemon** (optional)

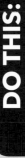

DO THIS:

1. Preheat the oven to 350°F with the rack in the middle position, and line a couple of rimmed baking sheets with parchment paper.

2. This is key: make sure the kale is super dry. I'm talking bone-dry, people. You don't want any traces of water on the leaves whatsoever. Pat them down with a paper towel if necessary.

3. Toss the dry leaves with the oil, using your hands to distribute it evenly. Arrange the kale in a single layer on the lined baking sheets, keeping some distance between the leaves. And make sure the leaves aren't folded over; otherwise, they won't crisp properly.

4. Bake each tray for 12 minutes or until crisp, but not burnt. Remove the kale chips from the oven and season to taste with fleur de sel (or your favorite seasoning salt) and lemon zest, if desired.

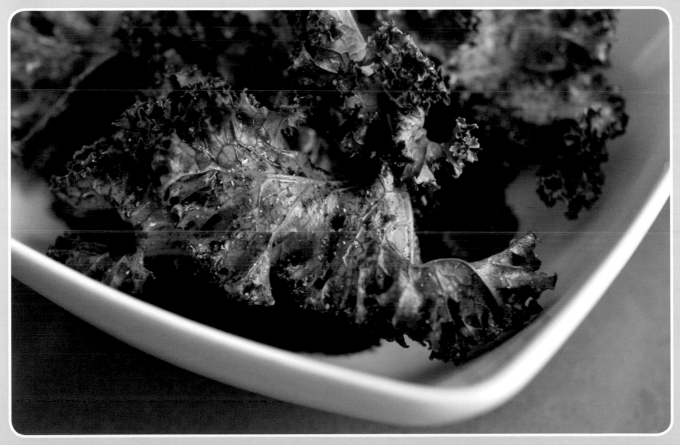

KALE CHIPS CAN BE A WONDERFULLY CRISP GARNISH FOR HEARTY WINTER SOUPS!

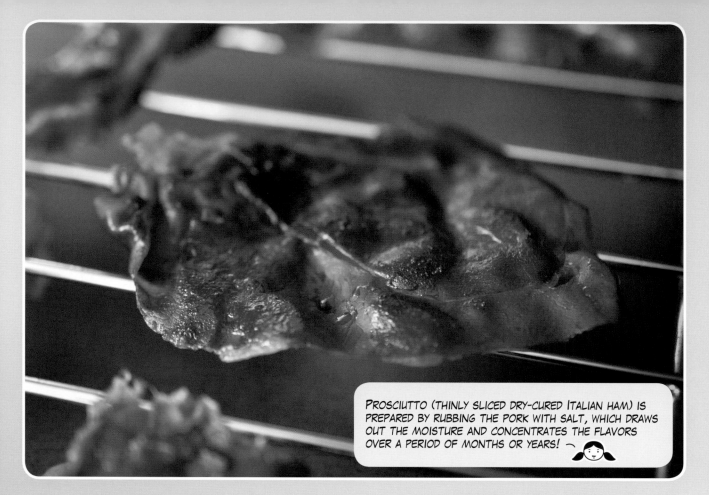

PROSCIUTTO (THINLY SLICED DRY-CURED ITALIAN HAM) IS PREPARED BY RUBBING THE PORK WITH SALT, WHICH DRAWS OUT THE MOISTURE AND CONCENTRATES THE FLAVORS OVER A PERIOD OF MONTHS OR YEARS! ~

PORKITOS (PROSCIUTTO CHIPS)

"Porkitos"—crunchy chips made of prosciutto—lend a wonderfully salty crunch to creamy soups, salads, and purées. Or you can just stuff your face with them. 'Cause really: Who doesn't love crispy pork chips?

Makes 2 servings
Hands-on time: 15 minutes
Total time: 15 minutes

3 ounces thinly sliced **prosciutto**

DO THIS:

1. Preheat the oven to 350°F with the rack in the middle position, and line a rimmed baking sheet with parchment paper. Arrange the prosciutto in a single layer on the lined baking sheets. Don't overcrowd the swine, or it won't crisp properly.

2. Bake for 10 to 15 minutes or until crunchy. Watch your chips like a hawk to make sure they don't burn. Porkitos will actually get crunchier as they cool, so err on the side of underbaking.

3. Transfer the chips to a wire rack to cool. Enjoy them as a salty snack or appetizer, or use them to dress up your salads. (But something tells me these chips'll be long gone before you've had time to whip up a salad.)

CRUMBLE AND SPRINKLE SOME PORKITOS ON A PLATTER OF CLASSIC EGG SALAD (PAGE 130)!

MUSHROOM CHIPS

Some folks don't like the soft, spongy texture of mushrooms. I'm not one of them, so I have no idea how they can pass up these meaty bursts of umami goodness. Still, I have to imagine that even the pickiest fungi-hater will fall madly in love with these crispity-crunchity oven-baked mushroom chips. To mere mortals like you and me, they're irresistible—like potato chips on flavor-enhancing steroids.

Makes 2 servings
Hands-on time: 20 minutes
Total time: 1½ hours

10 ounces king oyster **mushrooms**
2 tablespoons melted **ghee** or fat of choice
Kosher salt
Freshly ground **black pepper**

DO THIS:

1. Preheat the oven to 300°F with the rack in the middle position. Line a couple of rimmed baking sheets with parchment paper.

2. Use a mandoline slicer or knife to cut the mushrooms into ⅛-inch-thick slices. Arrange them in a single layer on the lined baking sheets. Make sure the mushrooms are super dry, and leave some space between the slices. Brush the melted ghee on both sides of the mushroom slices, and season with salt and pepper to taste.

3. Bake each tray for 45 minutes to an hour, or until the chips are golden brown and crispy. These chips won't continue to crisp after they leave the oven, so don't pull them out until they're crunchy.

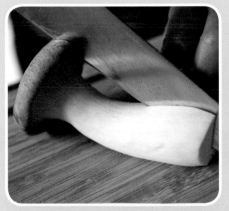
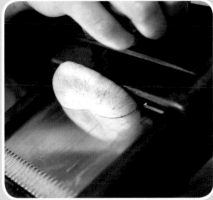
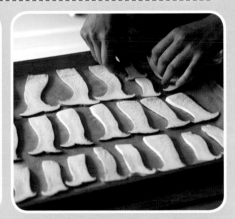

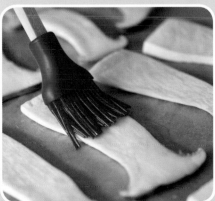
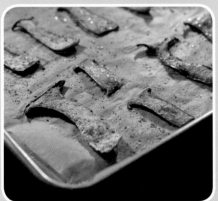
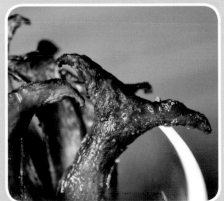

 CROUTONS ARE EVIL AND BLAND! TOSS THESE BABIES ONTO YOUR SALADS INSTEAD!

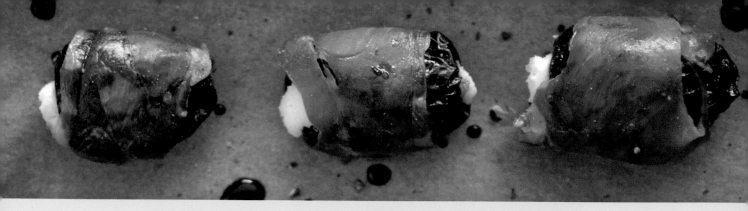

DEVILS ON HORSEBACK

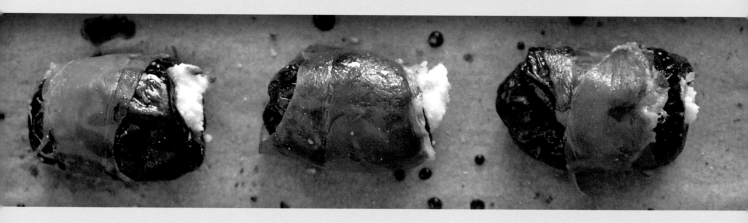

These little bites are sweet, savory, and delicious as sin.

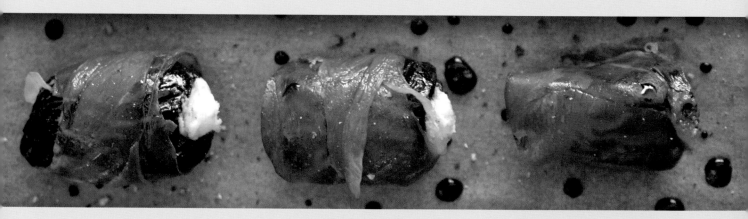

Makes 16 bites | Hands-on time: 10 minutes | Total time: 15 minutes

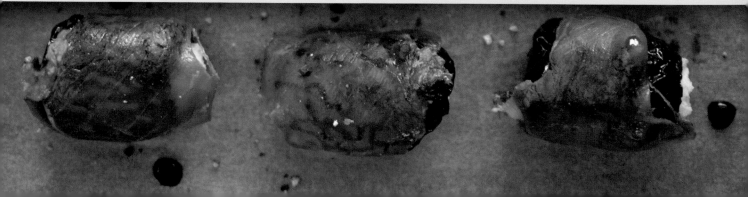

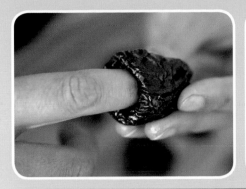
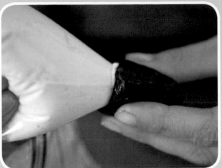
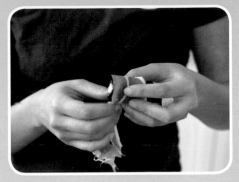

GET:

16   pitted **prunes**
½   cup **Macadamia Nut "Ricotta"** (page 46)
2   ounces thinly sliced **prosciutto**
Balsamic vinegar
Freshly ground **black pepper**

BAG IT!

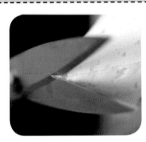

Don't have a pastry bag? Simply snip a ½-inch hole in the corner of a quart-sized plastic food storage or freezer bag, and you're good to go.

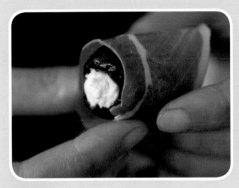
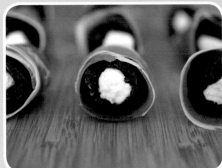
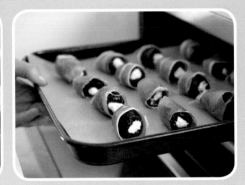

DO THIS:

1. Position an oven rack about 4 to 6 inches from the heating element, and preheat the broiler. Use your finger to carefully open up the cavity of each pitted prune. Then, with a pastry bag (or a sealable plastic food storage bag—see above), pipe the "cheese" into the prunes.

2. Wrap each prune in a thin layer of prosciutto, and arrange them in a single layer on a parchment-lined baking sheet. Broil for 2 to 4 minutes or until the prunes puff up and the prosciutto crisps and turns golden brown around the edges. Keep an eye on the prunes; they may be devils, but you don't want them to burn. Drizzle with balsamic vinegar and season with pepper to taste before serving.

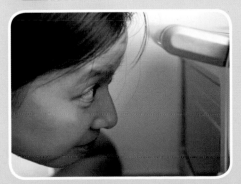
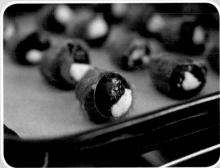
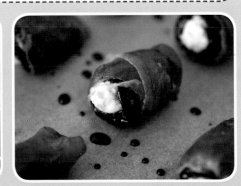

 ⌐ THROWING A BIG SHINDIG? BE SURE TO DOUBLE OR EVEN TRIPLE THE RECIPE!

CHOPPED LIVER + BACON

If you're like my friend Rebecca, "chopped liver" is synonymous with the gray mush forced upon you by your Jewish grandmother. I don't have a Bubbe, but if I did, I'm sure she'd cluck disapprovingly at this bacon-infused, highly non-kosher rendition of a classic. But don't let that stop you from making this savory, nutrient-dense spread for your next party. The combination of eggs, earthy chicken livers, caramelized onions, and crispy bacon will have you scraping the bottom of the bowl with your favorite crudités.

Makes 2 cups
Hands-on time: 45 minutes
Total time: 45 minutes

DON'T TURN YOUR NOSE UP AT ORGAN MEATS. LIVER IS PACKED WITH VITAMINS, MINERALS, AND FOLIC ACID, MAKING IT ONE OF THE MOST NUTRIENT-RICH FOODS AROUND!

- **3** slices thick-cut **bacon**, cross-cut into ¼-inch pieces
- **1** small **sweet onion**, thinly sliced
- **1** pound **chicken livers**
  Kosher salt
  Freshly ground **black pepper**
- **3** **Perfect Hard-Boiled Eggs** (page 120), quartered
- **2** tablespoons **balsamic vinegar**
- **¼** cup minced fresh **Italian parsley**

DO THIS:

1. Cook the bacon in a large skillet over medium heat. Stir occasionally to ensure even browning. Once it's crisp, transfer the crunchy bacon to a platter with a slotted spoon.

2. Add the onions to the bacon drippings in the pan. Cook over low heat for 30 minutes or until golden and translucent.

3. Trim the livers of any unsightly blood vessels or blobs of fat. Roughly chop the livers. Once the onions are caramelized, add the liver pieces to the pan with the onions.

4. Generously season the livers with salt and pepper, and sear them over medium-high heat for 2 to 3 minutes per side or until cooked through.

5. Toss the cooked livers and onions, eggs, and vinegar into the work bowl of a food processor, and pulse until combined. Taste for seasoning; if needed, adjust with salt, pepper, and/or balsamic vinegar.

6. Transfer the liver to a bowl and top with the reserved bacon bits and minced parsley. Serve with raw veggies.

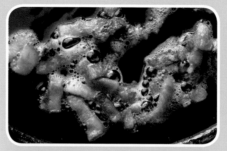
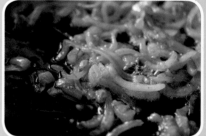
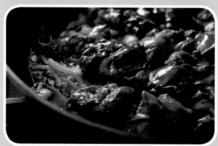
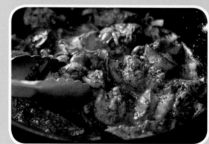
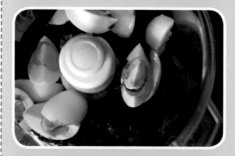
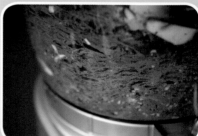
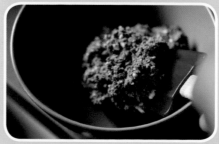
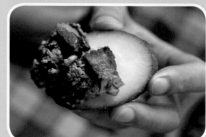

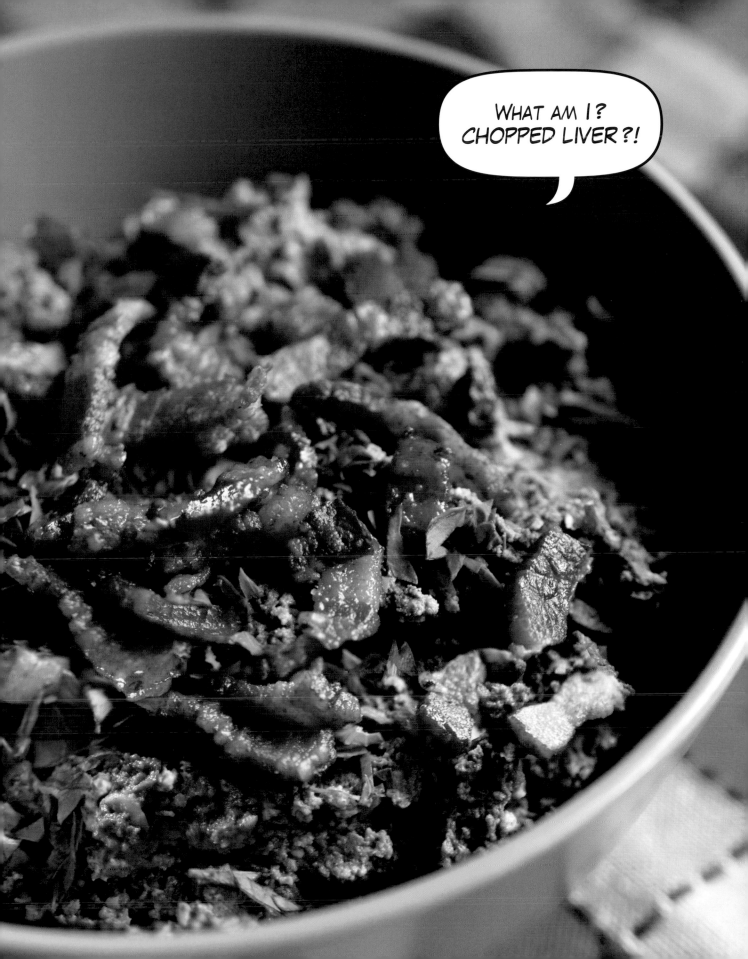

CRISPY GIZZARD CONFIT

Sure, gizzards can be tough and chewy when cooked over high heat, but if you take the time to braise them slowly in duck fat and crisp them up in a skillet, you'll be rewarded with tender, succulent nuggets. None of your dinner guests—or picky kids—will ever suspect that the meat they're happily eating is offal.

Makes 4 servings
Hands-on time: 10 minutes
Total time: 10 hours

1   pound cleaned **chicken gizzards**
¾   teaspoon **kosher salt**
1½ cups **duck fat**
3   **garlic cloves**, smashed and peeled
1   teaspoon whole black **peppercorns**
4   sprigs fresh **thyme**

DO THIS:

1. Season the gizzards with salt. Place them in a covered container and refrigerate for 8 to 24 hours.

2. When you're ready to cook, preheat the oven to 300°F. Melt the duck fat in a small ovenproof pot over medium heat. Toss the garlic, peppercorns, and thyme into the pot. Once the fat is fragrant from the herbs and garlic, add the gizzards. Stir to submerge the gizzards, and bring to a simmer.

3. Cut out a circle of parchment paper with the same diameter as the pot, and place it on top of the liquid. Cover with a lid and braise the gizzards in the oven for 2 hours or until fork-tender.

4. If desired, you can refrigerate the gizzards in the duck fat for up to a week. Just make sure you strain out the thyme, peppercorns, and garlic before storing because they're hard to pick out of the solidified fat. But if you're ready to eat, remove the gizzards from the fat and toss them into a skillet over medium-high heat. Fry the braised gizzards about 1 minute on each side, or until crispy. Transfer them to a plate and dig in.

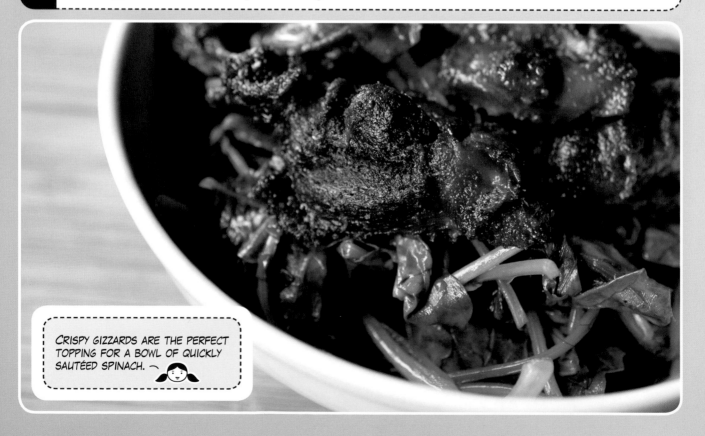

CRISPY GIZZARDS ARE THE PERFECT TOPPING FOR A BOWL OF QUICKLY SAUTÉED SPINACH. ⌐

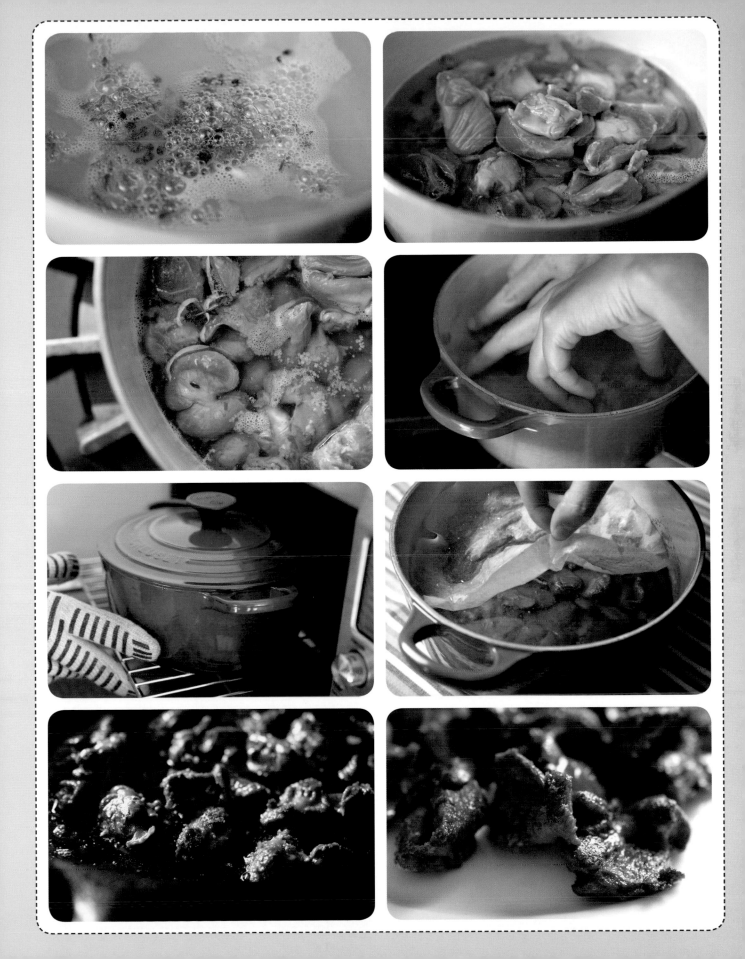

MAKIN' BACON

It's true: Paleo eaters can eat bacon. I'm not saying it should be the primary source of protein in your diet, but bacon's not the menacing artery-clogger it's been made out to be. So once again, we can enjoy unctuously mouth-filling slices of crunchy porkiness with our eggs or crumbled atop a salad. Hallelujah!

Of course, I know that Paleo doesn't give me license to gorge on the stuff, and that it's important to source my bacon from pastured pigs. That said, I can't resist the chewy-crisp texture and indelibly smoky punch that bacon imparts to dishes. Then again, who can?

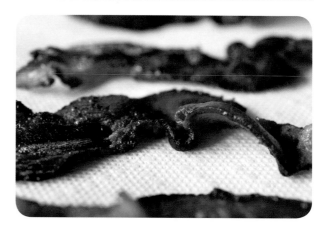

Here are my three favorite ways to cook bacon:

1. IN A MICROWAVE OVEN

Microwaving bacon is easy: just sandwich a few slices between sheets of paper towel, stick 'em on a plate, and nuke for 2 to 3 minutes, checking frequently. Of course, if you consider microwave ovens to be mini Three Mile Islands, you'll want to skip this method.

2. IN A SKILLET

Are you an old-school traditionalist? Arrange the bacon in a large, unheated cast iron skillet or griddle. Make sure the slices are in a single layer. Then, heat the pan and bacon together over medium heat. Cook for about 10 minutes before you flip the strips. Fry the bacon for another 5 to 10 minutes or until crispy, and then transfer the bacon onto paper towels or a wire rack. The only drawbacks? Skillet-fried bacon doesn't always cook evenly, and it tends to shrink in size dramatically.

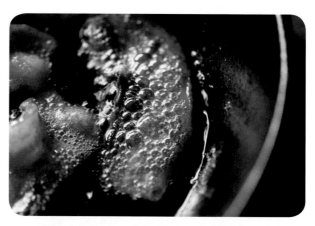

3. IN AN OVEN

My favorite way to cook bacon is in the oven. Place a wire rack atop a foil-lined rimmed baking sheet, and arrange the bacon slices on the rack in a single layer. Stick the tray on the middle rack of an unheated oven, and then set the oven to 400°F. Bake for 20 minutes or until the bacon reaches your desired level of crispness. Watch the bacon carefully to make sure it doesn't blacken and burn. Remove the bacon from the oven, and save the bacon drippings in a sealed container. The drippings will come in handy as a cooking fat, or as an ingredient for Five-Minute Bacon Aïoli (page 60).

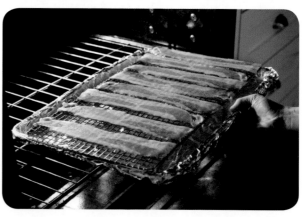

BACON + GUACAMOLE SAMMIES

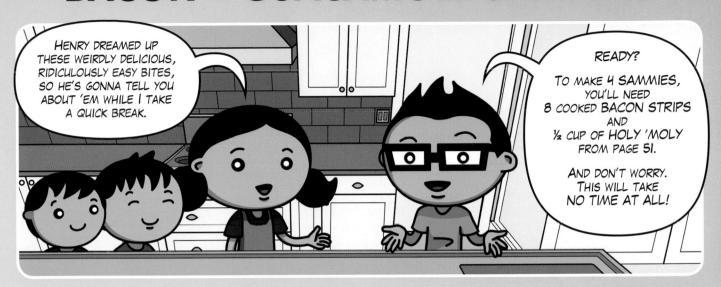

HENRY DREAMED UP THESE WEIRDLY DELICIOUS, RIDICULOUSLY EASY BITES, SO HE'S GONNA TELL YOU ABOUT 'EM WHILE I TAKE A QUICK BREAK.

READY?

TO MAKE 4 SAMMIES, YOU'LL NEED 8 COOKED BACON STRIPS AND ½ CUP OF HOLY 'MOLY FROM PAGE 51.

AND DON'T WORRY. THIS WILL TAKE NO TIME AT ALL!

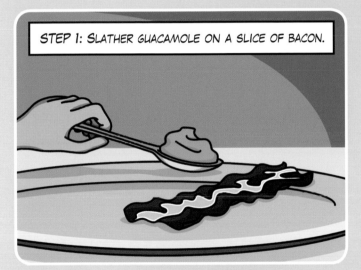

STEP 1: SLATHER GUACAMOLE ON A SLICE OF BACON.

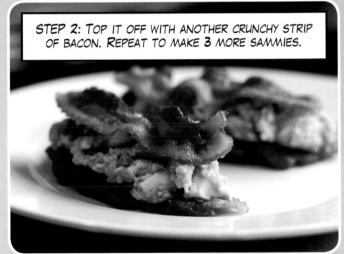

STEP 2: TOP IT OFF WITH ANOTHER CRUNCHY STRIP OF BACON. REPEAT TO MAKE 3 MORE SAMMIES.

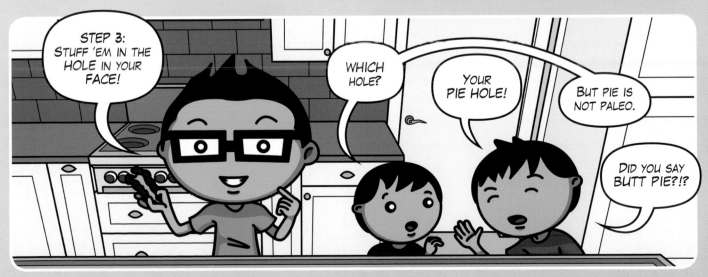

STEP 3: STUFF 'EM IN THE HOLE IN YOUR FACE!

WHICH HOLE?

YOUR PIE HOLE!

BUT PIE IS NOT PALEO.

DID YOU SAY BUTT PIE?!?

~ A WORD TO THE WISE: IF YOUR CRISPY BACON STRIPS ARE SUPER-LONG, SNAP 'EM IN HALF BEFORE YOU MAKE THESE SAMMIES, OR THE GUACAMOLE WILL SQUISH OUT WHEN YOU TAKE YOUR FIRST BITE.

THE BIG QUESTION:

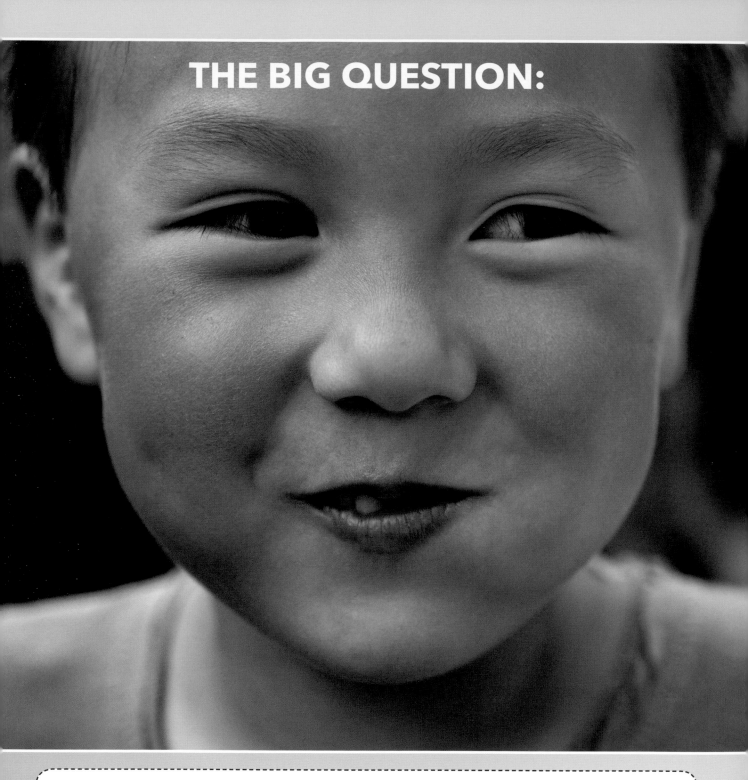

For the first few years of their lives—before Henry and I adopted a real-food-only approach to nutrition—our children ate what we ate: a low-fat diet with a heavy dose of factory-processed "healthy" snacks.

Smugly congratulating ourselves for feeding our kids as healthfully as possible, we kick-started each morning with homemade granola over low-fat yogurt or egg white omelets with whole wheat toast. Our family broke bread over nightly meals of "heart-healthy whole grains"—followed by desserts that were "naturally" sweetened with cane sugar or agave nectar. Never mind the digestive woes and sugar crashes.

DO THE KIDS EAT PALEO?

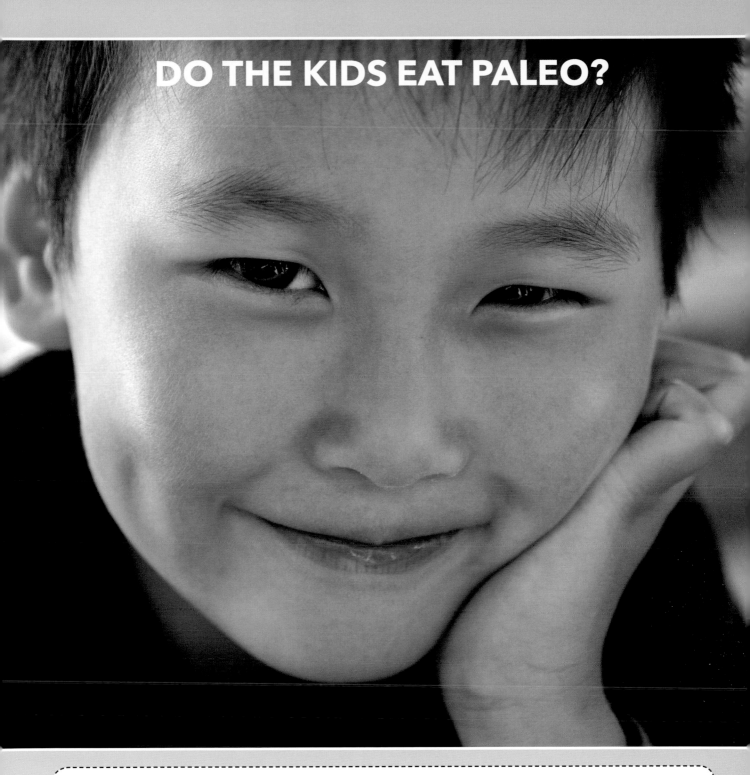

When I made the decision to stop eating hyper-processed, bad-for-you food products, it was tough to break the addiction—but at least I could appreciate the health benefits that came with the change. My kids? Not so much. They just wanted to know why we wouldn't have syrup-drenched waffles for breakfast anymore.

I envied the model Paleo parents out there who successfully took a cold-turkey approach to weaning their offspring. From what I could tell, they stood firm as their kids screamed and wailed in vain for their waffles and toast, their bean burritos and churros, their spaghetti and garlic bread, and their brownies and ice cream.

The theory was that once the junk food withdrawal symptoms subsided (and hunger took over), the kids would be good to go.

Sadly, our experience didn't go quite so smoothly.

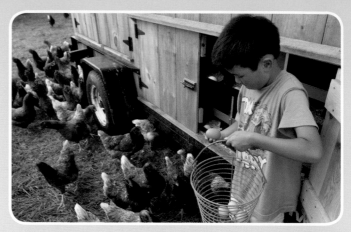

It all started promisingly enough. We did the big pantry/fridge/freezer purge. Breakfast cereals? Gone. Bagels? Gone. Organic cheddar goldfish crackers? Gone. Boxes of mac & cheese? Gone. For a while, the boys kept asking for cereal or waffles at breakfast. "Nope," I'd say. "But you can have eggs with bacon or sausage, and I'll cut you some strawberries."

"We'll just have the strawberries, then," they'd say.

Owen—three years older than his brother—handled the transition pretty well, all things considered. He didn't complain or demand grainy or sugary foods. But Big-O's never had much of a sweet tooth, and his palate is fairly broad; this is a kid who's always wolfed down Indian curries and dishes of *ankimo* (monkfish liver) at Japanese restaurants. While on a family trip to Mexico, he happily munched on a plate of deep-fried maguey worms.

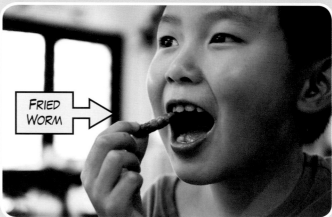

FRIED WORM ➡

These days, Owen eats pretty much whatever we put in front of him. He tends to be especially enthusiastic about Paleo dishes that he has a hand in making—even if all he does is help stir the pot.

Ollie, on the other hand, made abundantly clear that he was not on board with this Paleo business. This wasn't a surprise; our then-two-year-old was a "healthy" junk food addict of the highest order. Even before we made the switch to Paleo, Henry and I were concerned that Lil-O refused to eat anything but highly refined carbs: pasta, rice, bread, and sweets. He wouldn't touch meat, but we couldn't call him a vegetarian, either, because vegetarians eat vegetables.

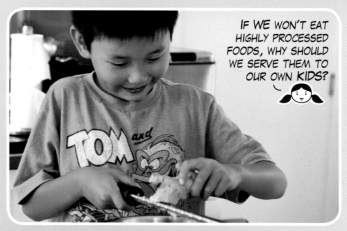

IF WE WON'T EAT HIGHLY PROCESSED FOODS, WHY SHOULD WE SERVE THEM TO OUR OWN KIDS?

One weekend soon after we started eating Paleo, Henry decided to serve Ollie only meat and vegetables until he was willing to try a bite. In response, our son went on a day-long hunger strike. Finally, desperate to get him to eat *something*, Henry tried to bribe Ollie with a new wooden toy train. "All you have to do is try one bite," my husband pleaded.

Ollie burst into tears.

"Kiddo," Henry reasoned with him, "in this house, we only have real food." My toddler stared at his dad, and then flung open the front door and ran outside.

"Then I don't want to live here anymore!" he yelled, tears coursing down his face.

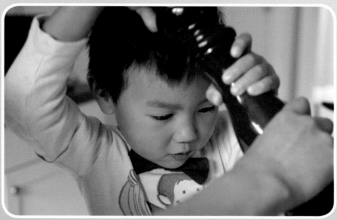

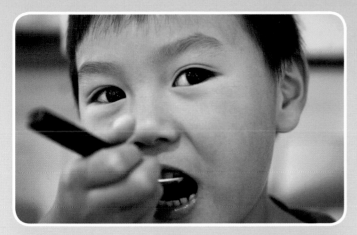

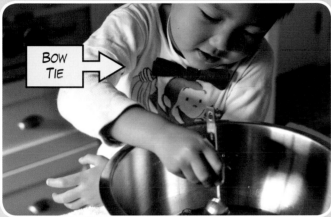

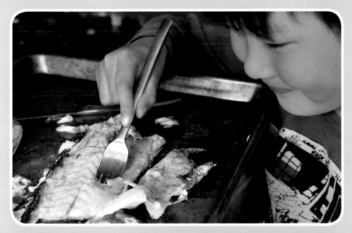

BOW TIE →

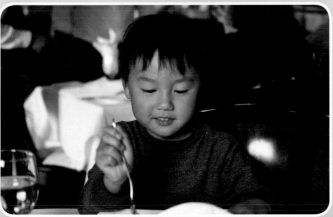

Alas, we declared our Great Meat & Vegetable Experiment a failure.

But we didn't give up. We continued to put real, whole foods on Ollie's plate. And slowly but surely, his once-narrow palate began to broaden. Our little guy is still no fan of my more exotic concoctions, but he now chows down on meat and fish, and no longer recoils at the sight of broccoli or asparagus.

The key, we discovered, was simple: model the food behaviors we want to see, and be persistent.

With no junk food in the house, the kids eventually got the message that no amount of rifling through our pantry was going to magically conjure up boxes of cookies or candy bars. We held firm when they flashed their puppy-dog eyes and begged for treats. And when supper was served, my boys knew not to demand their own separate "kid-friendly" meals of pizza bagels or processed chicken tenders like the ones seen on TV.

We eat what I make, and that's that. Yes, it would be easier to give in, but real food is non-negotiable in our house. It took some doing, but both of our kids are now aboard the Paleo train. I estimate that over 80 percent of their meals consist of whole, nutrient-dense foods. I know this because Henry and I prepare the vast majority of their breakfasts, lunches, and dinners.

Does that mean our children are perfectly Paleo? Nope. To really take hold, Paleo eating can't be forced. We've done our best to be good role models, explaining to our boys why they should stick with whole, nutrient-dense foods, and trusting them to make their own food choices when they're not at home. But that means they sometimes choose to eat stuff that's less than healthy. And we're okay with that. (Fortunately, our kids don't have any allergies or intolerances that make veering off Paleo more of an issue.)

So these days, when the kids are at school functions or playdates, we let them make their own food choices. Owen and Ollie are free to grab cupcakes at their pals' birthday parties (though Owen chooses to abstain more often than not). Henry and I don't force them to sit out the pizza parties at school, and we don't freak out (much) when grandma visits and sneaks each of them a breakfast pastry. But these are the exceptions rather than the rule.

And between you and me, I think that we've got 'em brainwashed already: one of Ollie's teachers recently told us that he's been telling the other kids at school that candy's not healthy.

I beamed with pride.

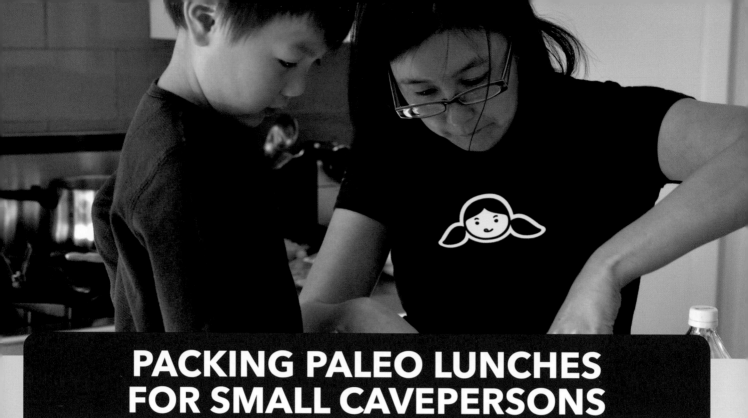

PACKING PALEO LUNCHES
FOR SMALL CAVEPERSONS

Nothing's easier than chucking pre-packaged trays of factory-made lunches into backpacks as we rush our children out the door…but I'm guessing none of us are eager to sacrifice our kids' health for the sake of convenience.

Of course, convenience still matters. Not many of us can devote hours each day to crafting five-star meals to cram into superhero lunch boxes. What we need are school lunches that are both easy *and* healthy.

Here are some lunch-packing tips that we've found particularly effective:

- Give your offspring a say in what goes into their lunchboxes. Even if you've packed the most delicious and nutritious meal possible for your kiddos, it'll all be for naught if it ends up in the garbage or traded away for a bag of chips and a can of soda. Encourage them to choose their own lunch items from your Paleo-friendly pantry and fridge. This way, the food you pack will actually stand a chance of being eaten.

- Some kids like variety, others like the same thing every day. But no matter what, the lunch you pack should contain some animal protein, vegetables, healthy fats, and fruit. Oh, and an occasional piece of dark chocolate makes for a nice treat, too.

- Invest in a few insulated containers and pack hot leftovers for your children. Owen's favorite lunches include leftover roast chicken and sautéed mushrooms sandwiched between slices of last night's steak.

- Sometimes, convenience foods aren't such a bad thing. Search out high-quality deli meat, mini sausages, dried fruit snacks, and jarred marinara sauce to throw together tasty lunches. Even better: use some of the building block recipes in this book to jazz up the noonday meal. Packing a small container of Paleo Ranch Dressing (page 62) is a surefire way to entice your little ones into finishing their vegetables.

Packing delicious lunch boxes with nourishing food that'll fuel your children's bodies and brains isn't rocket science. It may sound like a tall order, but just think of your young 'uns as miniature versions of you. Don't pack anything in their lunch boxes that you wouldn't happily eat.

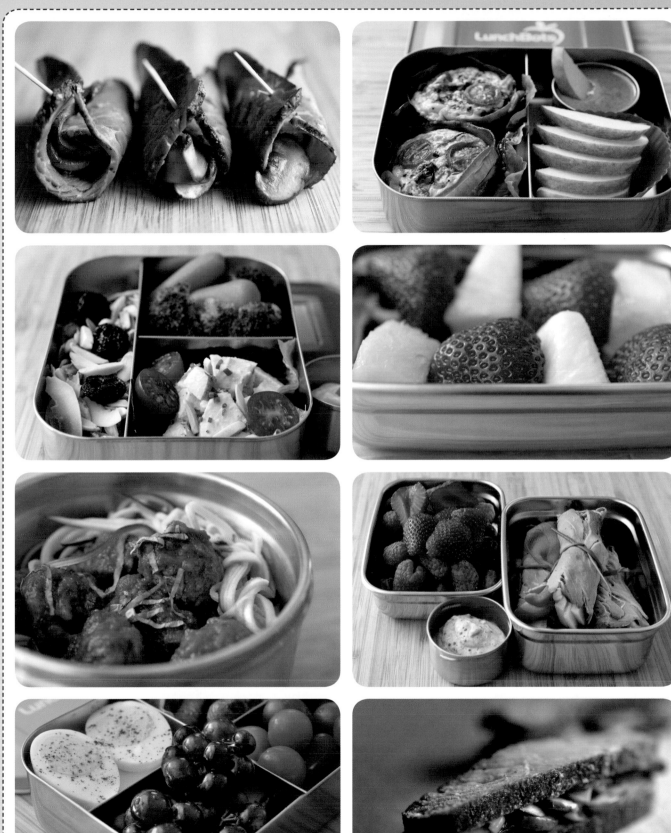

Digging these stainless steel food containers? Get them at lunchbots.com!

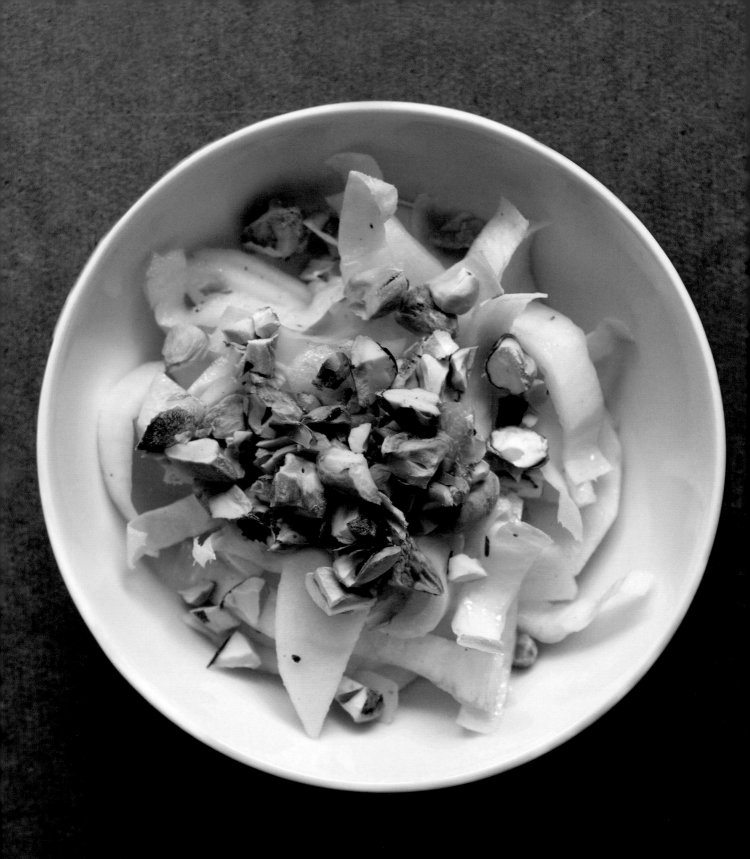

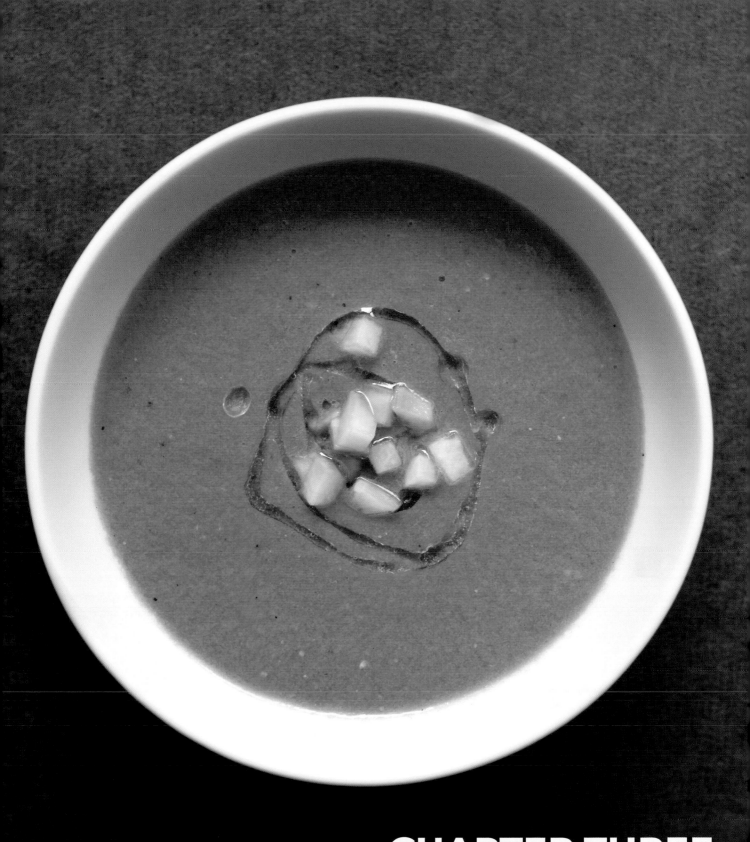

CHAPTER THREE:
SALADS + SOUPS

TOMATO + BASIL SALAD

I try to channel Chez Panisse's Alice Waters whenever I throw together a simple salad like this one, which means I get all up in your face (as nicely as possible, of course) about using high-quality ingredients. If you attempt this recipe with mealy, out-of-season tomatoes, you'll end up with a subpar salad. But if you start with juicy, ripe heirloom tomatoes, this little salad will explode with big flavor.

Makes 4 servings | Hands-on time: 10 minutes | Total time: 20 minutes

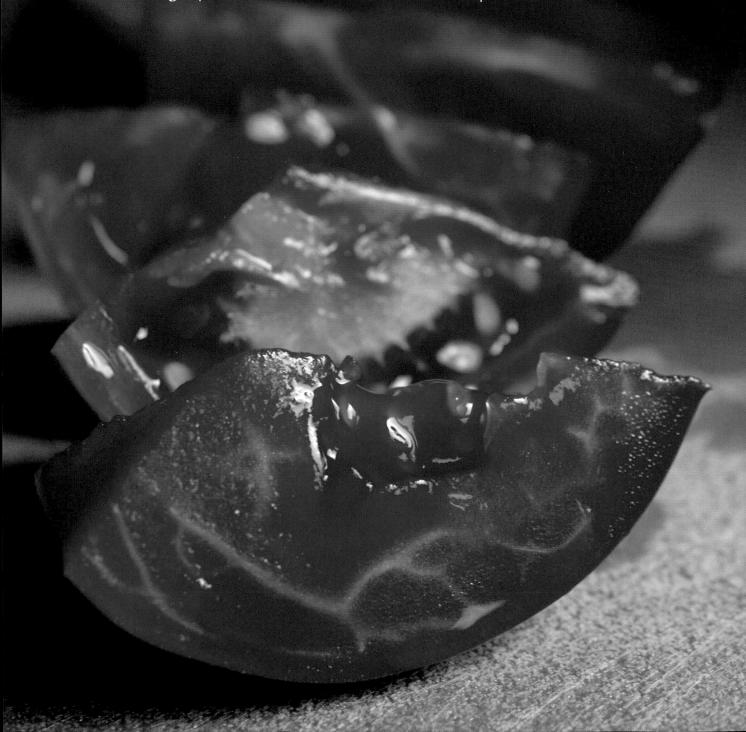

GET:

1. medium **shallot**, thinly sliced
2. tablespoons **balsamic vinegar**
3. ripe heirloom **tomatoes**, cut into wedges
   Fleur de sel
   Freshly ground **black pepper**
4. fresh **basil leaves**, cut into a chiffonade (see description below)
   Extra-virgin olive oil

DO THIS:

1. Mellow the bite of the sliced shallots by soaking them in a bowl of balsamic vinegar for at least 15 minutes.

2. Arrange the sliced tomatoes on a serving platter, and season with fleur de sel and pepper to taste. Top with the marinated shallots, basil, and a drizzle of extra-virgin olive oil. Serve immediately.

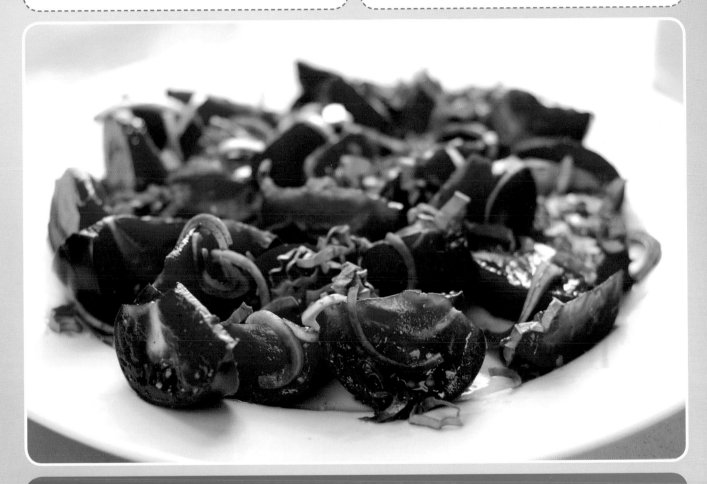

A CHIFFO-WHAT?

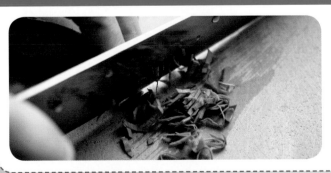

"Chiffon" is French for "rags," and a "chiffonade" simply refers to the process of making a thin, ribbonlike cut of greens or leafy herbs. It's an easy way to add an elegant garnish to your dishes.

The process is simple: Stack some leaves together, roll them lengthwise into a tight cylinder, and make thin, perpendicular slices with a sharp knife. You'll end up with a bright green pile of edible confetti.

 CRAVING MORE HEFT? TRY ADDING LUMP CRAB MEAT AND DICED HASS AVOCADO TO THIS SALAD.

WINTER KALE + PERSIMMON SALAD

This fruity, tangy salad is mega-tasty and super-nutritious. Plus, you can hastily assemble one to pack for lunch in the office or to accompany a hearty dinner on a cold night. And unlike many other salad greens, kale holds up beautifully and tastes even better the next day. What's not to love?

Makes 2 servings
Hands-on time: 5 minutes
Total time: 5 minutes

3 cups **baby lacinato kale**
1 medium **Fuyu persimmon**, peeled and thinly sliced
¼ cup **Citrus Vinaigrette** (page 59)
¼ cup **almond slivers**, toasted

DO THIS:

1. Cut the kale into a chiffonade (see page 93) by stacking the leaves, rolling them tightly, and cutting across the rolled leaves to produce fine ribbons.

2. In a large bowl, toss together the kale and persimmon slices. Dress with the vinaigrette to taste, and massage the dressing into the kale with your hands. Top with slivered almonds and serve.

CHEW ON THIS:

- How nutrient-packed is kale? On the Aggregate Nutrient Density Index scale, which measures nutrient density per calorie, kale's the only food with a perfect score of 1,000.

- For this recipe, use a tomato-shaped Fuyu persimmon—not an acorn-shaped Hachiya, which is bitter and astringent until it's in its softened, fully ripened state. In contrast, Fuyu persimmons have a crisp, apple-like texture, and add a floral sweetness and crunch to this salad.

- Kale salads aren't just for the winter. In the summer, substitute sliced stone fruit (peaches, plums, pluots, nectarines, or even pitted cherries) in place of the persimmon for a sweet and tangy variation.

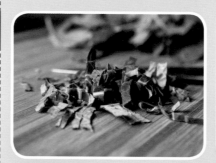
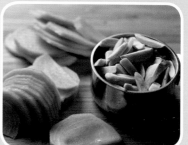
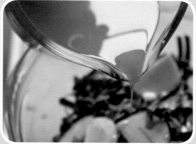
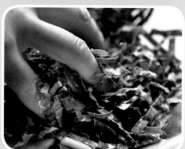
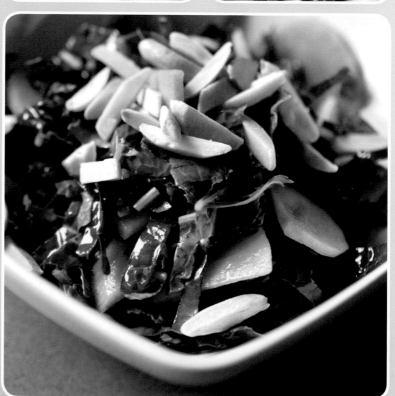

MADRAS CHICKEN SALAD

Don't you dare make a bland-tasting chicken salad tossed with plain old mayonnaise. Instead, punch it up with smoky, aromatic curry powder, crunchy apples, fresh herbs, and toasted almonds. With just a few pantry items, you can radically transform a ho-hum dish into an elegant and flavorful weeknight supper.

Makes 4 servings
Hands-on time: 15 minutes
Total time: 15 minutes

½ cup **Paleo Mayonnaise** (page 40)
¾ teaspoon **Indian curry powder**
1 teaspoon **kosher salt**
 Freshly ground **black pepper**
1 small Gala, Fuji, or Honeycrisp **apple**, peeled, cored, and cut into ½-inch dice
 Juice from ½ medium **lime**
1 pound cooked **chicken breast** or **thighs**
½ cup packed fresh **cilantro**, roughly chopped
2 **scallions**, trimmed and thinly sliced
¼ cup **almond slivers**, toasted

YOU CAN CHOOSE TO USE ANY INDIAN CURRY, BUT MY PERSONAL FAVORITE IS MADRAS CURRY, AN INTOXICATING BLEND OF OVER A DOZEN FRAGRANT SPICES!

DO THIS:

1. First, make the curried mayonnaise. In a small bowl, combine the Paleo Mayonnaise, curry powder, salt, and pepper to taste.

2. In a separate bowl, toss the apple chunks with the lime juice. This will ensure that your apples won't oxidize into brown, splotchy cubes—and the acid adds a nice zing to the salad, too.

3. Shred the chicken by hand, and toss it into the bowl with the acidulated apples. Add the cilantro, scallions, and curried mayonnaise, and mix well. Top with toasted almond slivers and serve.

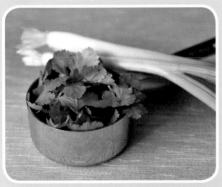
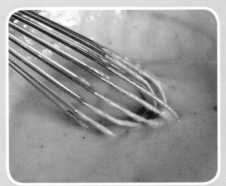
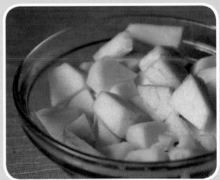
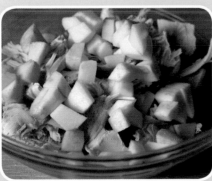
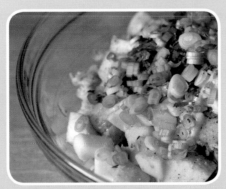
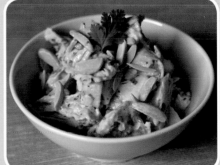

 MAKE THIS CHICKEN SALAD PORTABLE: WRAP IT IN BUTTER LETTUCE LEAVES!

SALADE LYONNAISE

For years, whenever we visited our favorite French bistro, I would always begin my meal with the same salad: wilted frisée with a soft-cooked egg and a generous sprinkle of smoky lardons. These days, I favor this homestyle variation, featuring peppery arugula and a drizzle of warm bacon dressing. Pop the yolk, and let all the components meld together for a rich, saucy salad.

Makes 2 servings
Hands-on time: 30 minutes
Total time: 30 minutes

4 slices **bacon**, cross-cut into ¼-inch pieces
2 **Poached Eggs** (page 128)
2 tablespoons **balsamic vinegar**
4 cups **baby arugula**
   Kosher salt
   Freshly ground **black pepper**

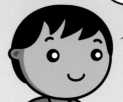

BACON!

DO THIS:

1. Arrange the bacon pieces in a single layer in a large cast-iron skillet, and slowly render the bacon over medium heat until crunchy, about 15 to 20 minutes. (Want more details? See page 49.)

2. In the meantime, if you don't already have poached eggs on hand, prepare them according to the instructions on page 128.

3. Transfer the bacon to a paper towel–lined plate. Once the remaining bacon fat has cooled slightly, carefully pour it into a small heat-resistant bowl or measuring cup. Add the balsamic vinegar to the bacon drippings, and stir briskly to mix.

4. Put the arugula in a salad bowl, and add as much of the warm bacon dressing as desired. Toss the salad by hand to evenly distribute the dressing, and season with salt and pepper to taste. Divide the greens among plates or large bowls. Top each portion with a poached egg and a shower of crispy lardons, and serve immediately.

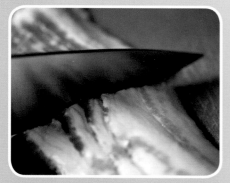
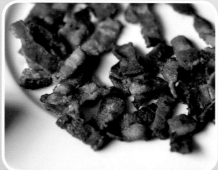
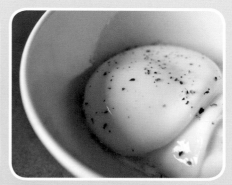
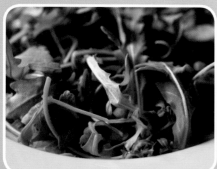
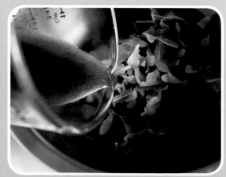
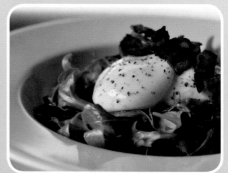

NOT A FAN OF BITTER SALAD GREENS? SUBSTITUTE FRESH BABY SPINACH FOR THE ARUGULA!

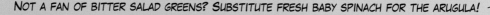

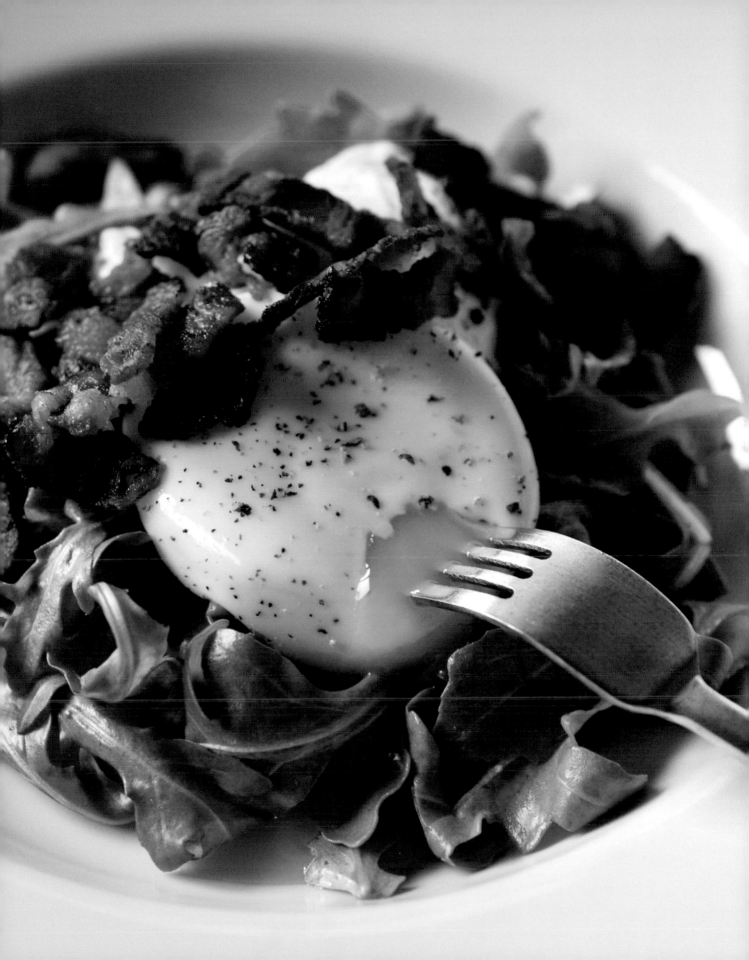

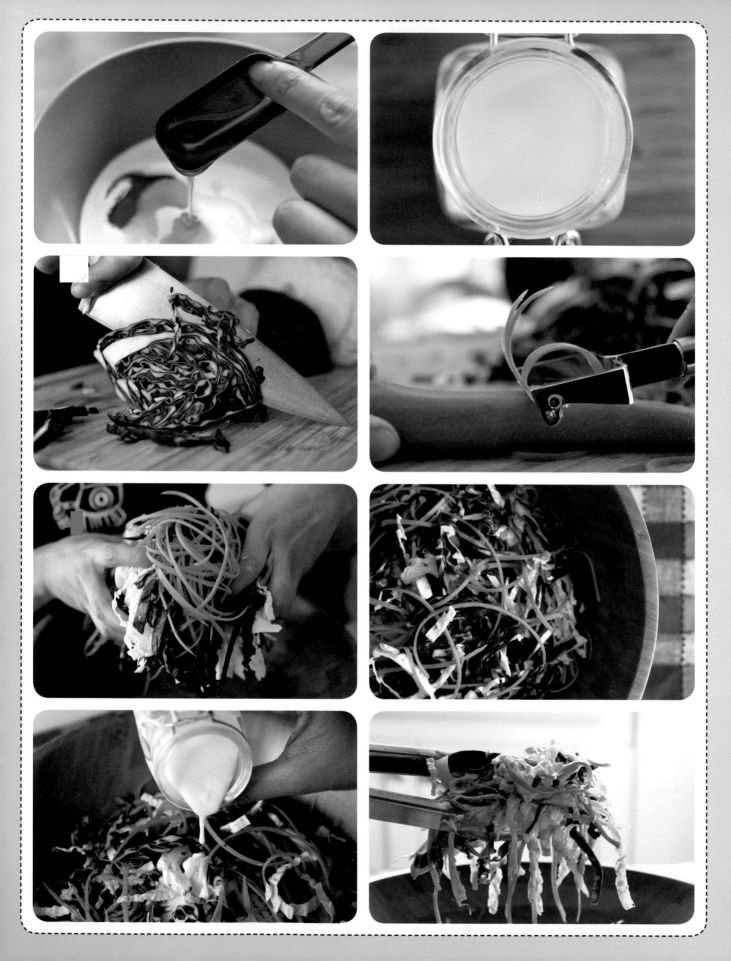

CLASSIC COLESLAW

Close your eyes and picture a cup of coleslaw. You're probably conjuring up a mental image of limp strands of cabbage drowning in bland, watery dressing, right? Sadly, modern coleslaw is often nothing more than a soggy mess, having lost much of the distinctiveness of its Dutch-American roots. (The name "coleslaw" is derived from the Dutch *koolsalade* or *koolsla*, meaning "cabbage salad"—though in its original eighteenth-century form, this tangy dish was dressed with hot melted butter and vinegar.)

Well, I've got a recipe that'll rehabilitate the reputation of this picnic staple for you. Once you get a taste of this Paleo coleslaw, you'll never look at this salad the same way again.

Makes 6 servings
Hands-on time: 20 minutes
Total time: 1½ hours

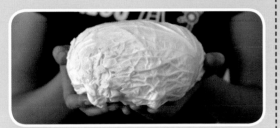

¼ cup **Paleo Mayonnaise** (page 40)
2 tablespoons full-fat **coconut milk**
2 tablespoons fresh **lemon juice**
1 tablespoon **honey**
   Kosher salt
½ head small **red cabbage**, finely chopped or shredded
½ head small **Savoy cabbage**, finely chopped or shredded
1 large **carrot**, shredded with a julienne peeler
   Freshly ground **black pepper**
2 tablespoons **sesame seeds**, toasted

DO THIS:

1. Make the dressing by vigorously stirring together the mayonnaise, coconut milk, lemon juice, honey, and ¼ teaspoon kosher salt in a small bowl. You'll end up with ½ cup of coleslaw dressing that can be refrigerated for up to 3 days in a covered container.

2. Toss the cabbage in a colander with 1 teaspoon of salt, and wait for an hour. The salt will draw the moisture out of the cabbage, softening it and preventing the liquid from waterlogging your dressed salad. Rinse the salt from the cabbage and pat it dry with a towel.

3. Mix together the cabbage and julienned carrot in a large bowl, and season with salt and pepper to taste. Toss the coleslaw with the dressing, and sprinkle with toasted sesame seeds before serving.

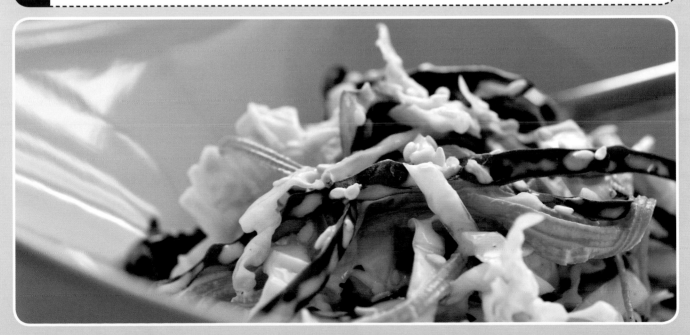

~ CLASSIC COLESLAW IS TERRIFIC, BUT DOESN'T ITALIAN COLESLAW SOUND EVEN BETTER? ADD THIN STRIPS OF PROSCIUTTO AND RED BELL PEPPERS TO MAKE INSALATA CAPRICCIOSA!

PISTACHIO APPLE SALAD

Can't decide whether to plate up something salty or sweet, crunchy or juicy, bitter or tangy, or nutty or fruity? Make this salad. It marries all of these contrasting yet complementary elements in one bright dish.

Makes 4 servings
Hands-on time: 15 minutes
Total time: 15 minutes

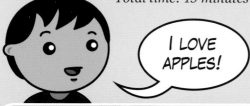

I LOVE APPLES!

3   medium **endive heads**, thinly sliced crosswise (about 3 packed cups)

2   medium Gala, Fuji, or Honeycrisp **apples**, peeled, quartered, cored, and thinly sliced

¼   cup **Honey Mustard Dressing** (page 58)
    Kosher salt
    Freshly ground **black pepper**

½   cup roasted and salted **pistachio nuts**, shelled and chopped

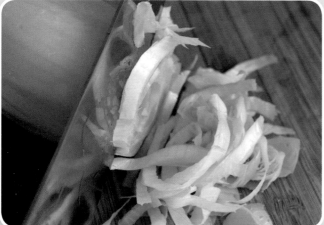

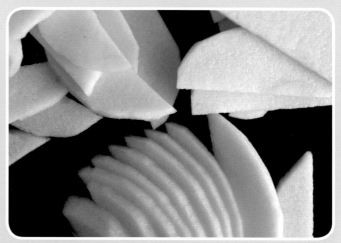

DO THIS:

Combine the endive and apple slices in a large bowl. Add enough dressing to suit your tastes, and gently toss the salad together with your fingers. Season with salt and pepper to taste, and divide among plates or bowls. Top with the chopped pistachio nuts before serving.

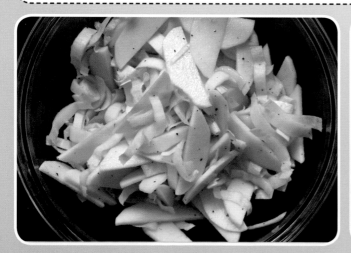

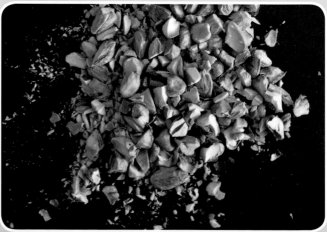

THIS SALAD IS THE PERFECT ACCOMPANIMENT FOR SAUSAGES, GRILLED PORK, OR BARBECUED MEATS!

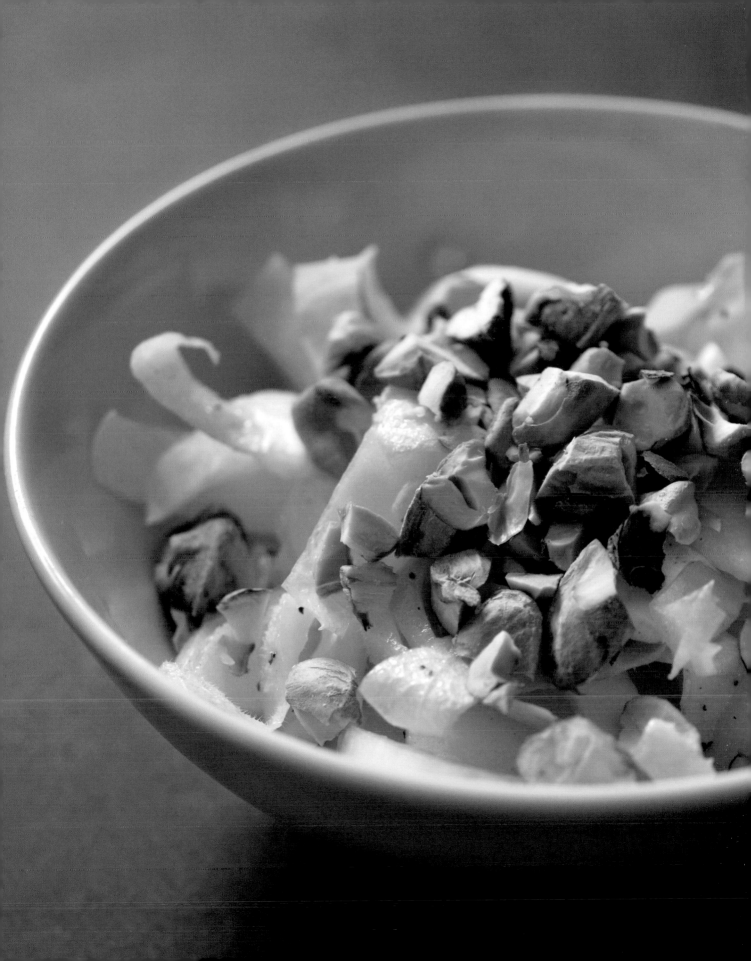

CRAB LOUIE

The classic Crab Louie originated in the early twentieth century somewhere on the West Coast, but the exact circumstances of its birth are lost to time. Some claim that this "King of Salads" was first served at Seattle's Olympic Club, while others insist that it was the invention of Solari's Restaurant in San Francisco's Union Square. Even James Beard and Helen Evans Brown—two of America's most esteemed food writers—could never quite see eye-to-eye on whether their beloved Crab Louie was a native son of Beard's Washington or Brown's California.

I'm a hometown gal, though, so my vote is for San Francisco. Besides, the centerpiece of this crisp, cool salad is fresh Dungeness crab—the very symbol of the city's two-hundred-year-old fishing industry. Piled atop lettuce and adorned with ripe tomatoes, hard-boiled eggs, and bright green asparagus, the succulent crab meat is what makes this simple salad one that's fit for a king.

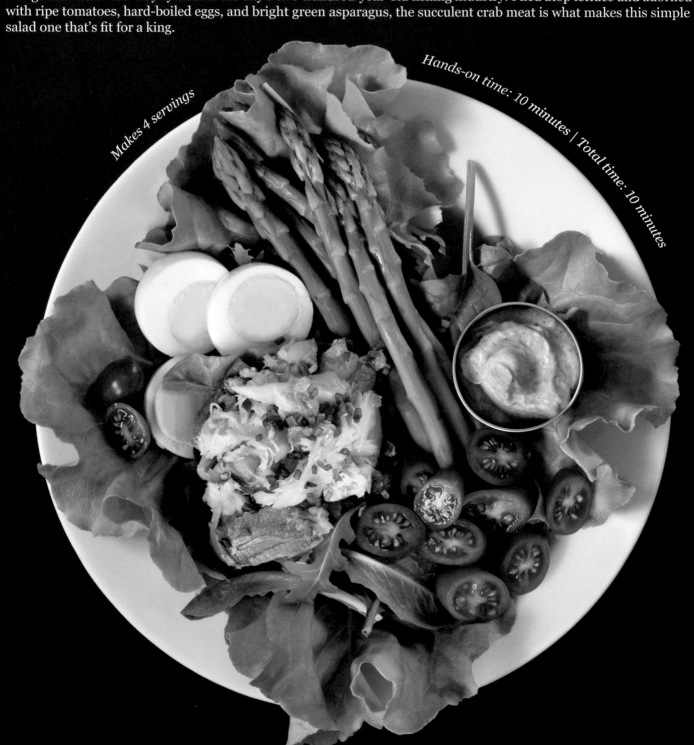

Makes 4 servings

Hands-on time: 10 minutes | Total time: 10 minutes

GET:

1 pound **asparagus**, trimmed

6 cups **lettuce leaves** or **salad greens**

1 pound cooked lump **crab meat** (see below)

4 **Perfect Hard-Boiled Eggs** (page 120), sliced in half

1 cup **cherry tomatoes**

¼ cup minced **chives**

½ cup **Louisiana Rémoulade** (page 63)

DO THIS:

1. Blanch the asparagus by cooking it in a pot of salted boiling water for 1 minute. Immediately transfer the asparagus to a bowl of ice water. Drain once the asparagus has cooled.

2. Divide the lettuce among 4 plates. Arrange the crab meat, asparagus, hard-boiled eggs, and tomatoes atop the lettuce. Garnish with chives, and serve with the rémoulade on the side.

HOW TO BRINE-BOIL A DUNGENESS CRAB

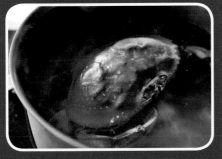

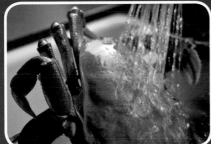

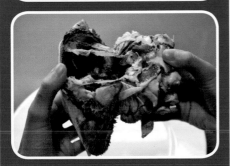

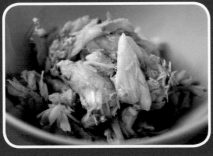

It's a snap to crack open a container of lump crab meat. But if you're in an ambitious mood, who am I to stop you from brine-boiling a live Dungeness crab? Fresh crustacean meat is a wonderfully delicate, sweet, and juicy reward that makes the effort more than worthwhile. Here's how to do the deed:

1. Bring 10 quarts of water to a roiling boil in a large stockpot. Then, add salt to the water 'til it tastes like sea water. Don't worry about over-salting the water; after all, the brine has to permeate through a tough shell.

2. Completely submerge the live crab in the water. Bring the water back up to a boil and cook for 20 minutes, or until the shell turns bright red-orange and the crab floats to the top. Remove the crab and run it under cold water until cool.

3. Carefully twist off the claws and legs, and use a crab cracker to snap them open. Remove as much meat as you can, but don't fret if there's not much in there. The real bounty's hidden in the body of the crab.

4. The bottom half of the crab's shell—the "apron"—can be easily pried open from the rear of the crab. Using your thumbs, find the crease between the upper and lower parts of the shell, and open the crab up like a book.

5. The upper half of the shell contains the gooey "crab butter." Some folks love it (hi, Mom!), but I don't, so I usually toss it.

6. The bottom, however, is chock-full of tender meat. To get at it, first remove and discard the long gill filaments on both sides of the crab. Then, firmly grasp what's left of the bottom shell with both hands, and break it in half.

7. Each side contains plenty of rich, juicy crab meat. Use a fork or some other sharp-and-pointy tool to pick out all the goodness.

Give yourself a round of applause. You've just brine-boiled a crab!

HEY, EAST COAST PEOPLE: THIS METHOD WORKS WITH ATLANTIC BLUE CRABS, TOO!

BONE BROTH

On a cold winter's day, nothing hits the spot like a steaming bowl of bone broth—especially when I'm feeling under the weather. Not only does it warm me from the inside out, it's also a terrifically nutritious superfood. Packed with health-promoting minerals like calcium and magnesium, bone broth is also loaded with collagen and gelatin, making it a magical elixir that boosts both intestinal and joint health.

And did I mention how wonderful it tastes? Done properly, bone broth reveals its divine depth and adds a robust, umami dimension to your soups and stews. Sure—broth made with bare bones can be less than appetizing, but that's why I always use meaty bones like cross shanks, oxtails, and short ribs to punch up the flavor. And to produce a gelatin-rich broth, make sure to include knuckles or chicken feet.

There are plenty of ways to make bone broth at home. I've simmered it on the stove and in a slow cooker, but when I want it pronto, I turn to my pressure cooker— an invaluable tool for quickly transforming a pile of bones into a rich, flavorful broth. Whichever method you choose, you'll love the rich, comforting flavors of this homemade stock.

Makes 8 cups
Hands-on time: 10 minutes
Total time: 1 to 24 hours

MAINTAIN A LOW SIMMER WHEN YOU'RE MAKING BONE BROTH, OR YOU'LL WIND UP WITH LOTS OF UNAPPETIZING (ALBEIT EDIBLE) GRAY SCUM ON THE SURFACE. IT MAY BE PACKED WITH PROTEIN (ALBUMIN), BUT I PREFER TO SKIM IT OFF 'CAUSE IT LOOKS NASTY.

2½ pounds assorted **beef**, **chicken**, and/or **pork bones** (see note on opposite page)

2 medium **leeks**, trimmed, cleaned (see note on page 219), and cut in half, or 1 small yellow **onion**, peeled, trimmed, and cut in half

1 medium **carrot**, peeled and cut into 3 pieces

8 cups **water**, plus more if needed

2 tablespoons Paleo-friendly **fish sauce**

1 teaspoon **apple cider vinegar**

¼ ounce dried **shiitake mushrooms** (optional)

4 **garlic cloves**, peeled and smashed (optional)

1 (1-inch) piece fresh **ginger**, peeled and cut into thick coins

Kosher salt or **Celtic sea salt**

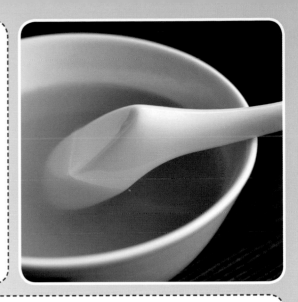

BONE BROTH THREE WAYS!

1. Place the bones and vegetables in a large (at least 6-quart) stockpot, slow cooker, or pressure cooker, depending on your desired method of cooking.

2. Add water to the pot, making sure the bones and vegetables are fully submerged. If you're using a pressure cooker, don't fill it beyond two-thirds capacity.

3. Pour in the fish sauce and apple cider vinegar. If desired, add dried shiitake mushrooms, garlic, and/or ginger to the broth. Then, cook using one of the three methods below.

4.

If cooking the broth in a stock pot:	**If cooking the broth in a slow cooker:**	**If cooking the broth in a pressure cooker:**
Cover and bring to a boil over high heat. Skim off the scum, and turn down the heat to maintain a low simmer. Cook, covered, for 12 to 24 hours, or until the bones are soft. Check occasionally and add water if needed to keep the bones and vegetables submerged. Cooking on the stovetop is the traditional way to make a pot of bone broth, but it takes a lot of babysitting. Patience is key!	Cover and set to cook on low for 8 to 24 hours. (You can actually simmer it for days; some say that the longer you cook your broth, the more nutrient-rich it becomes.) The advantage of using a slow cooker to make your broth is that you can leave the house without fear of burning it down to the ground. Still, you'll have to wait a long time before you can sip on a mug of broth, so plan ahead.	Lock the lid of the pressure cooker in place and cook over high heat. Once it reaches high pressure, immediately turn the burner down to the lowest possible setting ("simmer" usually works) that will still maintain high pressure. Set a timer for 45 minutes, and when it goes off, turn off the burner and remove the pot from the heat. Release the pressure naturally, about 10 to 15 minutes.

5. Strain the broth through a fine-mesh sieve (or cheesecloth-lined colander) to filter out the bones, veggies, and any remaining scummy bits. Season with salt to taste. Drink up.

6. This broth will keep in a covered container for a few days in the refrigerator (or for up to 6 months in the freezer). Once it's chilled, the bone broth should transform into a jiggly gel—a sure sign that it's loaded with gelatin. (And don't fret—it'll return to its liquid state once it's heated.)

 PRO TIP: YOU CAN ALMOST ALWAYS USE BONE BROTH WHENEVER A RECIPE CALLS FOR CHICKEN OR BEEF STOCK.

FAST PHỞ

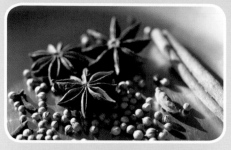
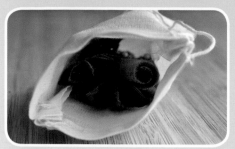
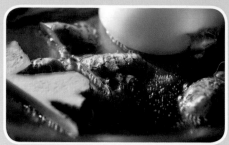
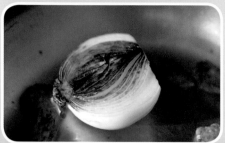
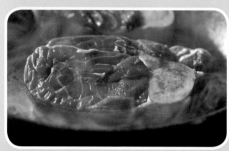
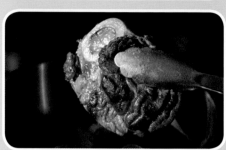
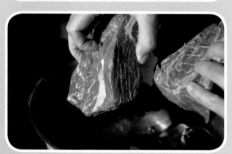
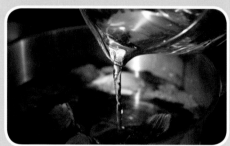
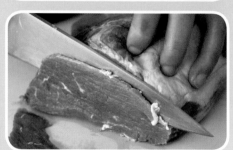

Phở bò—a classic Vietnamese rice noodle soup served with sliced rare beef and well-done brisket—occupies a special place in my heart. I cherish my childhood memories of slurping down steaming bowls of slow-cooked *phở* broth, savoring its aromatic spices and flavorings. My Paleo version omits the rice noodles, but leaves all the comforting beefiness intact. Plus, it takes just 2 hours to make!

Makes 4 servings
Hands-on time: 30 minutes
Total time: 2 hours

GET:

3	whole **star anise**
2	teaspoons whole **coriander seeds**
1	**cinnamon stick**
3	whole **cloves**
1	**green cardamom pod**
2	tablespoons **ghee** or fat of choice, divided
8	slices unpeeled **ginger**, each ½ inch thick
½	large **yellow onion**, peeled
2	(1-pound) **beef cross shanks**, 1½ inches thick
1½	pounds **oxtails**
1½	pounds **beef brisket**, cut in half along the grain

8	cups **water**
3½	tablespoons Paleo-friendly **fish sauce**
½	pound **beef eye of round roast**
8	cups **Zoodles** (page 143, optional)
2	**limes**, cut into wedges
3	**jalapeño peppers**, sliced
1	bunch fresh **cilantro**
1	bunch fresh **Thai basil**
1	bunch fresh **mint**
2	cups **bean sprouts**
	Paleo Sriracha (page 42)

PHỞ IS PRONOUNCED "FUH," AND WAS LIKELY NAMED AFTER POT-AU-FEU, THE CLASSIC FRENCH BEEF STEW, DURING FRANCE'S COLONIZATION OF VIETNAM.

DO THIS:

1. Heat a large frying pan over medium-low heat. Toss the star anise, coriander seeds, cinnamon stick, cloves, and cardamom pod into the dry pan and swirl them around until they're fragrant, about 2 to 3 minutes. Transfer the spices to an empty bouquet garni bag or loose tea leaf bag, and place it in a 6- or 8-quart pressure cooker. (This step's optional, but it beats having to fish out all the seeds when you're ready to eat.)

2. Crank up the burner to medium, and add 1 tablespoon of ghee to the pan. Once the fat has melted, add the ginger and onion, and cook for 3 to 5 minutes or until they're golden brown on both sides. Transfer the ginger and onion to the pressure cooker.

3. Add the remaining tablespoon of fat to the hot pan. Once it's sizzling, sear the beef cross shanks and oxtails in batches. Be careful not to overcrowd the pan; give the meat room to properly brown and develop the complex flavors necessary for the quick-cook broth. Resist the urge to frequently flip the meat. When the beef's nicely browned on the outside, transfer the pieces to the pressure cooker.

4. Lay the raw brisket on top of the seared meat in the pressure cooker. Add the water and fish sauce. The meat should be submerged, but make sure the contents of the pot don't exceed two-thirds of the cooker's capacity. Lock the lid onto the cooker, and bring it up to high pressure. (Be sure to follow the manufacturer's instructions. Remember: safety first!)

5. Turn down the heat to the lowest burner setting necessary to maintain high pressure, and cook for 50 minutes. Set a kitchen timer so you don't forget. While the soup is cooking, place the eye of round roast in the freezer for 20 to 30 minutes. Once the beef is partially frozen, cut it across the grain into thin slices.

6. When the timer goes off, take the cooker off the heat, and release the pressure naturally, about 10 minutes. Remove the lid, taste the broth, and season with more fish sauce if needed.

7. Remove the spice bag and strain the broth. Discard the bones, onions, and ginger, but reserve the meat. Cut the brisket across the grain and break up the large pieces of shank. Divide the meat into individual serving bowls. (I like to make this recipe sans noodles, but if you can't wrap your head around noodle-less phở, divide some zoodles into individual serving bowls, too.) Top the bowls with slices of raw eye of round.

8. Ladle the steaming broth into the serving bowls. The piping-hot phở broth will cook the raw beef (and zoodles, if you're using them). Arrange your garnishes—the lime wedges, sliced peppers, cilantro, Thai basil, mint, and bean sprouts—on a platter, and provide a squirt bottle of sriracha, too. Invite your guests to season their phở to their heart's desire.

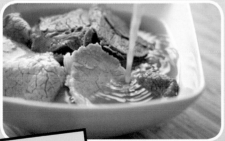 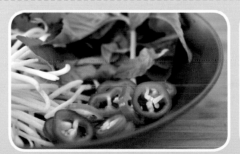 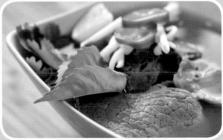

BONUS RECIPE!

SLOW PHỞ

If you're a classicist (or don't have a pressure cooker), you can prepare phở the traditional way: *slooowly*. After all, *phở* broth is traditionally slow-cooked for hours—or even days—to heighten the intensity of the beefy stock, and to infuse it with the steamy aroma of star anise, cinnamon, and cloves. Just follow the same steps as above, but use a slow cooker rather than a pressure cooker, and set it to cook on low for 12 hours. The only drawback to this method? It'll fill your house with a tantalizing fragrance that'll make your stomach growl for hours.

WEST LAKE SOUP

Makes 4 servings | Hands-on time: 30 minutes | Total time: 30 minutes

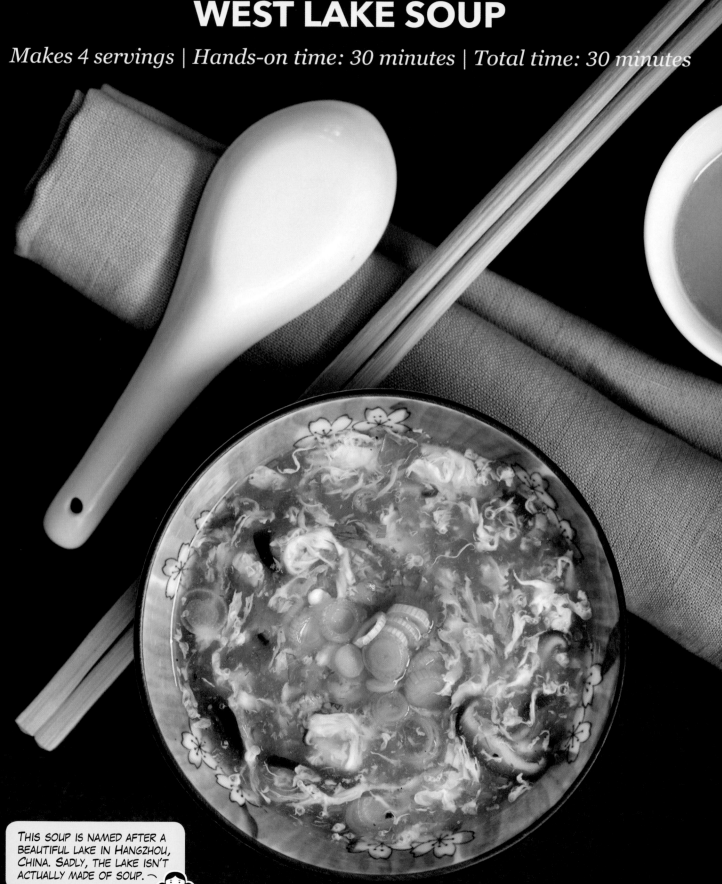

THIS SOUP IS NAMED AFTER A BEAUTIFUL LAKE IN HANGZHOU, CHINA. SADLY, THE LAKE ISN'T ACTUALLY MADE OF SOUP. ⌐

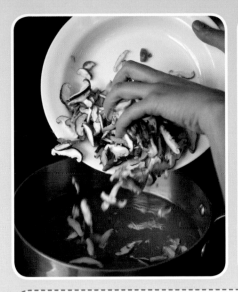
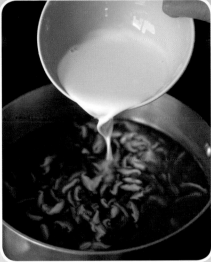
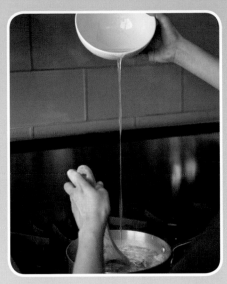

When I was a kid, a casual family meal at a Chinese restaurant could be a crapshoot. Some evenings, my grandfather would insist on ordering the most authentic dishes on the menu, many featuring odd bits that made my sister and me wrinkle our noses in disgust. Geoduck? Bitter melon? Bird spit? Like, actual bird *saliva*?

But if we were lucky, dinner would kick off with a beefy bowl of West Lake Soup. With bright green flecks of cilantro and cloudlike wisps of egg, this soup is both gorgeous and satisfying— which explains why we would gladly fill up on it before the slimy sea cucumber dish was served.

½ pound **flank steak**, finely minced
1 teaspoon **kosher salt**
2 teaspoons **rice wine vinegar**
1 teaspoon Paleo-friendly **fish sauce**
1 teaspoon **sesame oil**
Ground **white pepper**
6 cups **Bone Broth** (page 104) or **chicken stock**
¼ pound fresh **shiitake mushrooms**, stemmed and thinly sliced
¼ cup **arrowroot powder**, mixed with ¼ cup water to make a slurry
3 large **egg whites**, lightly beaten
1 cup packed fresh **cilantro**, finely minced
3 **scallions**, thinly sliced

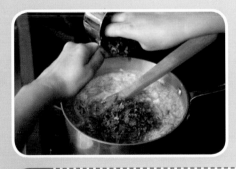
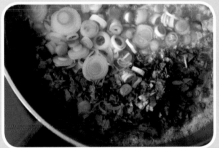
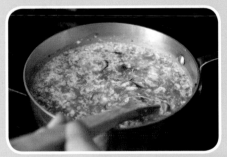

DO THIS:

1. Combine the beef, salt, vinegar, fish sauce, sesame oil, and ¼ teaspoon white pepper in a bowl.

2. Bring the broth and mushrooms to a boil over high heat in a saucepan. Lower the heat to maintain a simmer, and add the arrowroot slurry to thicken the soup, stirring well to incorporate.

3. Once the soup thickens, add the marinated meat and stir well. As soon as the meat is cooked through, about 30 seconds, turn off the heat. Season the soup with salt and white pepper to taste.

4. In a slow, steady stream, pour in the egg whites from high above the pot, stirring as the whites hit the liquid. The whites will cook upon contact with the hot soup, forming ribbon-like tendrils.

5. Mix in the cilantro and scallions. Ladle into bowls and serve immediately.

 YOU CAN SUBSTITUTE OTHER MEATS OR SEAFOOD FOR THE FLANK STEAK, BUT IF YOU USE GROUND MEAT, PARBOIL IT FIRST OR YOUR SOUP WILL END UP SCUMMY.

MULLIGATAWNY SOUP

"Mulligatawny" is the Anglicized word for the Tamil term *milagu thanni*—the fragrant "pepper water" invented to appeal to foreign palates when the British took over the Indian subcontinent in the nineteenth century. Mulligatawny's burgeoning popularity soon brought this rich curried soup across the seas to Westerners craving a taste of the exotic. These days, it's become a mainstay of Indian restaurants across the world, though few pause to remember its very British origins.

But even if you've never pondered why a Southern Indian soup has such an Anglo-sounding name, you can love mulligatawny for what it is: an assertively spiced curry soup that can be easily made with common ingredients found in any Paleo eater's pantry. It's versatile, too; throw in some emergency protein in the form of cooked chicken, lamb, or mutton, and your mulligatawny instantly becomes a complete meal.

Makes 4 servings
Hands-on time: 15 minutes
Total time: 45 minutes

2	tablespoons **ghee** or fat of choice
1	medium **yellow onion**, roughly chopped
1	teaspoon **tomato paste**
¼	cup shredded unsweetened dried **coconut**
2	**garlic cloves**, minced
1	(1-inch) piece fresh **ginger**, peeled and finely grated (about 1 tablespoon)
2	teaspoons **Indian curry powder**
3	cups **chicken stock** or **Bone Broth** (page 104)
1	**celery** stalk with fibrous strings removed, roughly chopped
1	**carrot**, peeled and roughly chopped
½	ripe **banana**, peeled
¼	cup diced Braeburn, Empire, McIntosh, or Cortland **apple**
2	tablespoons minced fresh **cilantro**

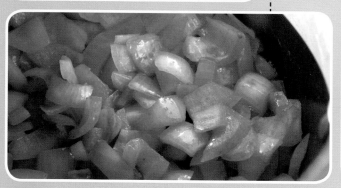

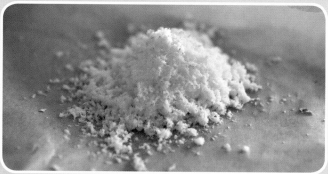

DO THIS:

1. Heat the ghee in a stockpot over medium heat. Add the onion and tomato paste and cook, stirring, until the onions soften, about 5 minutes.

2. Add the coconut, garlic, ginger, and curry powder to the pot, and stir to combine the ingredients. Then, pour in the broth, and add the celery, carrot, banana, and apple. Bring the contents of the pot to a vigorous boil.

3. Turn down the heat to low. Cover the stockpot and simmer for 30 minutes or until the vegetables and fruit are tender.

4. Use an immersion blender to blitz the ingredients together into a thick, fragrant soup. Garnish with minced cilantro and serve immediately.

SECRET INGREDIENT ALERT! MY SUPER-CHEF SISTER TAUGHT ME THAT DICED APPLE CAN ADD SWEETNESS AND TEXTURE TO PURÉED SOUPS!

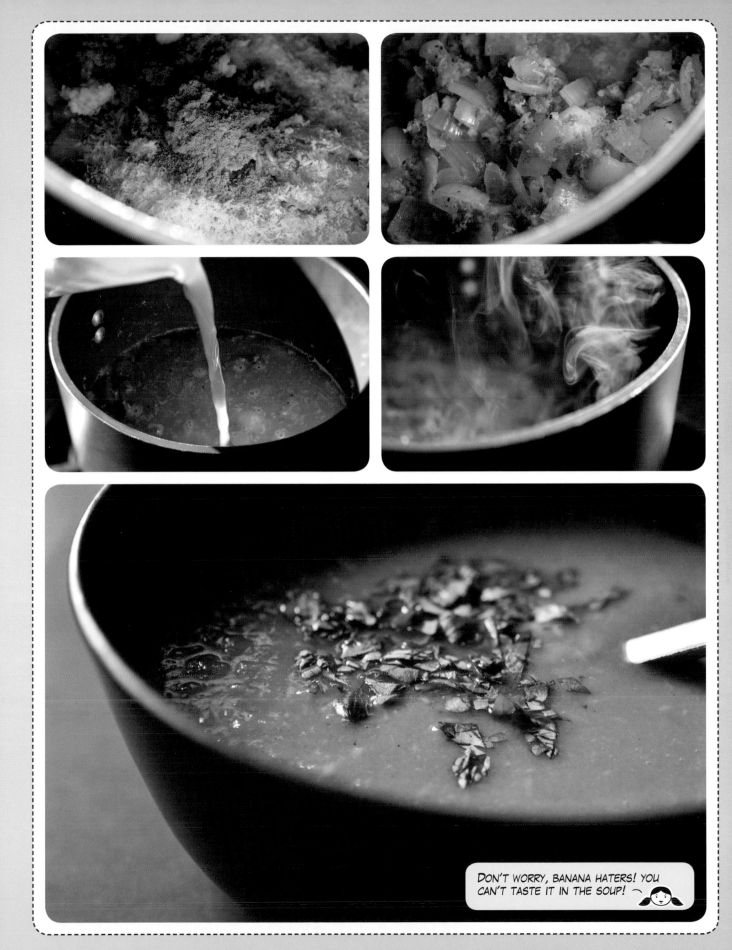

DON'T WORRY, BANANA HATERS! YOU CAN'T TASTE IT IN THE SOUP!

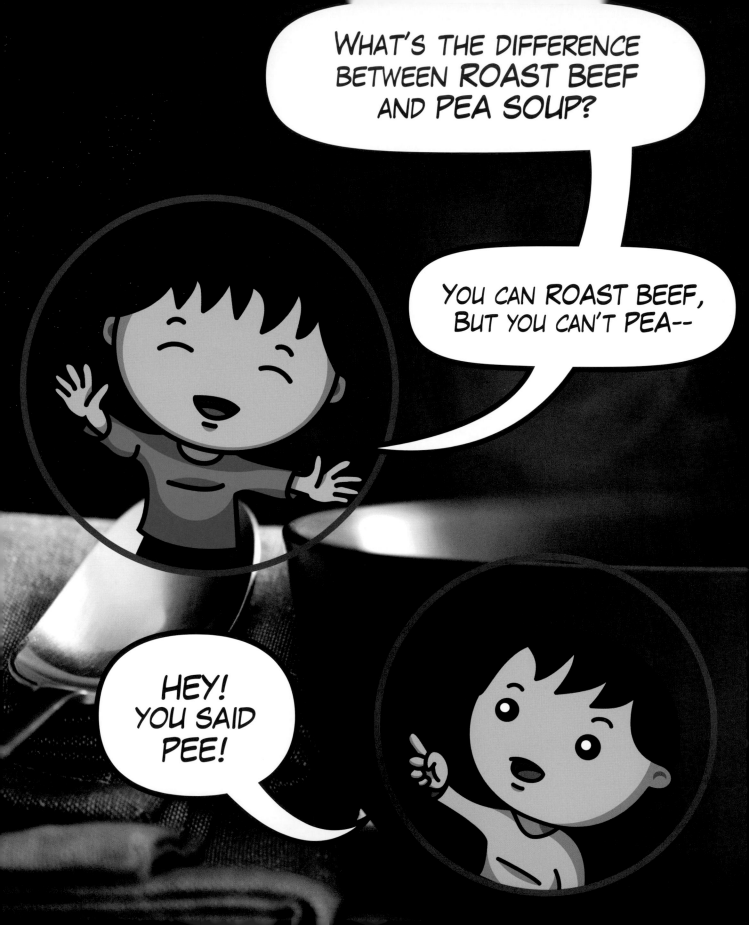

CURRIED CREAM OF BROCCOLI SOUP

This is a perfect example of what I call "garbage soup." On busy weeknights, I pull out whatever vegetables are languishing in my crisper and toss them in a pot with some pre-made broth. This formula works with just about any ingredients, but if you happen to have some broccoli florets and leeks in the fridge, give this recipe a go. The assertive curry spices and creamy texture of this soup make for a winning combination.

Makes 6 servings
Hands-on time: 20 minutes
Total time: 40 minutes

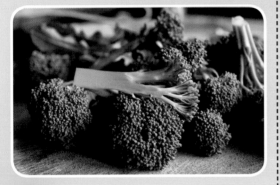

2 tablespoons **coconut oil** or fat of choice
4 **leeks**, white and light green ends only, cleaned, trimmed, and thinly sliced (see page 219)
1 large yellow **onion**, roughly chopped
3 medium **shallots**, roughly chopped
Kosher salt
1½ pounds **broccoli**, trimmed and cut into uniform-sized pieces
¼ cup diced Braeburn, Empire, McIntosh, or Cortland **apple**
4 cups **Bone Broth** (page 104) or stock of choice
1 tablespoon **Indian curry powder**
Freshly ground **black pepper**
1 cup full-fat **coconut milk**

DIRECTIONS

1. In a large stockpot, melt the coconut oil over medium heat. Add the leeks, onion, shallots, and a pinch of salt, and sauté until softened, 5 to 10 minutes.

2. Toss in the chopped broccoli and apple, and add the broth. Top off with some water if the vegetables aren't fully submerged. Crank the heat up to high.

3. When the soup boils, lower the heat to a simmer. Continue cooking on the stove for 20 minutes or until the vegetables are soft.

4. Add the curry powder and season with salt and pepper to taste. Turn off the stove and cool the soup slightly.

5. Use an immersion blender to blitz the ingredients together into a smooth, aromatic green broth. Add the coconut milk and stir to incorporate. Turn the heat up to high to bring the soup back up to a boil before serving.

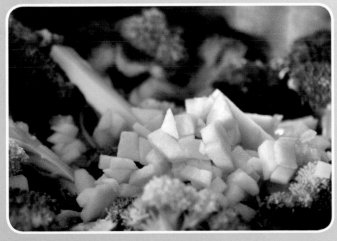

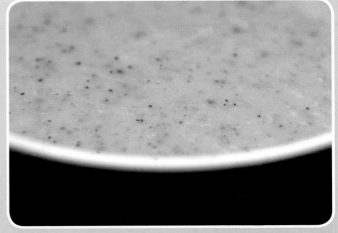

 SERVE THIS SOUP WITH A SIDE OF MUSHROOM CHIPS (PAGE 75)!

Makes 6 servings | Hands-on time: 15 minutes | Total time: 45 minutes

Nothing signals springtime like a bowl of sunshine-orange soup.

CARROT + CARDAMOM SOUP

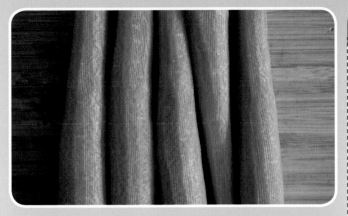

GET:

1 tablespoon **coconut oil**

2 large **leeks**, white and light green ends only, cleaned, trimmed, and thinly sliced
Kosher salt

1½ pounds large **carrots**, peeled and cut into ½-inch coins

¼ cup diced Braeburn, Empire, McIntosh, or Cortland **apple**

1 teaspoon minced fresh **ginger**

½ teaspoon ground **cardamom**

4 cups **chicken stock** or **Bone Broth** (page 104)

½ cup full-fat **coconut milk**
Freshly ground **black pepper**

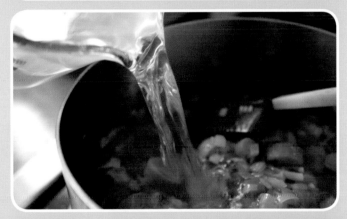

DO THIS:

1. Melt the coconut oil in a saucepan over medium heat. Add the leeks along with a generous pinch of salt, and sauté until translucent, about 5 minutes.

2. Toss in the carrot, apple, ginger, and cardamom, and stir until fragrant. Pour in the broth and bring to a boil over high heat.

3. Turn down the heat to low. Cover and simmer until the carrots are easily pierced with a fork, about 30 minutes. Mix in the coconut milk.

4. Transfer the soup in batches to a blender and process until smooth. Alternatively, purée the soup directly in the pot with an immersion blender. Season with salt and pepper to taste.

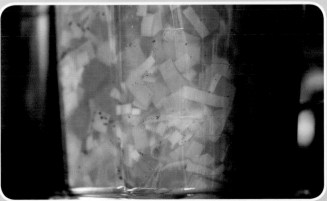

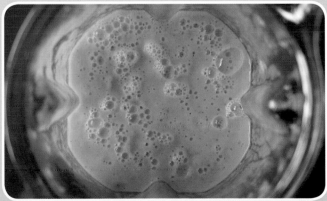

WATERMELON GAZPACHO

As a child, I despised gazpacho. Once I tasted the sharply acidic sludge my gastro-curious mom picked up at the neighborhood deli, I swore off chilled tomato soup for life. But years later, I sampled a bowl of Paul Bertolli's gazpacho at Oakland's Oliveto, and suddenly, my taste buds stood at attention. So *that's* what gazpacho tastes like when it's made with sun-ripened heirloom tomatoes and not watered-down vegetable juice mixed with metallic-tasting canned tomatoes! Who knew?

Nowadays, when the mercury rises, gazpacho's one of my favorite simple, make-ahead recipes—especially when combined with the bright flavors of juicy watermelon, cool cucumbers, and crisp red peppers. For this recipe, use the best tomatoes and sweetest watermelon you can find. And no, removing the skins from the tomatoes and cucumber is not optional. Make this soup when you're wilting under the sun, and you can thank me later. It's summertime in a bowl, people.

Makes 8 cups
Hands-on time: 30 minutes
Total time: 4½ hours

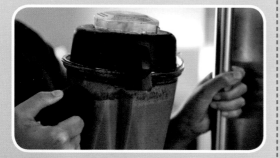

2	pounds ripe heirloom **tomatoes**
1	hothouse **cucumber** (approximately 1 pound), peeled
2	small **shallots**, coarsely chopped
1	medium **red bell pepper**, seeded, cored, and diced
4	fresh **cilantro** stalks with leaves
3	cups cubed and seeded **watermelon** (about 1 pound)
2	tablespoons **sherry vinegar**
⅓	cup **extra-virgin olive oil**, plus extra for garnish
1	teaspoon **kosher salt**
	Freshly ground **black pepper**
	Pinch of **red pepper flakes** (optional)

DO THIS:

1. Fill a large pot with water and bring it to a boil on the stove. In the meantime, fill a large bowl with water and ice.

2. Cut a small X on the bottom of each tomato with a sharp paring knife. Once the water reaches a rolling boil, carefully drop the tomatoes into the pot and blanch for 30 seconds. Transfer the tomatoes to the bowl of ice water.

3. After the tomatoes chill in the bowl for a minute or two, slide their skins off. Core and roughly chop them, reserving all the juice and seeds.

4. Finely dice one-third of the cucumber and set aside to garnish the finished soup. Roughly chop up the rest of the cucumber.

5. Toss the tomatoes, cucumber, shallots, bell pepper, and cilantro into a blender and purée until the vegetables are liquefied. Make sure to cover the lid with a towel to reduce splashes and splatters.

6. Add the watermelon, vinegar, olive oil, salt, pepper, and red pepper flakes (if desired) to the puréed vegetables, and blend until smooth. Taste and adjust for seasoning.

7. Refrigerate the soup in the blender cup for at least 4 hours or until fully chilled. The ingredients may separate while resting in the refrigerator, so just prior to serving, place the blender cup back on the base and blitz the soup again to recombine.

8. To serve, ladle the gazpacho into chilled cups or bowls. Top with a drizzle of olive oil, the reserved cucumber, and freshly cracked pepper.

IF YOUR BLENDER'S ON THE SMALL SIDE (WITH A CAPACITY OF LESS THAN 8 CUPS), BLITZ THE SOUP IN BATCHES.

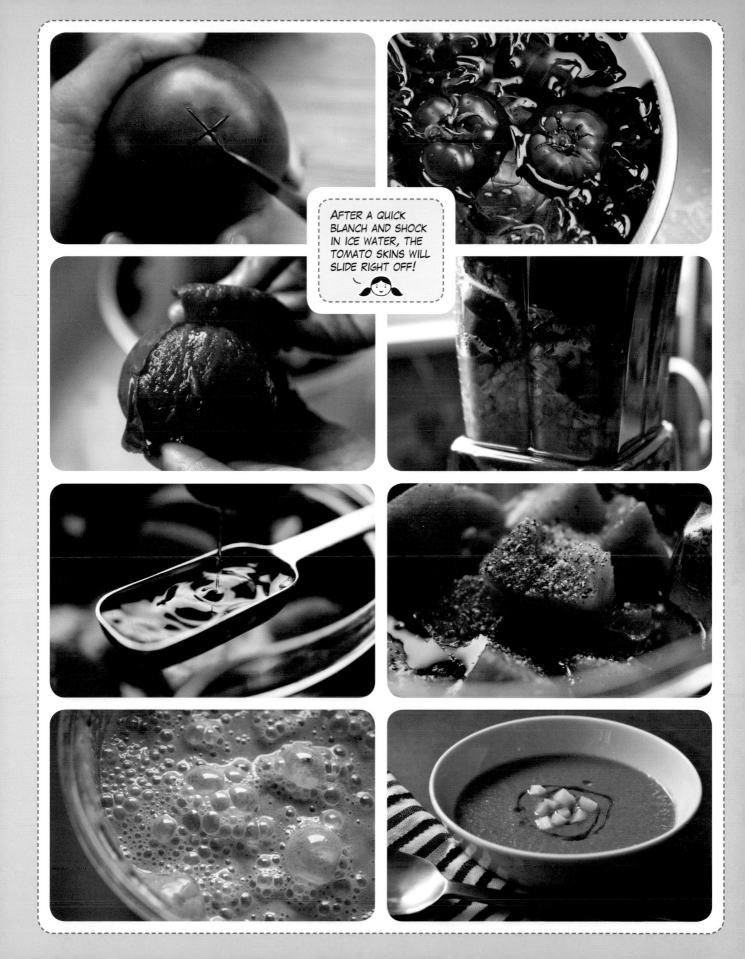

AFTER A QUICK BLANCH AND SHOCK IN ICE WATER, THE TOMATO SKINS WILL SLIDE RIGHT OFF!

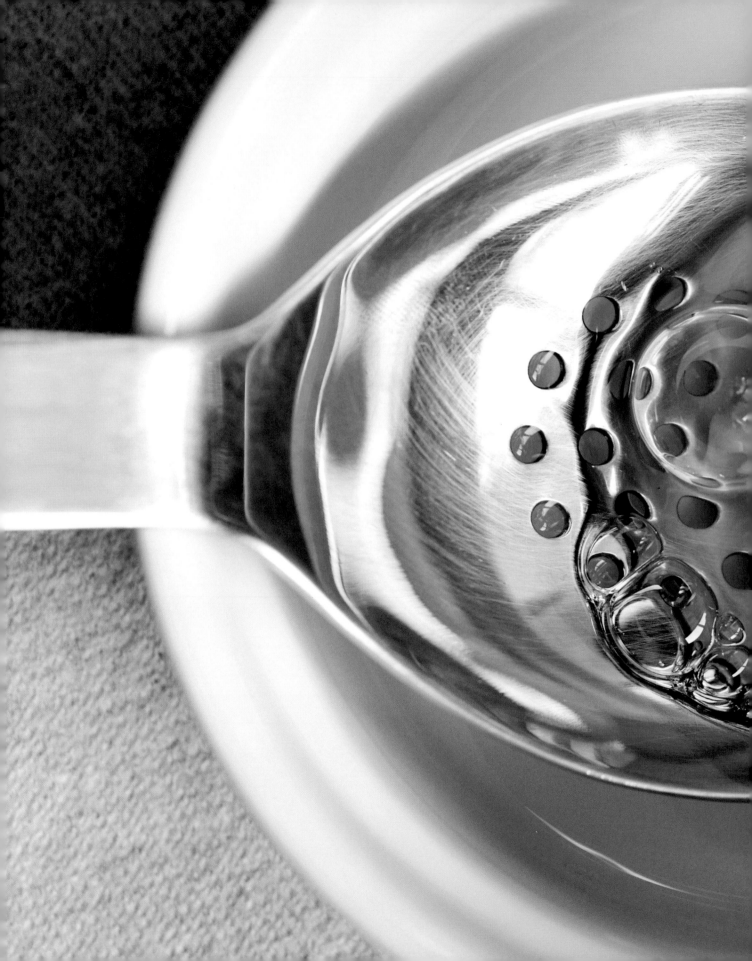

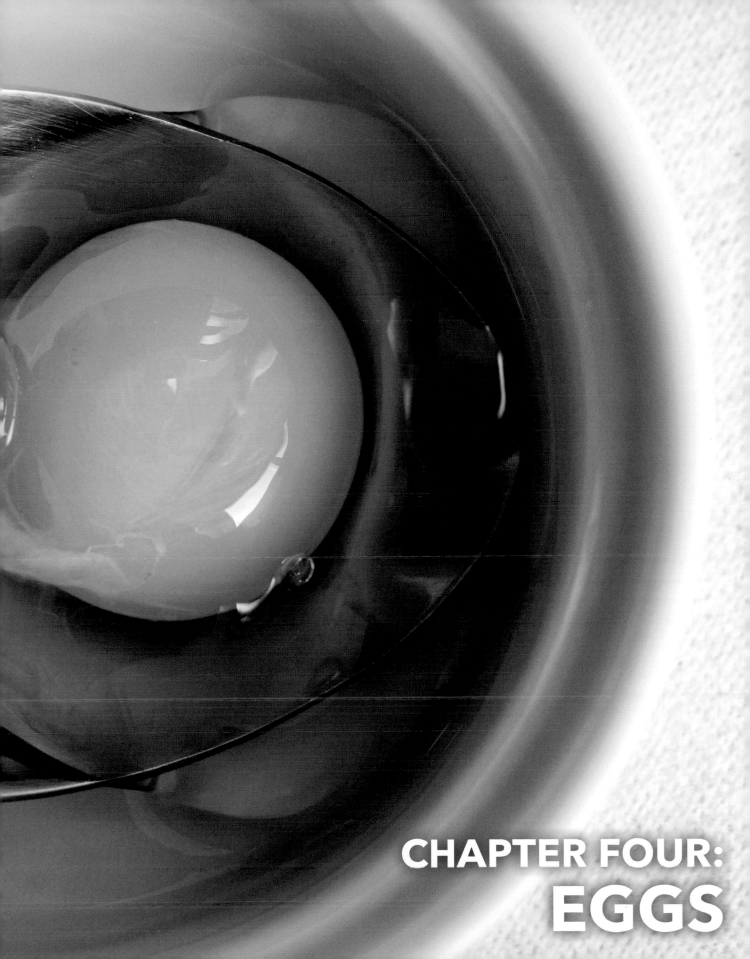

CHAPTER FOUR:
EGGS

PERFECT HARD-BOILED EGGS

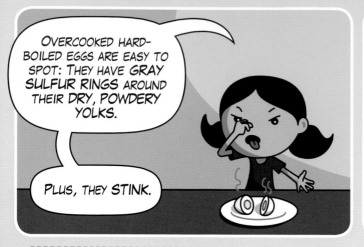

OVERCOOKED HARD-BOILED EGGS ARE EASY TO SPOT: THEY HAVE GRAY SULFUR RINGS AROUND THEIR DRY, POWDERY YOLKS.

PLUS, THEY STINK.

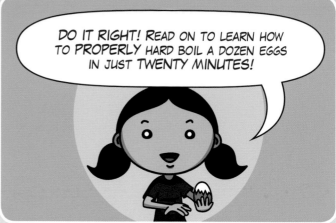

DO IT RIGHT! READ ON TO LEARN HOW TO PROPERLY HARD BOIL A DOZEN EGGS IN JUST TWENTY MINUTES!

Chemically speaking, when hard-boiled eggs are overcooked, the sulfur and hydrogen in the egg white form hydrogen sulfide, which in turn reacts with the iron in the yolks to form ferrous sulfide—a.k.a. the ugly, smelly, gray-green rings encircling the yolks. Overdone eggs are often also impossible to peel, leaving you with unsightly pockmarked disasters. Sure, these may be mere cosmetic flaws, but they make your eggs less than appetizing.

In contrast, properly cooked hard-boiled eggs are odorless and perfectly peelable, with vibrant, cheery yolks. And let's face it: to be a true kitchen ninja, you need to know how to consistently turn out perfectly formed hard-boiled eggs that everyone wants to pop in their mouths.

Makes 12 eggs
Hands-on time: 10 minutes
Total time: 20 minutes

12	large **eggs**, preferably ones that are at least a week old
6	cups **water**
1	teaspoon **baking soda**

DO THIS:

1. Using a pin or thumbtack, poke a hole on the wide bottom of each of the eggs.

2. Gently place the eggs in a wide saucepan in a single layer and add the water and baking soda. (The sodium bicarbonate will help the eggs separate from their shells, making them easier to peel.) Make sure the eggs are at least 1 inch below the surface.

3. Put the saucepan on the stove, and crank the heat to high. As soon as the water comes to a boil, set a timer for 1 minute. When the minute's up, take the pot off the heat, cover with a lid, and let the eggs sit in the hot water for 10 minutes. Don't forget to set a timer!

4. In the meantime, fill a large bowl with water and ice. Once the timer goes off, transfer the eggs to the ice water and submerge for 5 minutes.

5. Then, fish the eggs out of the icy water, gently rap them against a hard surface to crack the shells, and peel each egg starting from the bottom end (where you poked the pinhole). The shells should come right off, with no fuss or muss.

6. The result: perfectly cooked eggs, with no ugly gray-green rings around the yolks, no foul odor, and no telltale divots in the whites. If you aren't eating the eggs right away, store them in the fridge in a sealed container. They'll keep for up to a week.

ANOTHER WAY TO MAKE PERFECTLY HARD-COOKED EGGS: STEAM 'EM! ELISE BAUER OF
SIMPLY RECIPES RECOMMENDS STEAMING EGGS FOR PRECISELY 17 MINUTES. GIVE IT A GO!

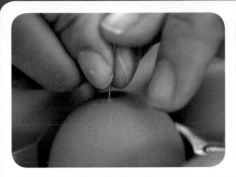
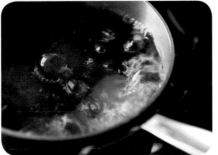
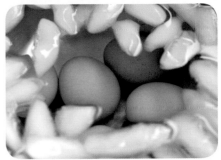

Why does this method work? Let's pull back the curtains.

1. **Older eggs are easier to peel—and a bit of baking soda also helps the shells slide off.**

   We all love farm fresh eggs, but as eggs age, they actually lose a bit of moisture through the pores in their shells, thus creating a bigger cushion of air between the inner and outer membranes of the egg. More important, the longer they sit, the more the eggs increase in pH level (in other words, it gets more basic as opposed to acidic), which results in a weaker attachment between the egg and the shell. As food science guru Harold McGee put it, "[t]he best guarantee of easy peeling is to use old eggs!"

   In the same way, baking soda helps to separate the egg from the shell. A little sodium bicarbonate in the cooking water makes it alkaline, which in turn draws some of the egg's water content out through the shell and into the pot.

2. **The pinholes help to further separate the eggs from their shells, and to keep the eggs from cracking during the cooking process.**

   Pricking a tiny hole in each egg allows the water to enter during the cooking process, which helps to separate the egg from its inner shell membrane. This also equalizes the pressure inside and outside the shell, which keeps it from cracking prematurely.

3. **By starting the eggs in cold water and icing at the end, you avoid overcooking.**

   Remember what I said about the danger of overcooking your eggs? If you plop eggs into water that's already boiling, you'll wind up cooking your eggs at 212°F—far too hot for a properly cooked egg. Plus, at that temperature, the insides of the eggs will come to a full boil, and the resulting bubbles will crack the shells. And we're not making egg drop soup, people.

   The far better approach is to heat the eggs along with the water. By removing the pot from the heat as soon as the water comes to a boil, the insides of the eggs don't go above 160°F or so—an ideal temperature for hard-boiled eggs.

   Lastly, the ice bath at the end also helps to ensure that the eggs don't continue (over)cooking. (Some say that the ice bath also helps "shrink" the eggs from the shell, making 'em easier to peel.)

Commit these tips to memory, and your hard-boiled eggs will always turn out perfectly!

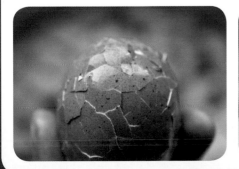
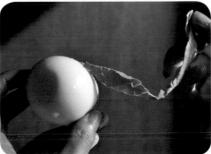
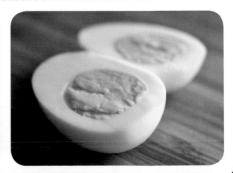

BACON-TOPPED DEVILED EGGS

Throwing a fancy shindig? Sometimes, it's worth going the extra mile to make deviled eggs—especially if there's bacon involved. If you can resist these porky, bite-sized morsels, you are not human, and we therefore can't be friends. Because I'm only friends with humans. Specifically, humans who love bacon.

Makes 24 pieces
Hands-on time: 25 minutes
Total time: 25 minutes

GO GRAB YOUR PITCHSPORKS!

12 **Perfect Hard-Boiled Eggs** (page 120)
½ cup **Five-Minute Bacon Aïoli** (page 60) or **Paleo Mayonnaise** (page 40)
2 **scallions**, thinly sliced (about 2 tablespoons)
1½ teaspoons **Dijon-style mustard**
1 teaspoon distilled **white vinegar**
Kosher salt
Freshly ground **black pepper**
½ cup **Crispy Lardons** (page 49)

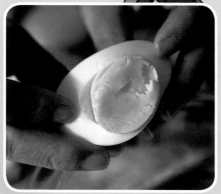 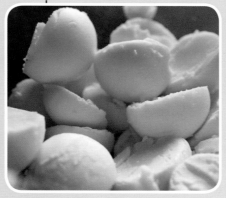 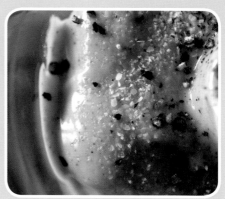

DO THIS:

1. Cut the hard-boiled eggs in half lengthwise, and carefully pop out the yolks from each egg. If necessary, use a small spoon to do the deed. Set aside the egg whites.

2. Toss the yolks and the aïoli or mayonnaise into the work bowl of a mini food processor. Add the scallions, mustard, and vinegar, and season with salt and pepper to taste. Pulse until the ingredients are thoroughly incorporated.

3. Scoop or pipe the yolk mixture into each egg white, and load it up with a generous amount of crispy bacon pieces before serving.

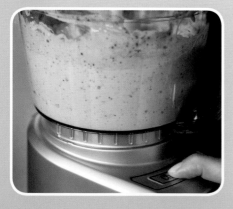 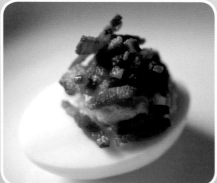 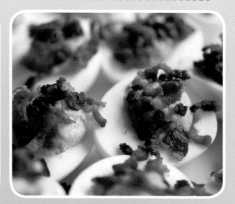

WHO SAYS YOU CAN'T SERVE BACON AND EGGS AT A DINNER PARTY?

LAZY DEVILS

I love deviled eggs, but for breezy, casual affairs (like lunch for myself), I'm just too lazy to go to all the effort. Whoops…Did I say "lazy"? I meant "busy." Whatever. You don't have to be Cinderella in the kitchen; with a spicy assist from Sriracha Mayonnaise, Lazy Devils look and taste even better than the real thing.

Makes 24 pieces
Hands-on time: 10 minutes
Total time: 10 minutes

12   **Perfect Hard-Boiled Eggs** (page 120)
½   cup **Sriracha Mayonnaise** (page 45)
4   ounces thinly sliced **prosciutto**
2   tablespoons minced **chives**
   Fleur de sel or whatever fancy artisanal finishing salt you've been saving up for that oh-so-special occasion

DO THIS:

1. Cut the hard-boiled eggs in half lengthwise. Use a butter knife to smear a generous dab of Sriracha Mayonnaise on the cut sides of the eggs, and arrange them on a platter.

2. Tear the prosciutto into ribbons, and use them to garnish the tops of each half-egg. Sprinkle the minced chives over the devils, and season each with a bit of sea salt immediately before serving.

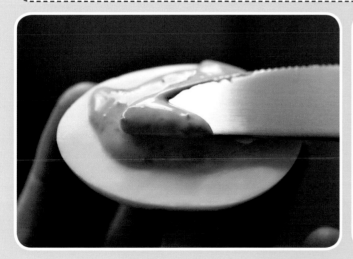

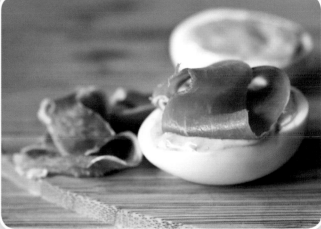

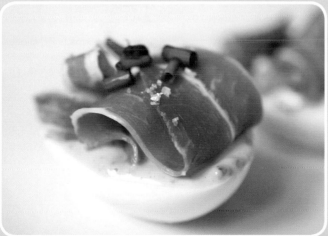

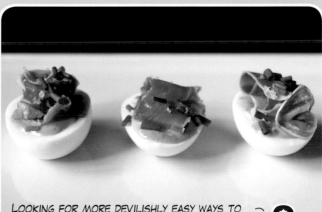

LOOKING FOR MORE DEVILISHLY EASY WAYS TO FLAVOR UP THESE EGGS? THEN TURN THE PAGE!

 ~ FLEUR DE SEL (FRENCH FOR "FLOWER OF SALT") OFFERS A MILD EARTHINESS AND DELICATE CRUNCH, MAKING IT ONE OF MY FAVORITE FINISHING SALTS.

HELLO
my name is
CLASSY DEVIL

Paleo Ranch Dressing (page 62)

Crispy Lardons (page 49)

Microgreens

Cherry tomatoes

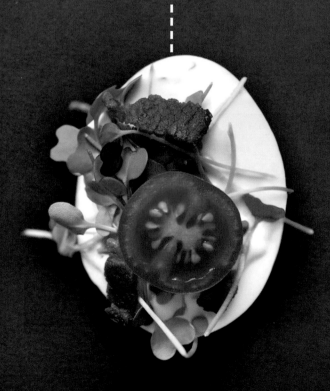

HELLO
my name is
ISLAND DEVIL

Paleo Mayonnaise (page 40)

Slow Cooker Kalua Pig (page 234)

Pineapple

Cilantro and sea salt

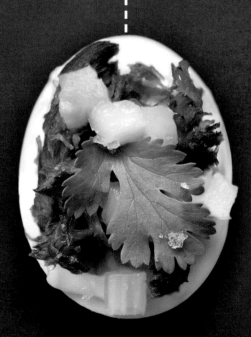

HELLO
my name is

LAZY
DEVIL

HELLO
my name is

CRABBY
DEVIL

Sriracha Mayonnaise (page 45)

Prosciutto

Chives

Fleur de sel

Holy 'Moly (page 51)

Crab

Apple and lime juice

Freshly ground black pepper

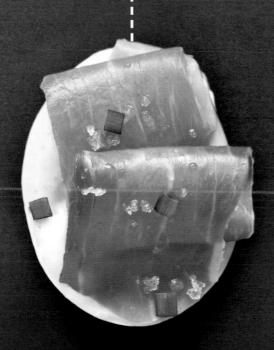

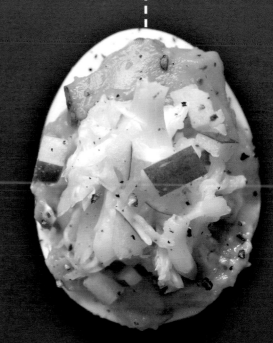

FURIKAKE, ASPARAGUS + EGGS

One of my favorite flavor enhancers is furikake—a traditional Japanese seasoning made of toasted sesame seeds, chopped seaweed, and dried bonito. (Be careful: most store-bought furikake contains added sugar and MSG, so read the labels carefully and stick to the brands with 100 percent real food ingredients.) Not only is furikake a good source of iodine, but its deep umami profile lends a crunchy brininess to any dish.

You can wake up your recipes with furikake in all sorts of ways. Here's a flavor-packed one-skillet meal of asparagus, eggs, and furikake (inspired by a dish from Chef Matt Abergel's Yardbird Restaurant in Hong Kong) that you can make for yourself in just five minutes. You heard that right: one skillet, five minutes. Go!

Makes 1 serving
Hands-on time: 5 minutes
Total time: 5 minutes

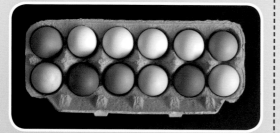

1   tablespoon **ghee** or fat of choice
6–8   thin **asparagus** stalks, trimmed
2   large **eggs**
      Kosher salt
      Freshly ground **black pepper**
      Juice from ½ small **lemon** (optional)
1   tablespoon **furikake seasoning**

DO THIS:

1. Arrange the oven rack 4 to 6 inches from the heating element, and preheat the broiler.

2. In an 8-inch cast-iron skillet, heat the ghee over high heat. As soon as it's sizzling, remove the skillet from the heat and toss in the asparagus. Shake gently to coat the spears with the melted fat.

3. Crack the eggs into the skillet next to the asparagus spears, and season with salt and pepper to taste.

4. Place the skillet under the broiler for 1 to 2 minutes, cooking the eggs to your desired doneness.

5. Remove the skillet from the broiler, and season with lemon juice.

6. Liberally sprinkle the furikake on the asparagus and eggs, and dig in.

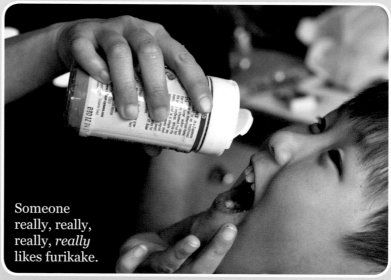

Someone really, really, really, *really* likes furikake.

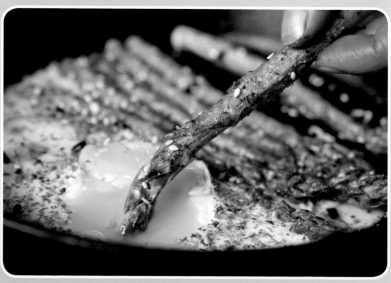

BUY YOUR FURIKAKE AT YOUR LOCAL ASIAN MARKET. WHAT? THERE AREN'T ANY IN YOUR NECK OF THE WOODS? MAKE YOUR OWN FURIKAKE BY MIXING TOGETHER TOASTED SESAME SEEDS, THIN STRIPS OF TOASTED NORI, AND A PINCH OF SALT! ⌐

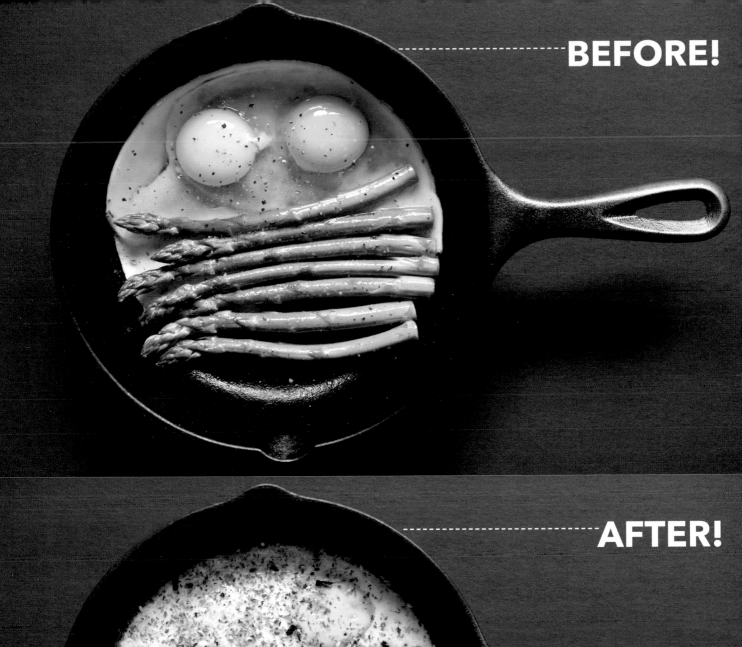

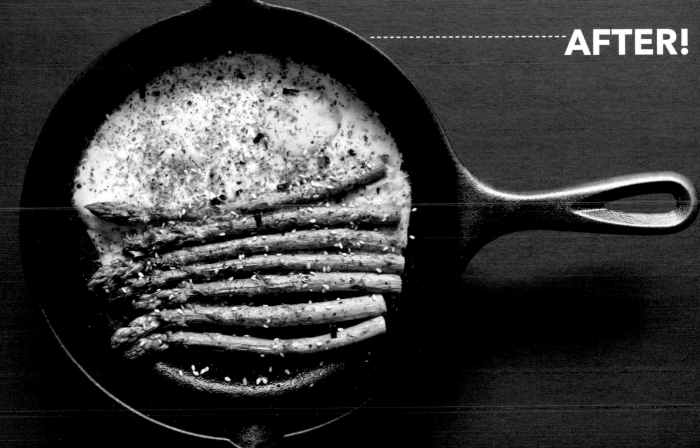

POACHED EGGS (THAT AREN'T UGLY)

Sick of omelets and scrambles? Then poach your eggs to produce a delicate, quivery oval of egg white. Pop it, and the creamy yolk becomes an instant sauce of its own. This is comfort food at its easiest, right?

Well...maybe. In Julia Child's *Mastering the Art of French Cooking*, she describes a perfect poached egg as "neat and oval in shape," with a white that "completely masks the yolk." Sadly, many of us struggle to achieve this standard. Our yolks end up overcooked, or our whites come out lumpy and misshapen. Or both.

But it doesn't have to be this way. With a few simple pointers and just ten minutes in the kitchen, we can all make beautifully poached *oeufs* that would make Julia proud.

GET:

2 large **eggs**
Kosher salt
Freshly ground **black pepper**

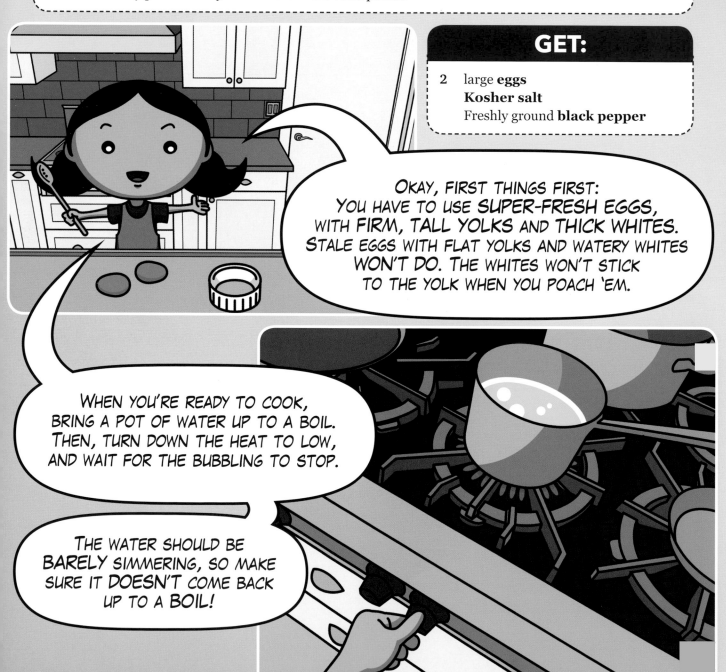

OKAY, FIRST THINGS FIRST: YOU HAVE TO USE SUPER-FRESH EGGS, WITH FIRM, TALL YOLKS AND THICK WHITES. STALE EGGS WITH FLAT YOLKS AND WATERY WHITES WON'T DO. THE WHITES WON'T STICK TO THE YOLK WHEN YOU POACH 'EM.

WHEN YOU'RE READY TO COOK, BRING A POT OF WATER UP TO A BOIL. THEN, TURN DOWN THE HEAT TO LOW, AND WAIT FOR THE BUBBLING TO STOP.

THE WATER SHOULD BE BARELY SIMMERING, SO MAKE SURE IT DOESN'T COME BACK UP TO A BOIL!

Makes 2 eggs
Hands-on time: 10 minutes
Total time: 10 minutes

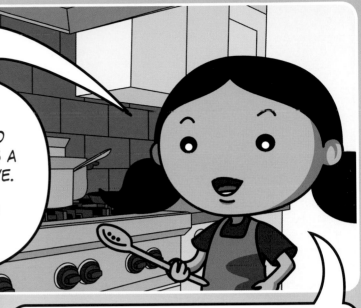

SOME FOLKS SWEAR THAT THE KEY TO A WELL-FORMED POACHED EGG IS TO ADD VINEGAR TO THE WATER. IT HELPS A LITTLE, BUT IT'S NOT TERRIBLY EFFECTIVE.

FRANKLY, VINEGAR'S MORE LIKELY TO MAKE YOUR EGGS TASTE SOUR.

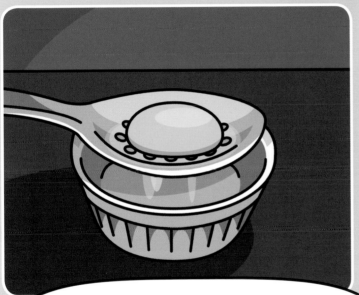

INSTEAD, THE SECRET (WHICH I LEARNED FROM HAROLD MCGEE) IS TO STRAIN EACH EGG WITH A LARGE PERFORATED SPOON TO GET RID OF ANY THIN, WATERY PART OF THE WHITE BEFORE COOKING. THE RESULT: NO WISPY EGG RIBBONS!

SLIP THE EGGS VERY GENTLY INTO THE HOT WATER, AND COOK 'EM JUST LONG ENOUGH FOR THE WHITE TO CONGEAL, ABOUT THREE MINUTES. THEN, REMOVE THE EGGS WITH A PERFORATED SPOON, AND ADD SALT AND PEPPER TO TASTE.

NOT EATING RIGHT AWAY? REFRIGERATE THE EGGS IN A CONTAINER OF COLD WATER. WHEN YOU'RE READY TO EAT, REHEAT IN BARELY SIMMERING WATER FOR A MINUTE OR UNTIL HOT.

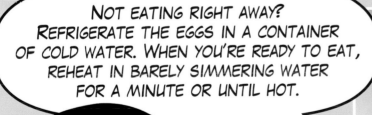

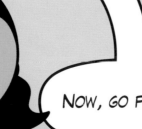

NOW, GO FORTH AND POACH!

CLASSIC EGG SALAD

No leftovers to pack for lunch? With some hard-boiled eggs and Paleo Mayonnaise on hand, a simple, creamy egg salad can be yours in less time than it takes for you to get dressed for work.

Makes 4 servings
Hands-on time: 10 minutes
Total time: 10 minutes

2 tablespoons minced **red onions** or **shallots**
8 **Perfect Hard-Boiled Eggs** (page 120)
¼ cup **Paleo Mayonnaise** (page 40)
½ medium **celery** rib, cut into ¼-inch dice
1½ tablespoons minced fresh **Italian parsley**
1 tablespoon fresh **lemon juice**
1 tablespoon **Dijon-style mustard**
½ teaspoon **kosher salt**
¼ teaspoon freshly ground **black pepper**

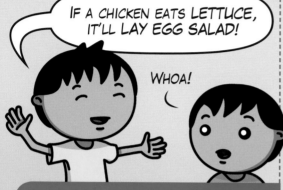

IF A CHICKEN EATS LETTUCE, IT'LL LAY EGG SALAD!

WHOA!

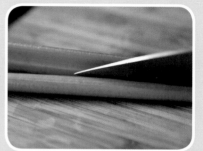
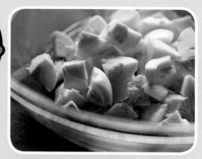

DO THIS:

1. Soak the minced onion or shallot in a small bowl of ice water for about 5 minutes to remove the bite. In the meantime, peel and dice the eggs.

2. Drain the onion and toss all the ingredients (minus the water, of course) into a large bowl, and mix to combine. Serve immediately, or store the egg salad in an airtight container for up to 3 days in the refrigerator.

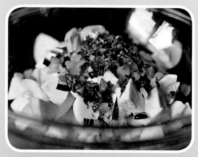
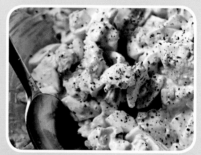

CHANGE IT UP:

Add a new twist to your egg salad!

- Use Sriracha Mayonnaise (page 45) in place of the Paleo Mayonnaise!

- Or add ¾ teaspoon red pepper!

- Or use 1 tablespoon capers and 1 tablespoon caper brine in place of the salt!

- Or add 2 tablespoons Crispy Lardons (page 49) to the salad!

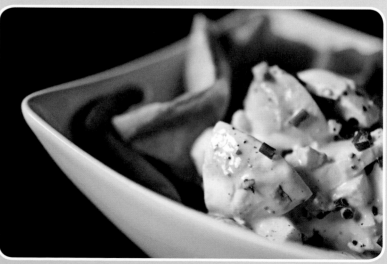

WANNA MAKE IT MORE EXOTIC? ADD A HALF TEASPOON OF CURRY POWDER AND SOME HALVED RED GRAPES!

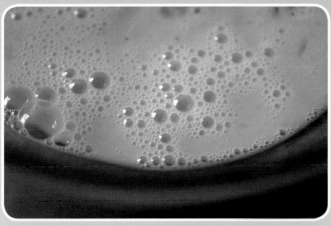
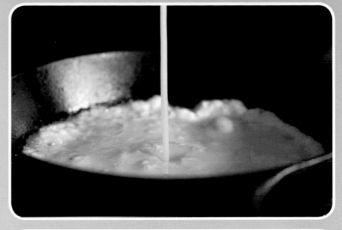
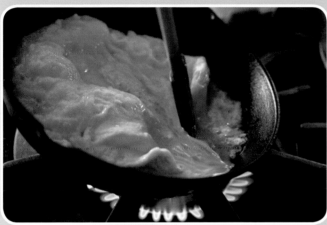
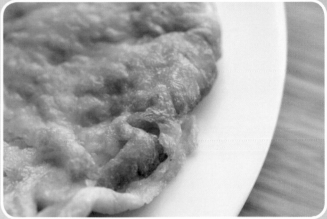

KAI JIAO (THAI OMELET)

Kai jiao is often described as a "Thai omelet," but unlike its Western counterpart, this egg dish is eaten at any time of day—usually atop a generous mound of rice and with a squirt of fiery sriracha. I often fry up a plain *kai jiao* for breakfast when I'm in a rush, but the first time you make this, do it right: prepare a batch of Easy Cauliflower "Rice" (page 156), plate it with *kai jiao*, and top it with Paleo Sriracha (page 42). Pow!

Makes 2 servings
Hands-on time: 10 minutes
Total time: 10 minutes

6	large **eggs**
2	tablespoons **tapioca flour**
1	tablespoon Paleo-friendly **fish sauce**
1	teaspoon fresh **lime juice**
3	tablespoons **ghee** or fat of choice, divided

DO THIS:

1. In a large bowl, beat together the eggs, tapioca flour, fish sauce, and lime juice until smooth.

2. Heat half the ghee over high heat in an 8-inch cast-iron skillet until it's sizzling-hot. Holding the bowl of egg mixture about 8 inches above the skillet, pour half of the batter in. This isn't just for theatrical effect; upon splashdown, the edges of the batter will puff up in the hot ghee, forming a crunchy frill. Cook for 30 seconds, and then flip and cook the other side for another 30 seconds.

3. Transfer to a plate, and repeat with the remaining ghee and egg mixture to make a second *kai jiao*. This crisp-on-the-outside, fluffy-on-the-inside egg dish is best when served hot off the stove.

 THROW IN A GENEROUS PINCH OF THINLY SLICED GREEN ONIONS AND MINCED CILANTRO FOR SOME EXTRA COLOR AND TEXTURE!

UOVA IN PURGATORIO

I wish I could tell you that I discovered "eggs in purgatory" in my explorations of southern Italy, but the sad truth is that most of my (pre-Paleo) time in the mezzogiorno was spent hunting for pasta and gelato. It wasn't until a lazy weekend brunch at New York's Dell'Anima that I discovered *uova in purgatorio* and fell head over heels. Dell'Anima's upscale version of this fiery Neapolitan classic features smoky pancetta, but I also love the nostalgia-inducing combination of sausage and mushrooms.

Uova in purgatorio is rustic comfort food at its finest. Use a fork to swirl the oozy yellow yolks into the spicy, meaty tomato sauce, and your taste buds'll be transported—not to purgatory, but to paradise. (Man, that was super-corny. Please accept my apologies.)

Makes 4 servings
Hands-on time: 30 minutes
Total time: 30 minutes

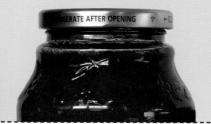

- **1** tablespoon **ghee** or fat of choice
- **½** medium **yellow onion**, cut into ¼-inch dice
- **¼** pound cremini **mushrooms**, thinly sliced
- **Kosher salt**
- Freshly ground **black pepper**
- **1** pound loose **Italian pork sausage**
- **2** cups **marinara sauce**
- **1** teaspoon **red pepper flakes**
- **4** large **eggs**

DO THIS:

1. Preheat the oven to 400°F with the rack in the upper-middle position.

2. Melt the fat in a large skillet over medium heat. Add the onions and sauté until translucent, about 5 minutes. Toss in the mushrooms and season with salt and pepper. Cook for 5 minutes or until the moisture released by the mushrooms evaporates.

3. Add the sausage to the pan, breaking it up with a spatula. Cook until it's no longer pink. Pour the sauce onto the meat and add the red pepper flakes. Stir to combine the ingredients, and cook until the sauce simmers.

4. Divide the saucy mixture into four 8-ounce ovenproof ramekins or mini cocottes. Make a small well in the center of each, and crack an egg in it. Sprinkle salt and pepper on the eggs. Place the ramekins on a tray in the oven, and bake until the eggs are done to your desired consistency, about 10 to 15 minutes. Serve immediately.

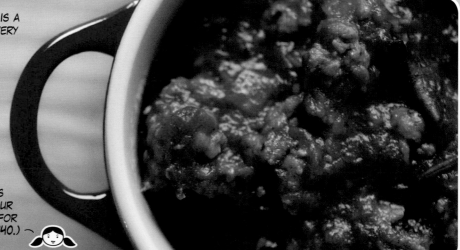

LOOSE SAUSAGE (OR BULK SAUSAGE) IS A MAINSTAY IN MY KITCHEN. IT'S THE VERY EPITOME OF EMERGENCY PROTEIN: FLAVORFUL, VERSATILE, AND SIMPLE TO PREPARE.

KEEP SOME IN YOUR FREEZER, AND THAW IT ON DAYS WHEN YOU'RE CRUNCHED FOR TIME. IT'S EASY TO FORM THE SAUSAGE INTO PATTIES OR MEATBALLS, OR TO STIR-FRY IT WITH VEGETABLES.

BUT REMEMBER: QUALITY MATTERS, SO MAKE SURE YOUR SAUSAGE COMES FROM A GOOD SOURCE. (OR MAKE YOUR OWN! FOLLOW STEP 1 OF MY RECIPE FOR MAPLE SAUSAGE PATTIES ON PAGE 240.)

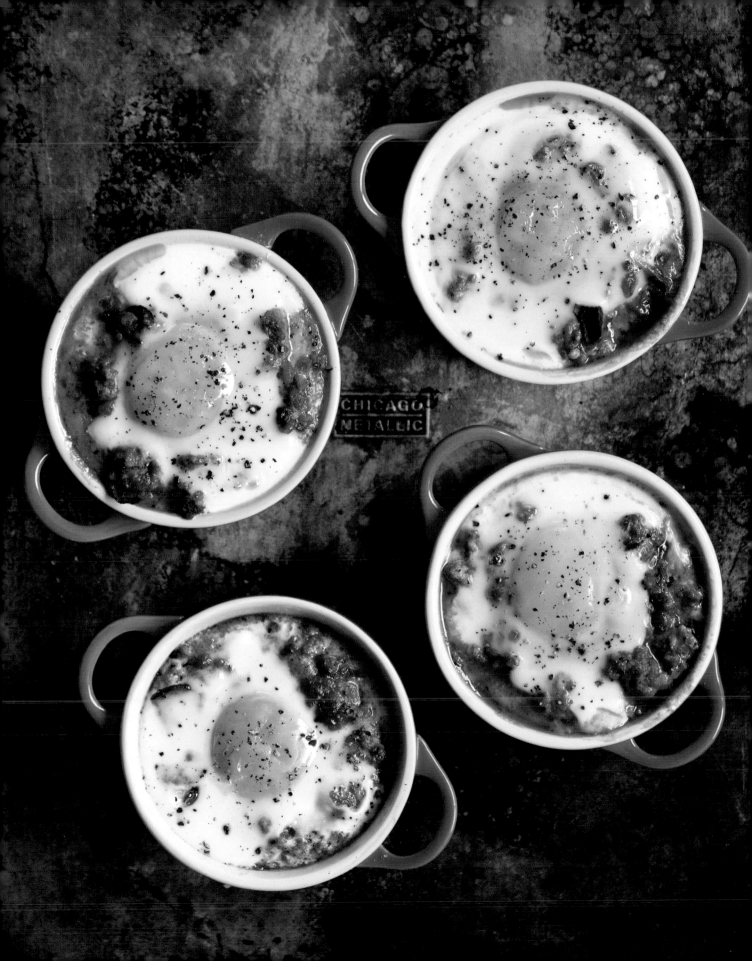

PROSCIUTTO-WRAPPED FRITTATA MUFFINS

Frittatas are a staple for any Paleo eater, but they can be challenging to eat on the go—especially during the morning rush. To solve this problem, I make muffin-sized frittatas, wrapped in savory prosciutto shells. Sorry, gang: you no longer have an excuse for stopping at the donut shop on your way to work.

Makes 12 muffins
Hands-on time: 20 minutes
Total time: 50 minutes

- 4 tablespoons **coconut oil** or fat of choice, divided
- ½ medium **yellow onion**, minced
- 3 **garlic cloves**, minced
- ½ pound **cremini mushrooms**, thinly sliced
  Kosher salt
  Freshly ground **black pepper**
- 8 large **eggs**
- ¼ cup full-fat **coconut milk**
- 2 tablespoons **coconut flour**
- ½ pound frozen chopped **spinach**, thawed and squeezed dry
- 5 ounces thinly sliced **prosciutto**
- 1 cup **cherry tomatoes**, halved

DO THIS:

1. Preheat the oven to 375°F with the rack in the middle position. Heat 2 tablespoons of coconut oil over medium heat in a large cast-iron skillet, and sauté the onions with a pinch of salt until they're soft and translucent, about 5 minutes.

2. Add the garlic and mushrooms and cook until the moisture from the mushrooms evaporates. Season with salt and pepper to taste, and transfer to a plate to cool.

3. Beat the eggs in a large bowl. Add the coconut milk and coconut flour to the beaten eggs. Whisk until the batter's thoroughly mixed, and then stir in the mushrooms and spinach.

4. Brush a 12-cup muffin tin with the remaining 2 tablespoons of melted coconut oil, and line each cup with a layer of prosciutto. Cover the bottom and sides completely. Spoon the frittata batter into each cup, and top with the halved cherry tomatoes.

5. Bake for about 20 minutes, rotating the tray from back-to-front halfway through the cooking process. The muffins are done when an inserted toothpick comes out clean.

6. Cool the muffins in the pan for a few minutes before transferring them to a wire rack to cool.

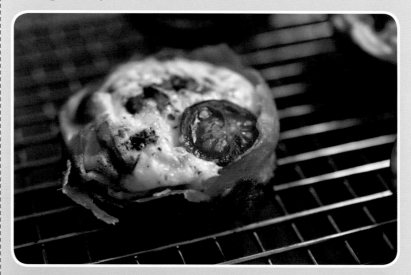

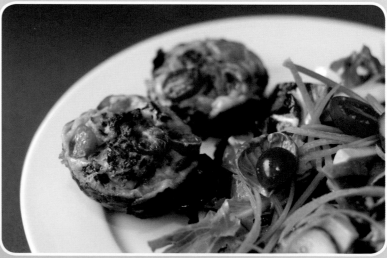

A PROPER FRENCH OMELET

Unlike the rubbery clumps of eggs that pass for omelets at the corner diner, French omelets are all about the technique. They're rapidly whipped throughout the cooking process, and taken off the heat before the eggs stiffen, producing a much softer and fluffier omelet that melts in your mouth.

Makes 2 servings
Hands-on time: 5 minutes
Total time: 10 minutes

6   large **eggs**
    Kosher salt
    Freshly ground **black pepper**
1   tablespoon finely chopped fresh **chives**, **Italian parsley**, or **chervil** (optional)
2   tablespoons **ghee** or fat of choice, divided

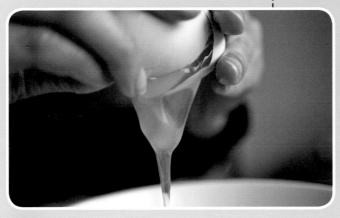 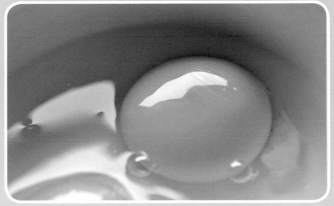

DO THIS:

1. Crack the eggs into a large bowl, and add a generous pinch of salt, some freshly ground pepper, and if desired, fresh herbs. Thoroughly beat the egg mixture with a fork.

2. Heat 1 tablespoon of ghee in a small cast-iron skillet over high heat. Once the fat is shimmering, lower the heat to medium, and pour half of the egg mixture into the skillet.

3. Stir vigorously and continuously with a fork while shaking the pan with your other hand for about 2 minutes. Rapidly whisk the egg base as it comes in contact with the skillet so that the egg sets as tiny, bubbly strands rather than a dense yellow blob.

4. As soon as most of the egg is solid, stop stirring for about 10 seconds, and then carefully fold the omelet over. Transfer to a plate, and repeat with the remaining mixture to make a second omelet.

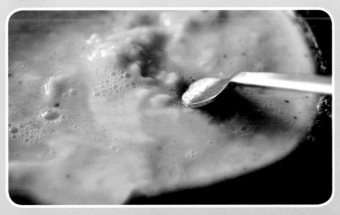 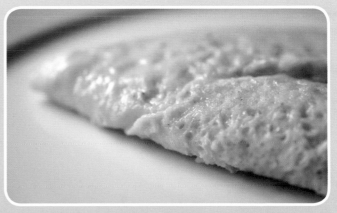

 FORGET TO ADD HERBS TO YOUR EGG MIXTURE? DON'T WORRY YOUR PRETTY LITTLE HEAD. JUST USE 'EM TO GARNISH YOUR FINISHED OMELET!

CHINESE EGG FOO YOUNG

For decades, my in-laws owned a Chinese restaurant in the San Francisco Bay Area, serving up the Westernized dishes that many Americans know so well: pot stickers, chow mein, deep-fried wontons, sweet-and-sour pork. My husband grew up in the restaurant's kitchen, and egg foo young was a childhood favorite.

I didn't encounter egg foo young until after I met Henry in college and he took me to visit his family's restaurant. But as soon as I took my first bite of these savory egg patties, I knew I had to have the recipe.

Egg foo young, which means "lotus flower egg," is enduringly popular and infinitely flexible; one Japanese-Chinese variant called *kani-tama* is stuffed with crab meat, and in parts of Missouri, folks slather egg foo young with mayonnaise and sandwich it between slices of white bread. (It's called a St. Paul sandwich, named after the Chinese-American inventor's hometown in Minnesota.)

Not surprisingly, my version of egg foo young isn't served with bread or the traditional accompaniment of soy-based brown gravy—but as a finishing touch, I can never resist a spicy squirt of Paleo Sriracha.

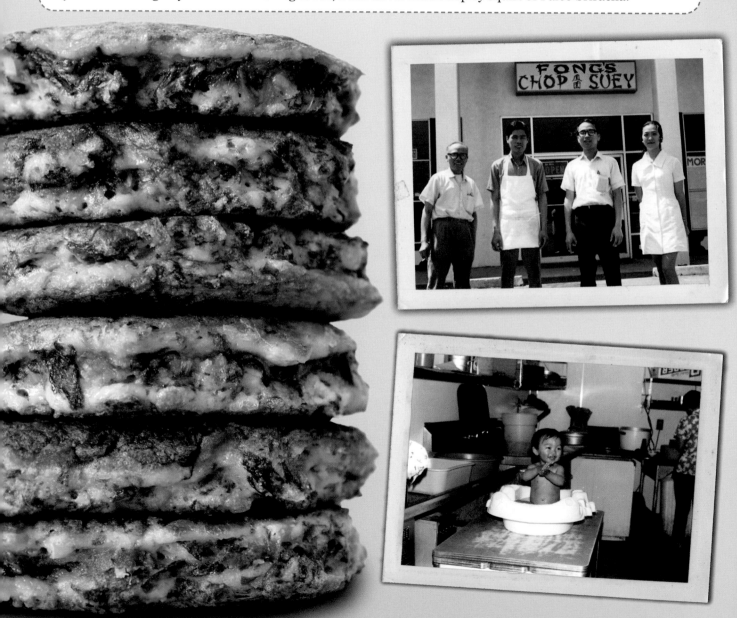

GET:

6	large **eggs**
¼	cup **coconut flour**
1	teaspoon Paleo-friendly **fish sauce** (or kosher salt to taste)
½	teaspoon **apple cider vinegar**
1	cup diced **ham** or cooked meat of choice
10	ounces frozen **spinach**, thawed and squeezed dry
2	**scallions**, thinly sliced
1	tablespoon minced fresh **cilantro**
½	teaspoon **baking soda**
	Freshly ground **black pepper**
	Ghee, for frying
	Paleo Sriracha (page 42) (optional)

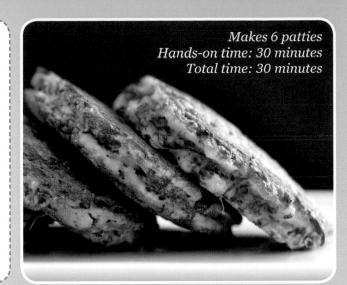

Makes 6 patties
Hands-on time: 30 minutes
Total time: 30 minutes

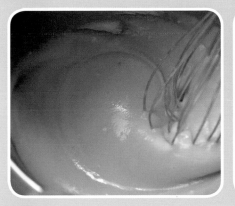
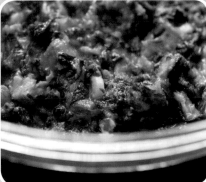
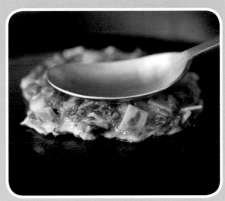

DO THIS:

1. In a large bowl, whisk together the eggs, coconut flour, fish sauce, and apple cider vinegar until smooth and lump-free. Stir in the ham, spinach, scallions, cilantro, and baking soda, and season with pepper to taste.

2. In a large skillet or griddle, heat a tablespoon of ghee over medium heat until shimmering. Scoop a quarter-cup of batter onto the skillet, and flatten with the back of a spoon until it's about ½ inch in height. Let it cook undisturbed for 3 minutes, until golden brown. Using a spatula, carefully flip over the egg foo young, and fry for another 2 to 3 minutes or until cooked through.

3. Transfer the patty to a wire rack, and repeat Step 2 to cook up the remaining pancakes. (If you have room in the skillet, you can fry up more than one at a time, but don't overcrowd the patties.)

4. Serve with Paleo Sriracha if you're feeling spicy. (Or break out the leftover gravy from page 198!)

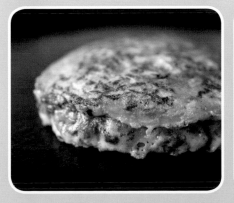
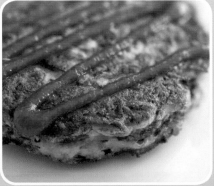
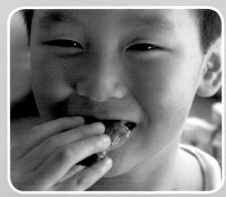

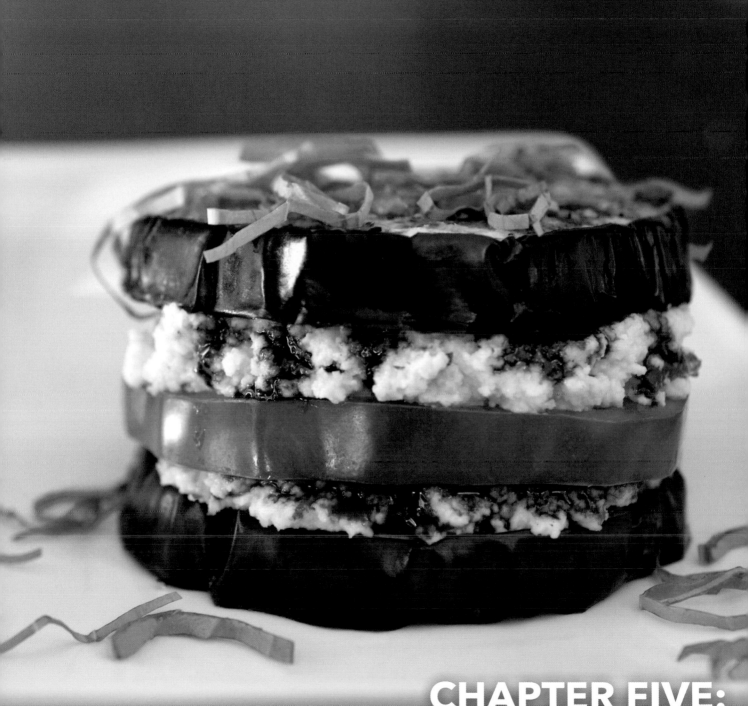

CHAPTER FIVE:
PLANTS

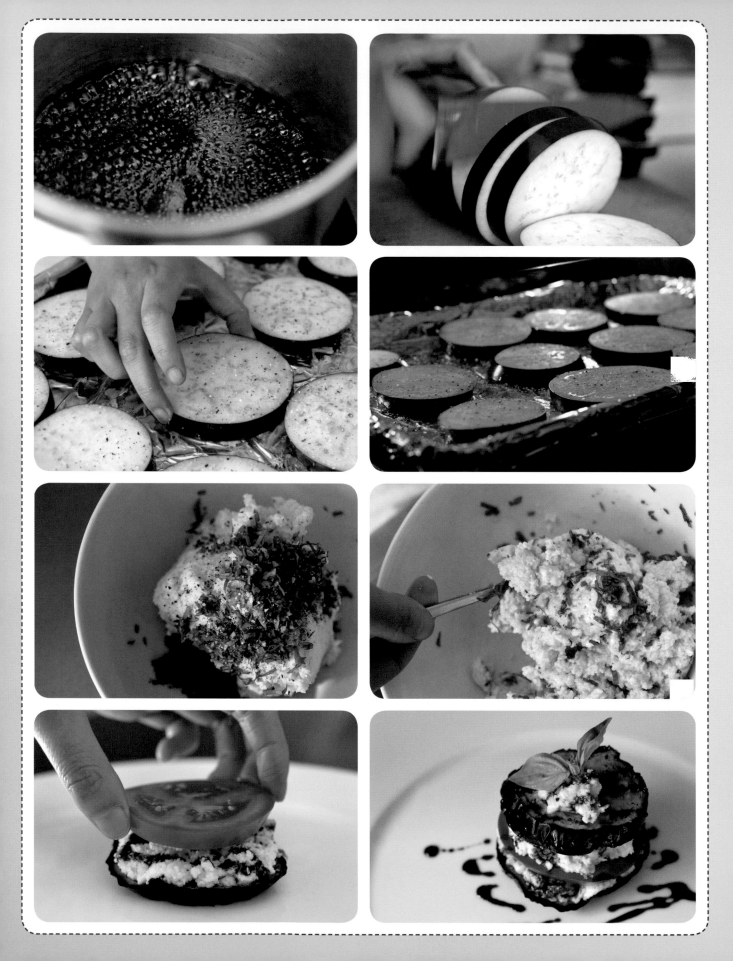

EGGPLANT "RICOTTA" STACKS

When I'm busy prepping for a dinner party, I don't have the time or energy to straighten up the house before guests arrive. Instead, I conscript my husband to put away the avalanche of laundry and accumulated clutter that threaten to bury us in our own home. (But don't feel *too* sorry for him; I still do all the dishes.)

Thankfully (for Henry), I've found ways to prep fanciful, Paleo-friendly dishes by quickly assembling premade components. These Eggplant Ricotta Stacks, for example, require minimal effort but deliver maximum flavor. Punctuated with the penetrating tang of a balsamic reduction, these "cheesy" vegetable stacks will excite your palate like nothing else…and free up some time so you can help with the laundry.

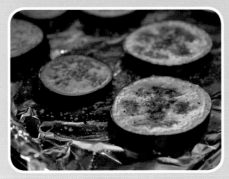 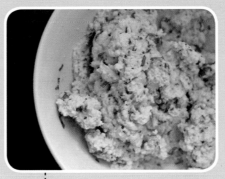 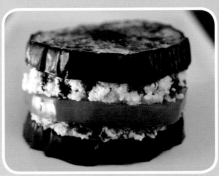

Makes 6 servings
Hands-on time: 30 minutes
Total time: 30 minutes

THIS RECIPE REQUIRES COOKING, BUT IT WAS INSPIRED BY AN EYE-OPENING MEAL AT ONE LUCKY DUCK, A RAW VEGAN JOINT IN NEW YORK CITY!

1 cup **balsamic vinegar**
1 medium **shallot**, minced (about ¼ cup)
2 tablespoons melted **ghee** or fat of choice
2 **globe eggplants** (approximately 1 pound each), sliced crosswise into ½-inch rounds
Kosher salt
Freshly ground **black pepper**
1½ cup **Macadamia Nut "Ricotta"** (page 46)
2 tablespoons minced fresh **basil**, plus more for garnish
1 tablespoon **extra-virgin olive oil**
2 large heirloom **tomatoes**, sliced into 1-inch rounds

DO THIS:

1. In a small saucepan, bring the balsamic vinegar and shallots to a rolling boil over high heat. Lower the heat to medium, and continue cooking until the liquid is syrupy and reduced by half, about 15 minutes.

2. While the balsamic reduction is cooking, place a wire rack 6 inches from the heating element in the oven, and turn on the broiler. Coat a foil-lined baking tray with the melted ghee, and arrange the eggplant slices on top. Season liberally with salt and pepper, and flip the eggplant slices over to season the other side.

3. Broil the eggplant rounds for 2 to 3 minutes. Using tongs, flip each slice over, rotate the tray, and broil for another 2 to 3 minutes or until golden brown. Set aside to cool.

4. In a bowl, combine the Macadamia Nut "Ricotta," basil, and olive oil. Season with salt and pepper to taste, and then stir to thoroughly incorporate.

5. Assemble the stacks by spreading generous spoonfuls of the herbed "ricotta" and drizzles of balsamic reduction between layers of eggplant and tomato slices.

6. Garnish with basil and a final splash of balsamic reduction before serving.

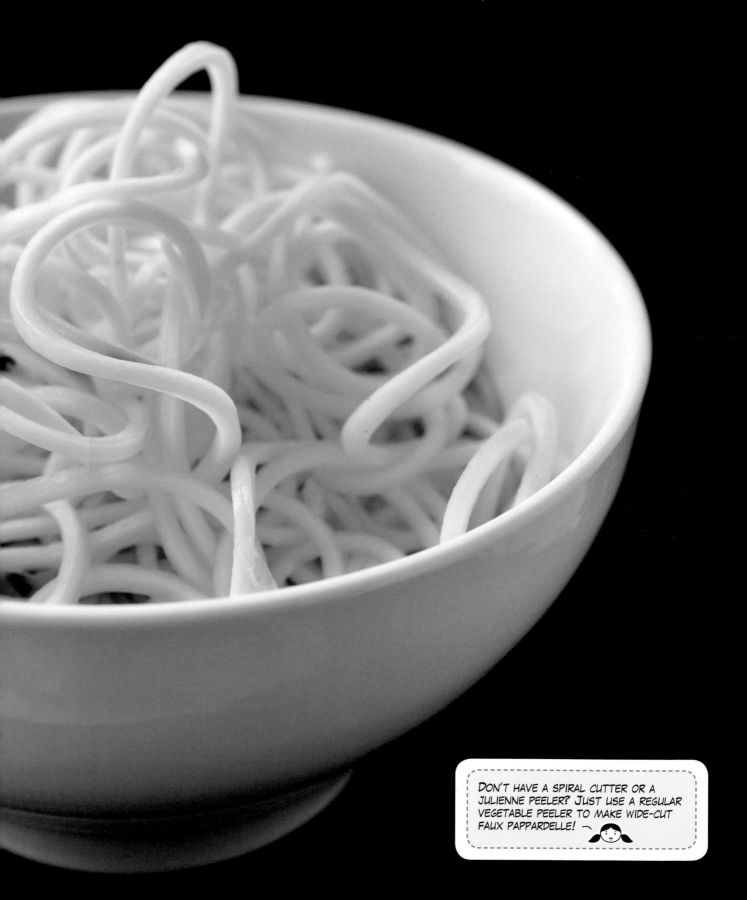

DON'T HAVE A SPIRAL CUTTER OR A JULIENNE PEELER? JUST USE A REGULAR VEGETABLE PEELER TO MAKE WIDE-CUT FAUX PAPPARDELLE!

ZOODLES

Got a craving for noodles? Rather than giving in to your carb-loving demons, grab some zucchini and cut them into thin, julienned strings. With their mild taste and excellent slurpability, zoodles are an amazingly adaptable stand-in for pasta, soaking in the flavors of your favorite sauces and broths.

But beware: cook 'em too long, and you'll end up with a waterlogged dish and limp, mushy zoodles. My recommendation is to toss the raw zucchini strands in warm sauce or soup just before serving; that way, the zoodles will be perfectly al dente by the time you and your sweetie reenact the candlelit spaghetti dinner scene from *Lady and the Tramp*. All together now: *Awwwww!*

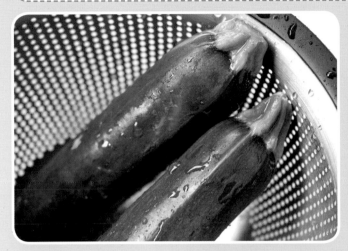
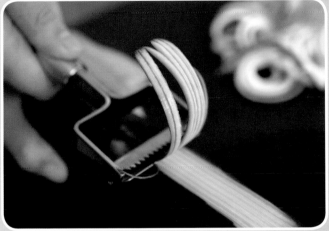

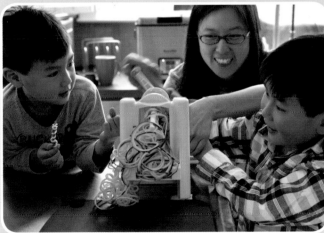
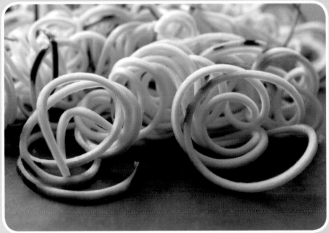

GET:

6	medium **zucchini**

AND:

A julienne peeler, spiral cutter, or mad knife skillz

DO THIS:

I feel kind of silly calling this a recipe, as it involves little more than julienning a bunch of zucchini. There are, however, a number of ways to quickly produce an overflowing pile of zoodles. My two favorite methods? Use a julienne peeler or a spiral cutter. (Of course, if you're a certified kitchen ninja, feel free to hand-cut your zoodles.)

Yes, both are specialty kitchen tools, but they're not one-trick ponies. You can use them to shred all kinds of fruits and vegetables. Plus, they'll entice your gadget-crazy kids into helping you crank out your zoodles. Isn't child labor a wonderful thing?

 CUT UP MORE ZUCCHINI THAN YOU THINK YOU'LL NEED. ZOODLES SHRINK WITH HEAT!

ROASTED PORTOBELLO MUSHROOMS

The beefiness of roasted portobello mushrooms make for a hearty side, but I hate taking the time to marinate them—especially when I'm in a rush. Luckily, there's a swift and simple way to prep these meaty caps. Add a drizzle of citrus or balsamic vinegar and *presto!* An easy, flavorful vegetable dish is yours. Bonus: portobello mushrooms are a wonderfully sturdy and Paleo-friendly alternative to burger buns, too!

Makes 2 servings
Hands-on time: 10 minutes
Total time: 25 minutes

- 4 large **portobello mushrooms**, wiped clean with a damp cloth or paper towel
- 2 tablespoons melted **ghee** or fat of choice
  Kosher salt
  Freshly ground **black pepper**
- 1 teaspoon dried **thyme** or **basil** (optional)
  Juice from ½ small **lemon**

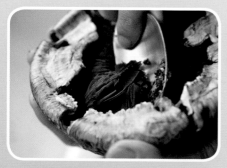 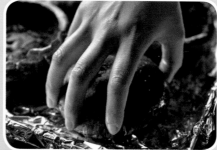 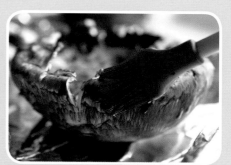

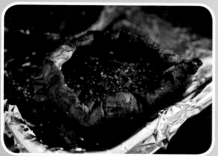 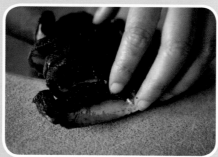 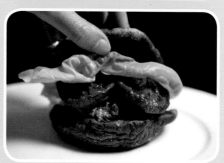

DO THIS:

1. Arrange the rack in the middle position in the oven, and preheat the oven to 400°F. Line a baking sheet with foil. Remove the stems from the mushrooms, and scrape out the gills with a spoon. Flip the caps gill-side down, and use a small knife to cut a shallow X on the top of each mushroom.

2. Arrange the mushrooms on the foil-lined sheet, and brush each cap—top and bottom—with melted fat. Season with salt and pepper to taste, and, if desired, dried herbs. Roast the mushrooms gill-side up in the oven for 10 minutes.

3. After 10 minutes, most of the juices in the upturned caps should have evaporated. Flip the mushrooms over, and cook for an additional 10 minutes. Once the mushrooms are tender and cooked through, transfer them to a cutting board, slice 'em up, and add a squirt of lemon before serving. (But don't slice the cooked caps if you're using them as burger patties!)

 THE ONLY DIFFERENCE BETWEEN BUTTON MUSHROOMS, CREMINI MUSHROOMS, AND PORTOBELLO MUSHROOMS IS AGE. BUTTONS ARE THE BABIES, AND CREMINIS ARE THE REBELLIOUS TEENAGERS, WHILE PORTOBELLOS ARE THE FULLY MATURE VERSION OF THIS UMAMI-PACKED MUSHROOM.

KABOCHA WEDGES

To Cambodians, it's *abóbora*. Koreans call it *danhobak*. In Thailand, it's *fak thong*, while Aussies and Kiwis refer to it as Japanese squash. But I've always known this winter squash by its Japanese name: *kabocha*.

If you're getting tired of butternut squash, give *kabocha* a shot. It's perfect in cold weather, but *kabocha*'s available year-round, so pick a heavy one at the market and lug it home. Don't be superficial and choose one that's shiny and bright green; unlike a lot of other vegetables, this squash tastes better with age.

When you're ready to cook, make sure you have a sharp knife and strong arms, because cutting into this hearty (and hardy) squash ain't easy. But once you breach the *kabocha*'s tough green skin, you'll discover a bright orange interior that—when roasted—yields a subtly nutty sweetness. The delicate crunch of these colorful wedges will give way to a creamy flesh that's lighter and fluffier than baked yam or pumpkin.

Makes 4 servings
Hands-on time: 10 minutes
Total time: 40 minutes

1 medium **kabocha squash**
2 tablespoons melted **ghee** or fat of choice
Kosher salt
Freshly ground **black pepper**
Balsamic vinegar (optional)

DO THIS:

1. Preheat the oven to 400°F with the rack in the middle position, and line a rimmed baking sheet with foil. If desired, peel the squash with a vegetable peeler. (The skin is edible, so peeling's optional.)

2. Muster up some brute strength and cut the squash in half. The best way to attack it is to first cut off the top and bottom. Once the flesh is exposed, slicing through the kabocha should be a breeze.

3. Scrape out the seeds and stringy stuff with a spoon, and cut the squash into uniform wedges. Toss the kabocha with melted ghee, and season with salt and pepper to taste.

4. Arrange the wedges in a single layer on the baking sheet. Roast for 30 minutes, flipping halfway through the cooking time. You'll know the squash is ready when the pieces are slightly crunchy on the outside but still soft and fluffy on the inside.

5. Drizzle with balsamic vinegar, if desired, before serving.

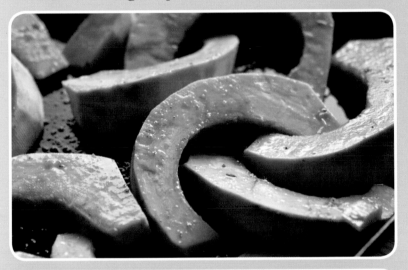

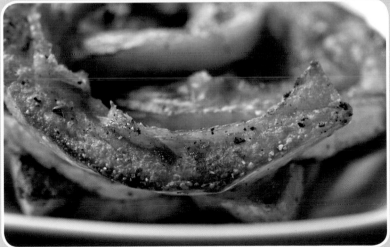

 THESE THICK 'N CRISPY WEDGES ARE A GREAT ALTERNATIVE TO STEAK FRIES!

CAVOLINI AL FORNO

Makes 6 servings | Hands-on time: 30 minutes | Total time: 1 hour

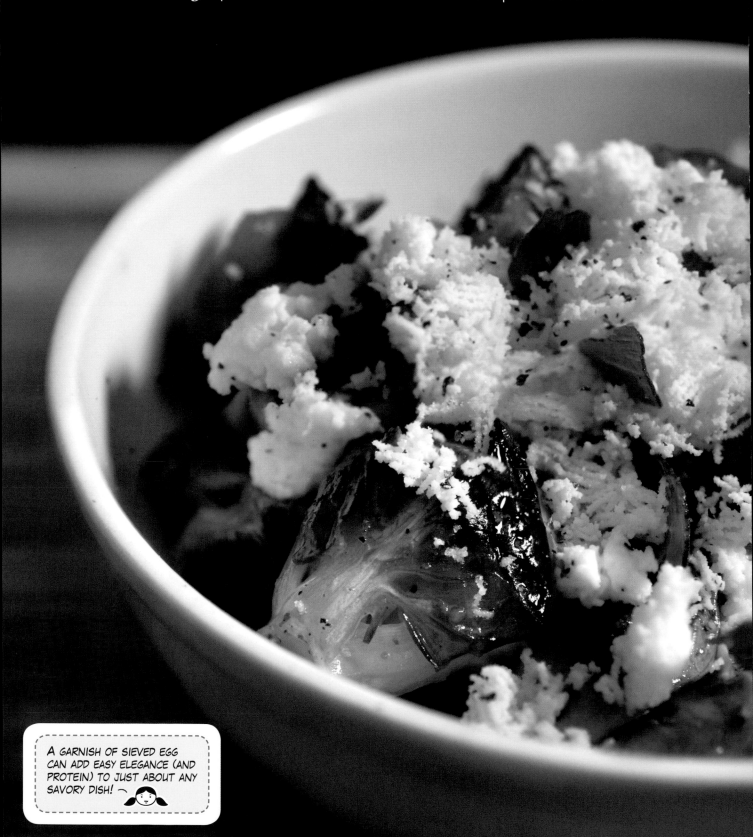

A GARNISH OF SIEVED EGG CAN ADD EASY ELEGANCE (AND PROTEIN) TO JUST ABOUT ANY SAVORY DISH!

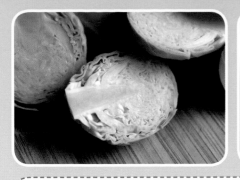
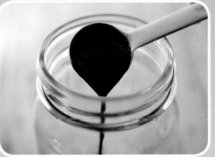
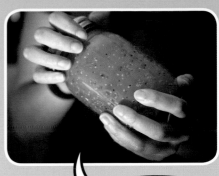

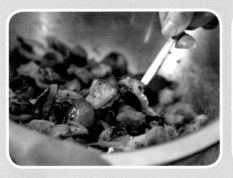
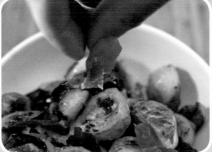
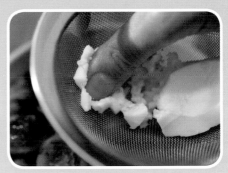

As the name suggests, Brussels sprouts hail from Belgium, where these tender buds have been cultivated for centuries. But sadly, they're nowhere near as popular as their culinary compatriot: Belgian waffles. I get it: most people prefer syrup-drenched breakfast cakes to vegetables.

But obviously, they haven't yet tried roasted Brussels sprouts tossed in a sharp mustard vinaigrette and topped with prosciutto chips and sieved egg. This hearty Italian side will convert even the staunchest sprouts hater. Personally, I can't get enough of *cavolini al forno*—I often add extra Porkitos and eggs so I can enjoy an entrée-sized portion of this dish.

Mustard Vinaigrette

- ¼ cup **extra-virgin olive oil**
- 2 teaspoons aged **balsamic vinegar**
- 2 teaspoon **Dijon-style mustard**
- 2 teaspoons minced **shallot**
- ½ teaspoon **kosher salt**
  Freshly ground **black pepper**

Brussels Sprouts

- 2 pounds **Brussels sprouts**, trimmed and halved
- 3 tablespoons melted **ghee**
  Kosher salt
  Freshly ground **black pepper**
- 4 **Porkitos** (page 74), crumbled
- 2 **Perfect Hard-Boiled Eggs** (page 120), peeled and pushed through a sieve

SHAKE IT!

DO THIS:

1. If you haven't made a batch of Porkitos yet, hop to it—especially if you've only got one oven.

2. Preheat the oven to 400°F with the rack in the middle position. Then, combine all the vinaigrette ingredients in a jar. Seal tightly and shake well. (Yes, you can whisk 'em together in a bowl instead, but where's the fun in that?)

3. Toss the Brussels sprouts with melted ghee, and season with salt and pepper to taste. Arrange the sprouts in a single layer on a foil-lined baking sheet and roast for 35 minutes or until browned on the outside and tender on the inside, rotating the tray and flipping the spouts at the midpoint. (If you don't have Perfect Hard-Boiled Eggs handy, now's the perfect time to make some.)

4. Toss the Brussels sprouts with the vinaigrette in a large bowl. Plate the sprouts, add a sprinkle of crumbled Porkitos, and garnish with the sieved eggs. Taste and adjust for seasoning, and serve immediately.

 DON'T YOU DARE THROW AWAY THE OUTER LEAVES OF THE BRUSSELS SPROUTS. SAVE 'EM TO MAKE BRUSSELS SPROUTS CHIPS (PAGE 70)!

BROCCOLI BAGNA CÀUDA

Even a simple vegetable side can take on a deep, layered flavor profile when you add umami and heat to the mix. That's why I'm a big fan of bagna càuda, a simmered Piedmontese "hot bath" of garlic, anchovies, red pepper flakes, and olive oil. Thankfully, you don't have to zip around the streets of Turin on a scooter to get a taste of this mouth-filling, savory sauce. Tossed with lemony, oven-roasted broccoli, spicy bagna càuda brings full-bodied heat to any dinner table. Besides, it's just plain fun to yell BAHN-yah COW-dah!

Makes 4 servings
Hands-on time: 20 minutes
Total time: 40 minutes

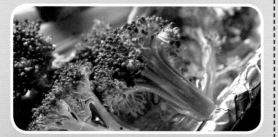

2   bunches **broccoli** (about 2 pounds), cut into florets, with stems peeled and cut into uniform pieces

2   tablespoons **macadamia nut oil** or fat of choice

     Kosher salt

     Freshly ground **black pepper**

6   **anchovy fillets** packed in olive oil (about half of a 2 ounce can), drained and minced

¼   cup **extra-virgin olive oil**

2   **garlic cloves**, minced

½   teaspoon **red pepper flakes**

     Finely grated zest and juice from 1 medium **lemon**

DO THIS:

1. Preheat the oven to 400°F with the rack in the middle position.

2. In a large bowl, toss together the broccoli and macadamia nut oil, and season generously with salt and pepper. Arrange the broccoli in a single layer on a foil-lined rimmed baking sheet.

3. Roast the tray of broccoli for 30 to 35 minutes, or until tender and toasty, tossing the broccoli and turning the baking sheet halfway through the cooking time.

4. In the meantime, make the bagna càuda. Cook the minced anchovies and olive oil in a small saucepan over low heat. Stir until the anchovies melt into the oil, which should take 3 to 5 minutes. Remove the pan from the heat, and stir in the garlic and red pepper flakes.

5. When the broccoli's done roasting, transfer it to a large bowl, and mix it with the garlic-anchovy sauce, lemon zest, and lemon juice.

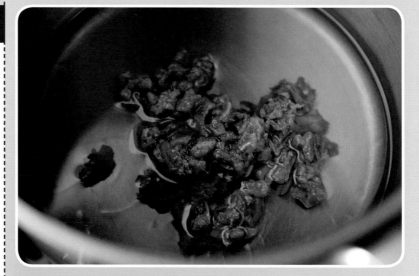

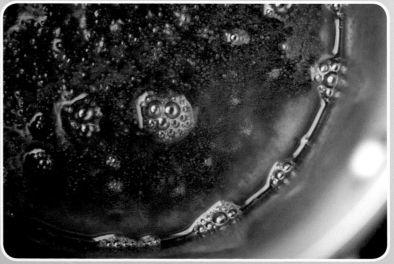

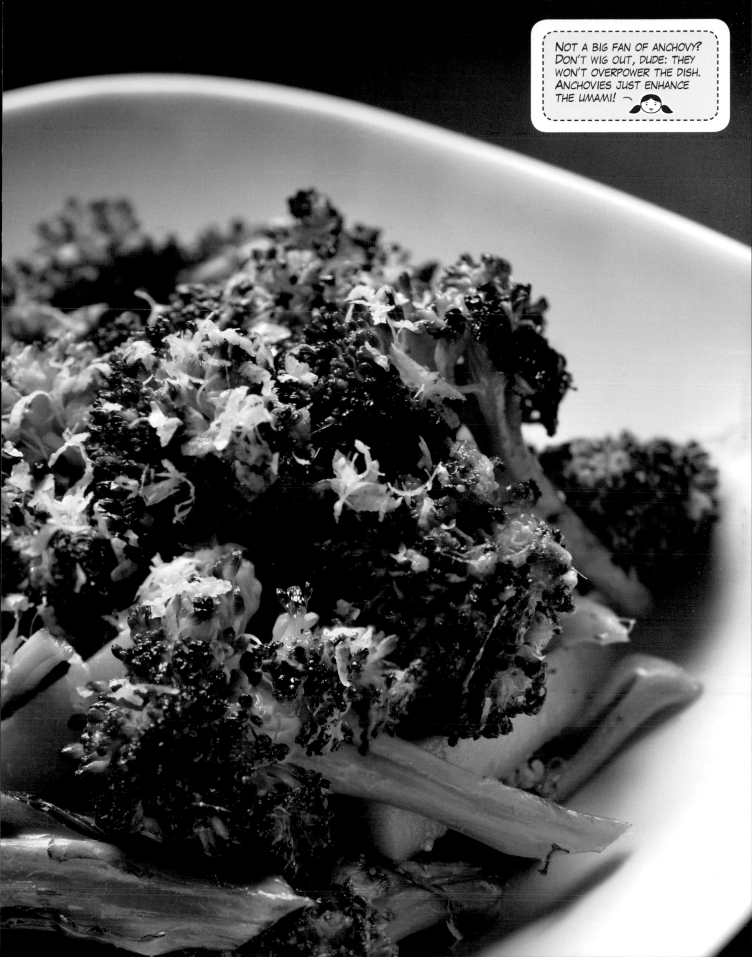

NOT A BIG FAN OF ANCHOVY?
DON'T WIG OUT, DUDE: THEY
WON'T OVERPOWER THE DISH.
ANCHOVIES JUST ENHANCE
THE UMAMI!

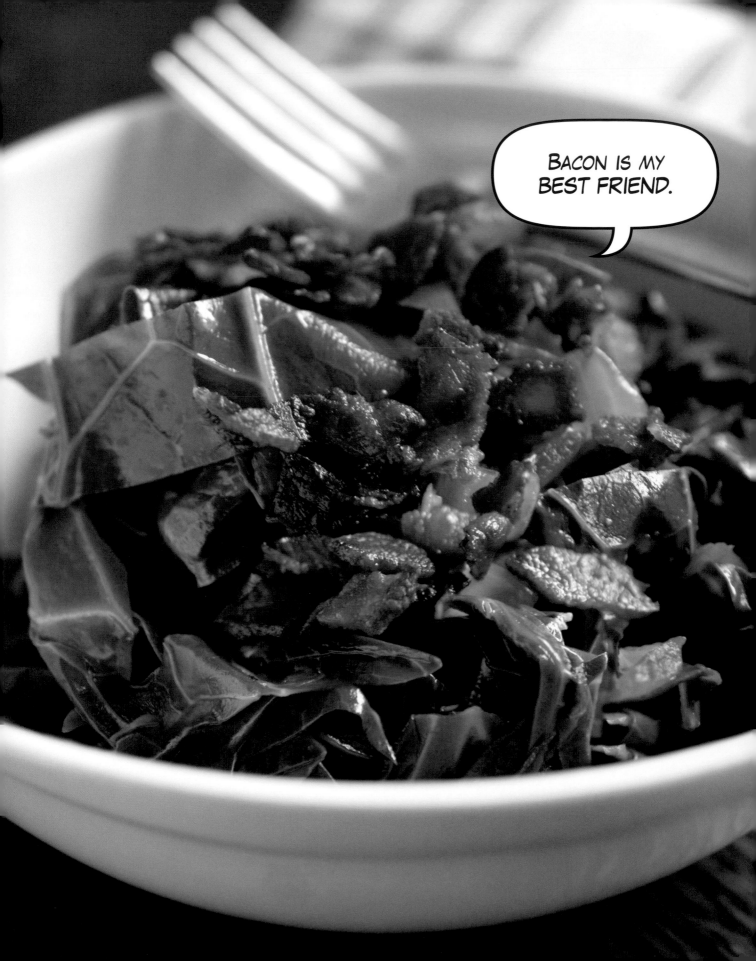

PRESSURE-COOKED
SPICY COLLARDS + BACON

If you hail from south of the Mason-Dixon line (like Henry's family, which put down roots in Louisiana long ago), you're no doubt accustomed to slow-cooked collard greens. For generations, Southern grandmothers have insisted that collards become silky only after hours of cooking—but sometimes, when the lid comes off the pot, the overcooked greens have taken on the color and texture of bayou mud.

There are ways around this problem. The food nerds over at *Cook's Illustrated* suggest shallow-blanching collards before sautéing them to achieve the proper tenderness—but who has the time or energy to cook their greens twice? Instead, I use a pressure cooker to achieve slow-food results in fast-food time.

The crispy bacon isn't optional, by the way. The porky bits add a crunchy, salty contrast to these spicy collard greens. Besides, once you add bacon, I'm sure you'll be hailed as a true Southern hero.

Makes 4 servings
Hands-on time: 20 minutes
Total time: 30 minutes

GOT LEFTOVERS? REPURPOSE YOUR COLLARDS AS THE SPICY FILLING IN A VEGGIE-PACKED FRITTATA!

- 3 slices **bacon**, cross-cut into ¼-inch pieces
- 1 small **yellow onion**, cut into ½-inch dice
  Kosher salt
- 2 bunches **collard greens**, stems removed and leaves roughly chopped into ribbons
- ½ cup **Bone Broth** (page 104) or chicken stock
- 2 tablespoons **apple juice**
- 1 tablespoon **apple cider vinegar**
- ¼ teaspoon **red pepper flakes**
  Freshly ground **black pepper**

DO THIS:

1. Toss the bacon in a 6-quart (or larger) pressure cooker, and crank up the heat to medium to slowly render the grease. Remove the crispy bacon bits with a slotted spoon and set aside.

2. Toss the onions and a sprinkle of salt in the bacon drippings, and sauté until translucent, about 5 minutes. Add the greens, broth, juice, vinegar, and pepper flakes, and stir to incorporate. Securely fasten the lid of the pressure cooker, and increase the heat to high.

3. Once the pot reaches high pressure, decrease the heat to low to maintain high pressure for 8 minutes. Release the pressure naturally, and remove the lid.

4. Season with salt and pepper to taste. Plate the collards and top with the crispy bacon bits.

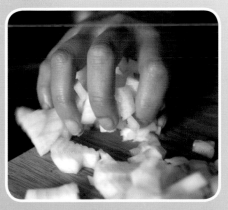
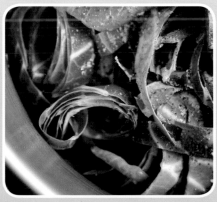
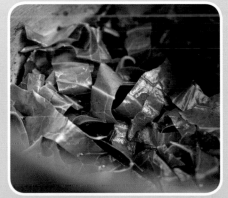

 IF YOU'RE LUCKY, YOU'LL HAVE SOME POT LICKER LEFT IN THE PRESSURE COOKER. "POT LICKER" (OR "POT LIQUOR") REFERS TO THE RICH JUICES REMAINING AT THE BOTTOM OF A POT AFTER REMOVING THE COOKED FOOD. POUR THE SPICY, FRAGRANT BROTH INTO A BOWL AND SLURP AWAY!

SWEET POTATO HASH

If you've got a food processor, this sweet and savory plate o' carbs can be in your craw in 10 minutes. With a few simple mods, you can transform this side dish into a fast, complete meal: top it with a couple of fried eggs for breakfast, or mix in some cooked meat for a satisfying supper. This hash is incredibly versatile, so feel free to adjust the seasonings and ingredients to your heart's desire.

Makes 2 servings
Hands-on time: 15 minutes
Total time: 15 minutes

1   large **garnet yam**, peeled
     Kosher salt
     Freshly ground **black pepper**
½   teaspoon **garlic powder**
½   teaspoon **onion powder**
½   teaspoon dried **rosemary**, **thyme**, or **chives**
2   tablespoons **ghee** or fat of choice
     Aleppo pepper (optional)

DO THIS:

1. Cut the yam lengthwise so the pieces fit in the feeding tube of a food processor, and shred using the machine's julienne slicer blade. Don't have a food processor? Manually shred it with the large holes of a box grater. Transfer the shredded yams to a large bowl and season with salt, black pepper, garlic powder, onion powder, and herbs.

2. Heat the ghee in a large cast-iron skillet over medium heat. When the oil is shimmering, add the seasoned yam and stir-fry for a minute. Cover with a lid and continue cooking for 3 to 5 more minutes or until the hash is soft and tender and some crispy brown bits appear. If desired, add a dash of Aleppo pepper before serving.

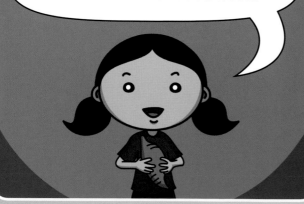

KNOW WHAT? MOST "YAMS" SOLD IN THE U.S. AREN'T TRUE YAMS AT ALL. THEY'RE SWEET POTATOES!

ORANGE-FLESHED SWEET POTATOES ARE JUST CALLED YAMS TO DISTINGUISH 'EM FROM THEIR YELLOW-FLESHED COUSINS.

SO WHEN I SAY "YAMS," I'M ACTUALLY TALKING ABOUT SWEET POTATOES!

FEEDING A LUMBERJACK? THROW A COUPLE OF JUICY BIG-O BACON BURGERS (PAGE 226) ON TOP FOR GOOD MEASURE!

EGG IT UP!

When in doubt, add an egg. Split the hash into two servings and top each pile with a couple of sunny-side-up eggs. The addition of eggs makes this a full and well-balanced meal with plenty of fat and protein to accompany the healthy carbohydrates.

Try this: Melt a tablespoon of ghee in an 8-inch cast-iron skillet over medium-low heat. When it foams, crack 2 large eggs into a bowl and pour 'em gently into the hot pan. Season the eggs with salt and pepper, and cover with a lid for 2 to 3 minutes, depending on how runny you like your yolks.

Once they're done, carefully slide them out of the skillet and on top of a mound of hash. Repeat with the remaining eggs. Sprinkle more Aleppo pepper on top, and dig in.

OR:

Try this bacon-y variation: When you're stir-frying the hash, add ½ cup of Caramelized Onions (page 38), and before serving, top with ¼ cup of Crispy Lardons (page 49).

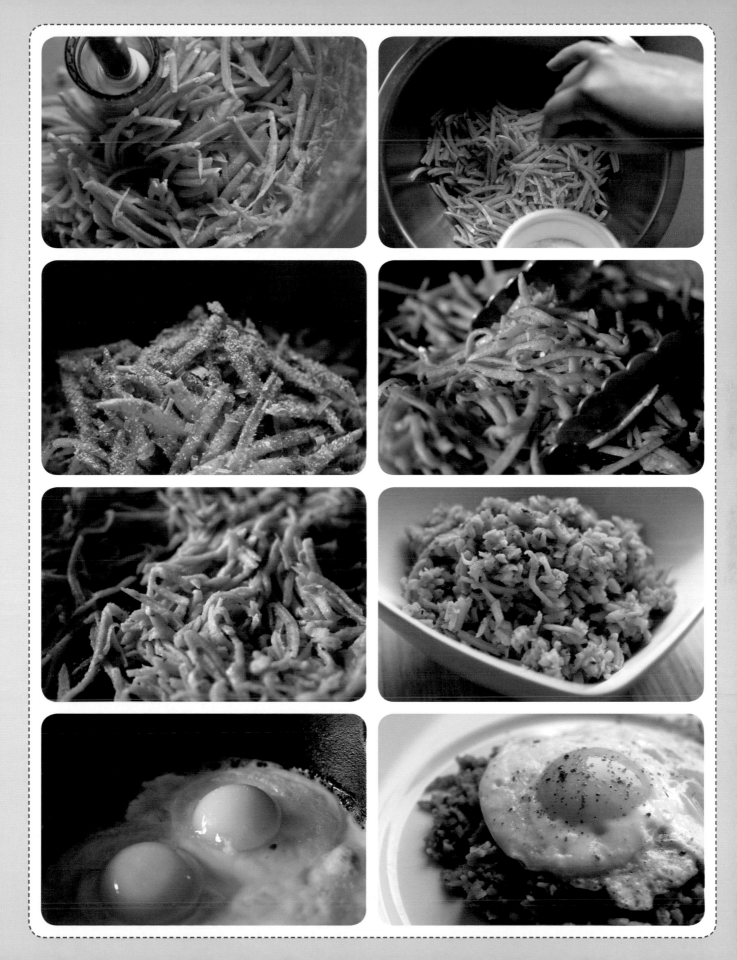

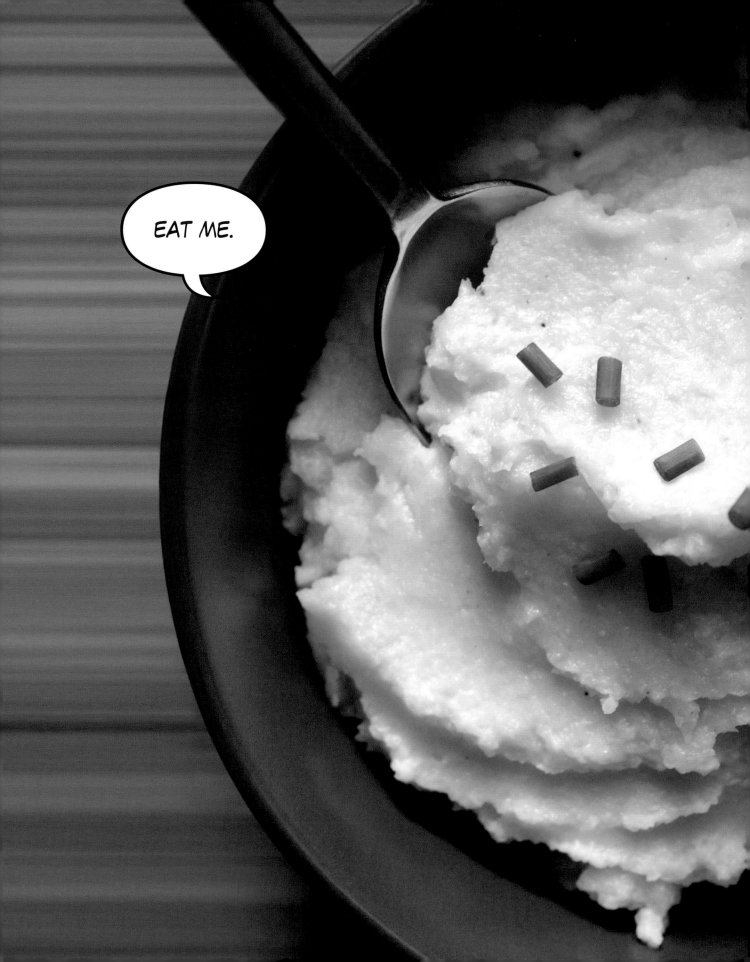

GARLIC MASHED CAULIFLOWER

It's almost obscene how easy it is to whip up a batch of garlicky, creamy mashed cauliflower—or as I like to call it, mashed *faux*-tatoes. (Rim shot! Somewhere, my pun-loving husband is cracking up.) But unlike potatoes, cauliflower cooks up in a flash, and it's nowhere near as finicky—or starchy. Trust me, folks: once you try this recipe, you'll find yourself coming back to it again and again.

Makes 8 servings
Hands-on time: 10 minutes
Total time: 20 minutes

1 large **cauliflower** head, cut into uniform pieces
Kosher salt
5 **garlic cloves**
2 tablespoons **ghee** or fat of choice
Freshly ground **black pepper**
¼ teaspoon freshly grated **nutmeg** (optional)

DO THIS:

1. Fill a large stock pot with an inch or two of water and fit a steamer insert in the pot. Cover the pot and place it on a burner set on high.

2. Season the cauliflower pieces liberally with salt. When the water comes to a boil, place the cauliflower and garlic onto the steamer insert. Put a lid on it, and steam for about 10 minutes or until the cauliflower is easily pierced with a knife. Don't worry: you won't overcook it. Just make sure there's enough water in the bottom of the pot, and you'll be fine.

3. Drain the cauliflower and garlic in a colander, and then toss them into a food processor outfitted with a regular chopping blade. Add the ghee, pepper to taste, and nutmeg, if desired. Pulse everything until smooth—but don't overdo it, champ. We're not making soup.

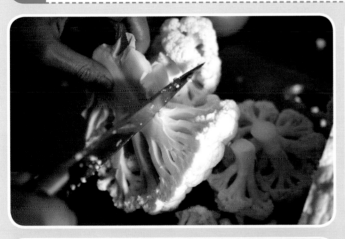
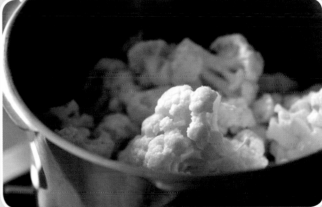
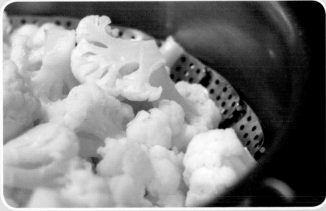
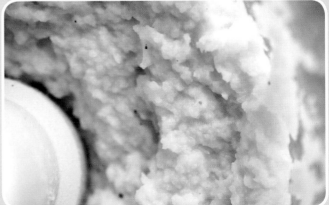

EASY CAULIFLOWER "RICE"

When I first went Paleo, I bid good-bye to my rice cooker. (All three of them, actually. What can I say? I have a nasty habit of hoarding kitchen appliances.) It was a symbolic thing—an official farewell to my grain-gobbling ways. But in my heart of hearts, I knew I was still the Asian girl who grew up shoveling down bowl after bowl of white rice at my parents' kitchen table. If it's true that "you are what you eat," then I'm made of 55 percent rice. So to make a grain-free existence sustainable for me, I was desperate for a rice substitute. Luckily, it wasn't long before I came up with a foolproof recipe that's even tastier than the real thing.

Makes 6 cups
Hands-on time: 20 minutes
Total time: 20 minutes

1   medium **cauliflower** head, cut into uniform pieces
2   tablespoons **ghee** or fat of choice
1   small **yellow onion**, minced
    Kosher salt
    Freshly ground **black pepper**

DO THIS:

1. Toss the cauliflower into a food processor, and pulse until it's the size of rice grains.

2. In a large skillet, melt the ghee over medium heat, and sauté the onion along with a pinch of salt for 5 minutes or until translucent.

3. Add the cauliflower and stir to evenly distribute the onions. Season with salt and pepper to taste. Cover and cook for 5 to 10 minutes longer or until tender.

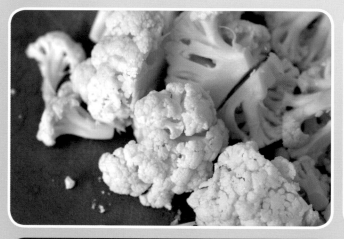

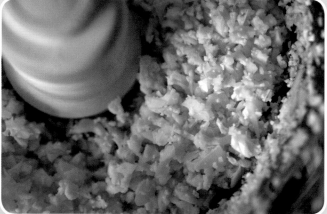

CHANGE IT UP:

Ready to flex your creative muscles? This versatile side is a blank slate that can be mixed and matched with any number of ingredients to form new combinations. Need examples?

Stir ½ cup of Salsa Roja Asada (page 54) into the "rice" in Step 2 before covering to cook, and you'll have Spanish rice in no time. In the mood for something more tropical? Then check out the next page. Just turn your head a little to the right.

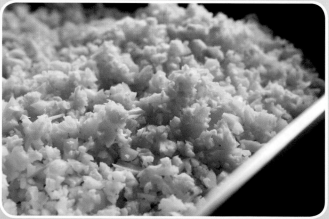

COCONUT PINEAPPLE "RICE"

Is plain old cauliflower "rice" too boring for you? Then hold on to your grass skirts and tiki torches, 'cause this recipe's *da kine*, brah! It's going to send a bombin' flavor wave crashing over your head!

Okay, that was kind of over-the-top. But paired with a savory main, this "rice" really will hit the spot.

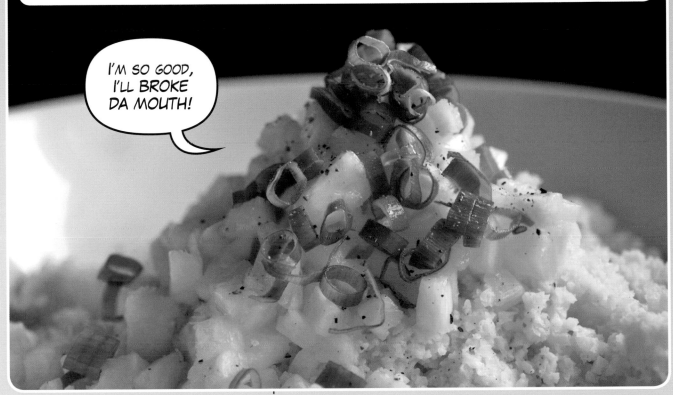

I'M SO GOOD, I'LL BROKE DA MOUTH!

Makes 6 servings
Hands-on time: 30 minutes
Total time: 30 minutes

THIS TROPICAL "RICE" IS TASTY ON ITS OWN, BUT IT'S EVEN BETTER WHEN PAIRED WITH SLOW COOKER KALUA PIG (PAGE 234).

1   medium **cauliflower** head, cut into uniform pieces
2   tablespoons **coconut oil** or fat of choice
1   small **yellow onion**, finely minced
    Kosher salt
½   cup full-fat **coconut milk**
1   cup fresh **pineapple**, cut into ¼-inch dice
1   **scallion**, thinly sliced
    Freshly ground **black pepper**

DO THIS:

1. Toss the cauliflower into a food processor, and pulse until it's the size of rice grains.

2. In a large skillet, melt the coconut oil over medium heat, and sauté the onion with a sprinkle of salt for 5 minutes or until translucent. Add the cauliflower and coconut milk to the skillet, and stir to evenly distribute the ingredients. Season with salt to taste. Cover and cook for 5 to 10 more minutes or until the "rice" has absorbed the coconut milk and the texture is tender and fluffy.

3. Transfer the "rice" to a large bowl. Add the pineapple and scallion, and gently mix to incorporate. Taste and adjust the seasoning with salt and pepper.

 THIS TROPICAL "RICE" IS THE PERFECT ACCOMPANIMENT FOR GRILLED MEATS AND THAI CURRIES.

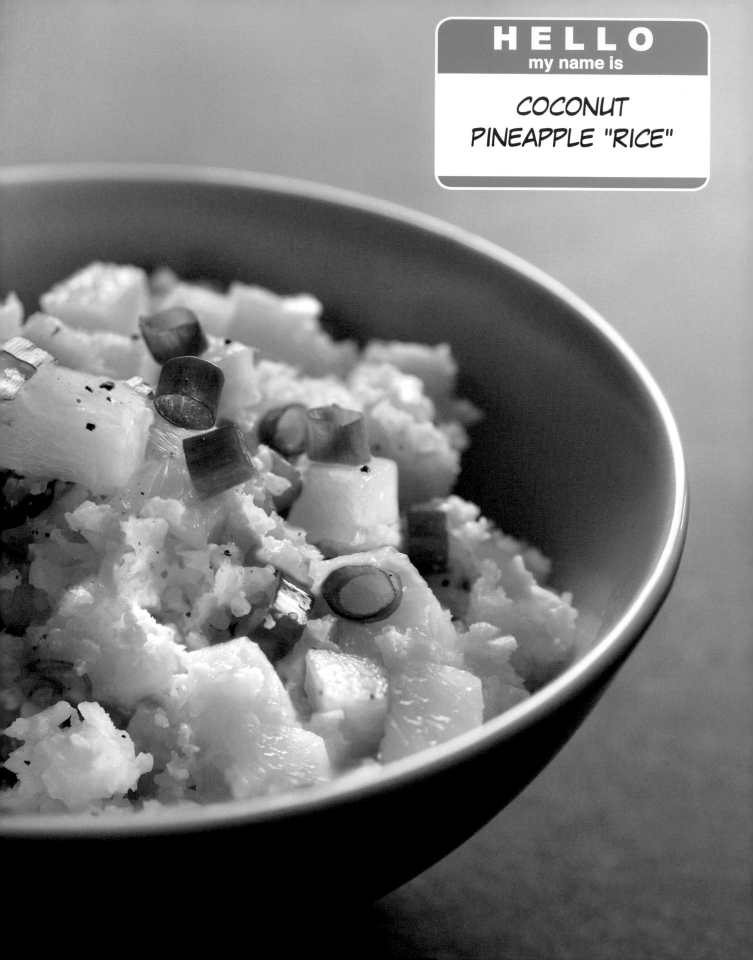

HELLO
my name is

COCONUT
PINEAPPLE "RICE"

HELLO
my name is

ASIAN CAULIFLOWER FRIED "RICE"

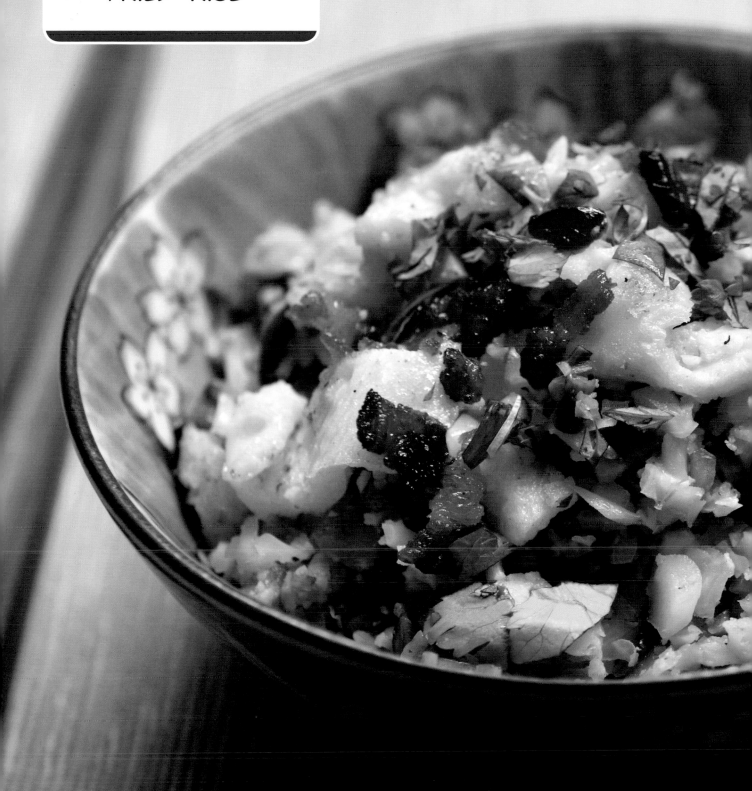

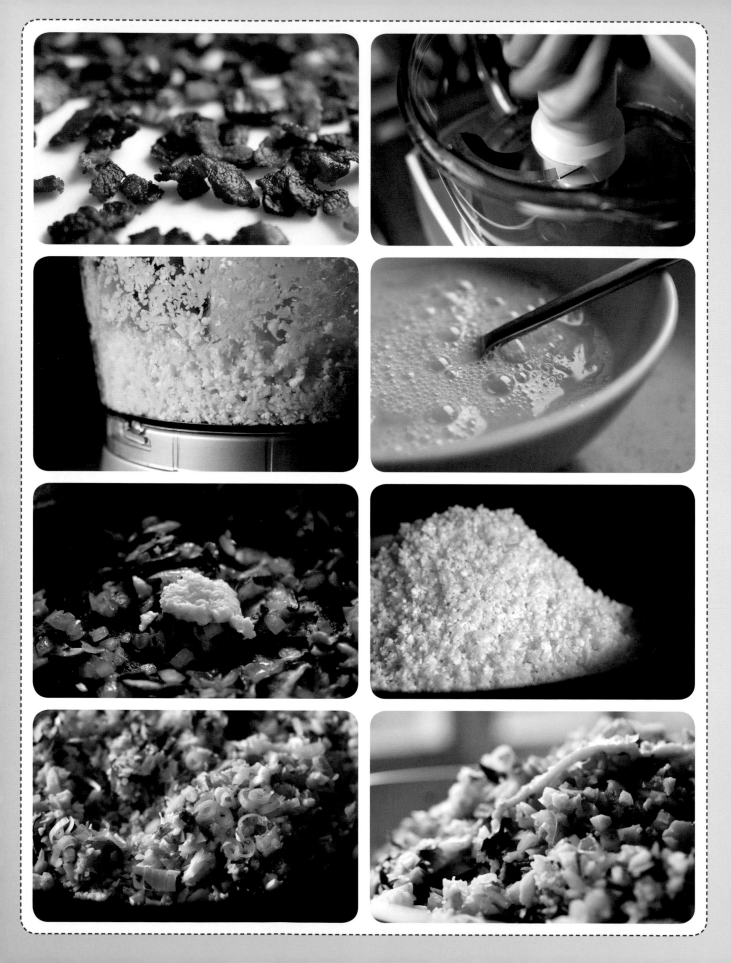

ASIAN CAULIFLOWER FRIED "RICE"

In Chinese homes, rice is almost always eaten in its steamed form. Shoveled from bowl to mouth, fluffy white rice is a staple food for billions—a fragrant, starchy companion to wok-charred dishes of meat and vegetables. But with the vast quantities of rice that's steamed in every Chinese kitchen, there's bound to be leftovers—and the need to repurpose them in new and appetizing ways.

Enter *fried rice*. With a red-hot pan, a resourceful cook can easily whip up a well-seasoned platter of fluffy fried rice tossed with spring onions and springy ribbons of sunny yellow egg.

Thankfully, grain-free eaters can indulge in a bowl (or three) of fried rice, too. I daresay my Asian Cauliflower Fried "Rice" easily trumps the greasy, soy-drenched stuff peddled by your local Chinese restaurant. Sure, this recipe takes a bit of time and effort to prepare, but once you taste it, you'll be hooked for life on this deeply satisfying one-wok meal.

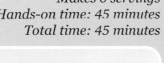

Makes 6 servings
Hands-on time: 45 minutes
Total time: 45 minutes

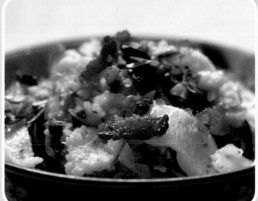

3	slices **bacon**, cross-cut into ¼-inch pieces
1	medium **cauliflower** head, cut into uniform pieces
2	large **eggs**
	Kosher salt
	Freshly ground **black pepper**
2	tablespoons **ghee** or fat of choice
1	small **yellow onion**, minced
4	ounces **cremini mushrooms**, thinly sliced
1	(1-inch) piece fresh **ginger**, peeled and finely grated (about 1 tablespoon)
2	tablespoons **coconut aminos**
1	teaspoon **coconut vinegar**
1	teaspoon Paleo-friendly **fish sauce**
2	**scallions**, thinly sliced
2	tablespoons chopped fresh **cilantro**

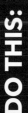

DO THIS:

1. Cook the bacon in a large skillet over medium heat, stirring occasionally. Once it crisps up, about 15 minutes, transfer the crunchy bacon to a paper towel–lined plate with a slotted spoon.

2. While you're crisping the bacon, toss the cauliflower into a food processor, and pulse until it's the size of rice grains. Pro tip: don't overdo it. We don't want liquid cauliflower.

3. In a small bowl, whisk the eggs together with salt and pepper to taste. Pour the eggs into the hot bacon drippings, and fry up a thin egg omelet. Remove the omelet from the pan, slice it into ribbons, and set aside.

4. Melt the ghee in the skillet over medium-high heat, and add the onions along with a sprinkle of salt and pepper. Once the onions are soft and translucent, about 5 minutes, throw in the sliced mushrooms. When the mushrooms are browned, add the grated ginger and stir for 30 seconds to incorporate.

5. Add the cauliflower "rice," season with a bit more salt and pepper, and mix the ingredients together. Place a lid on the skillet, turn the heat down to low, and cook for about 5 minutes with the skillet covered. The "rice" is ready when it's tender but not mushy.

6. Season with the coconut aminos, coconut vinegar, and fish sauce. Before serving, mix in the scallions, cilantro, omelet slices, and the reserved crispy bacon.

WANT MORE PROTEIN? TOP THE "RICE" WITH *SLOW COOKER KALUA PIG* (PAGE 234) OR LEFTOVER STEAK!

A DAY IN THE LIFE

(OF A DRUG-DEALING, NIGHTSHIFT-WORKING, FOOD-BLOGGING MOM)

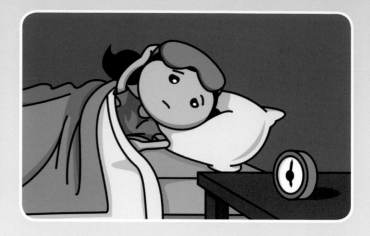

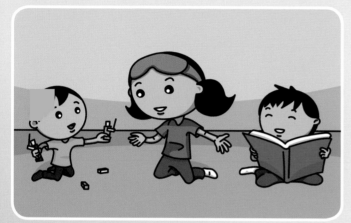

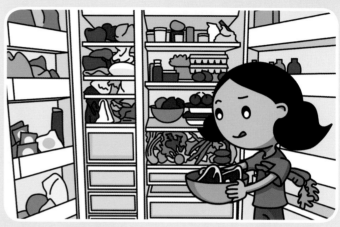

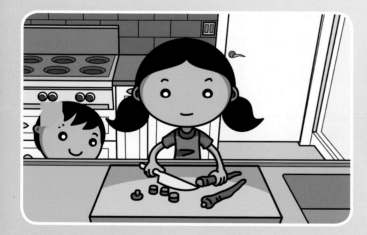

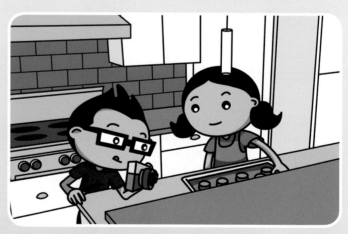

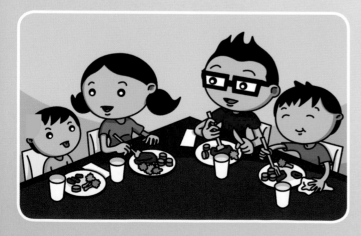

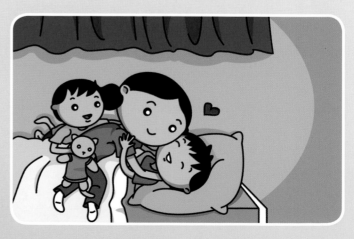

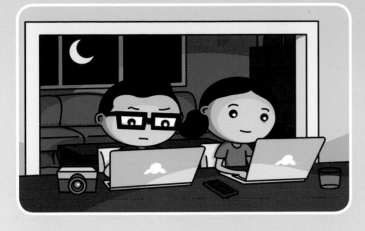
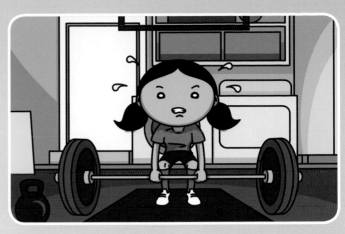
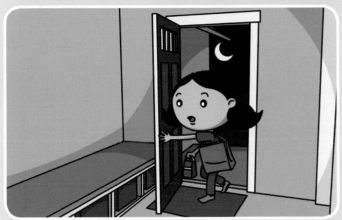
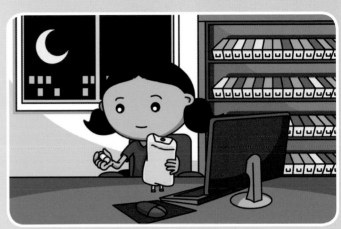
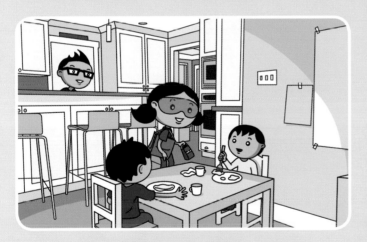
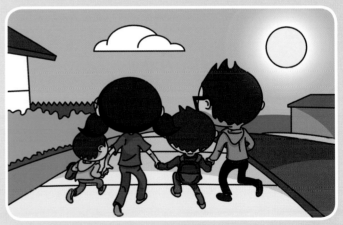
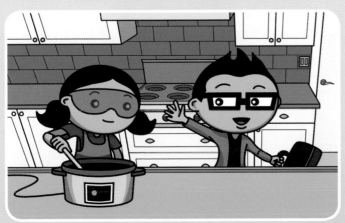
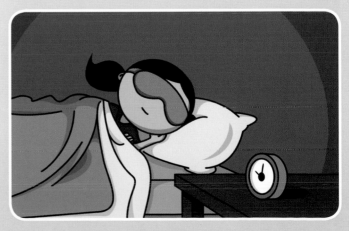

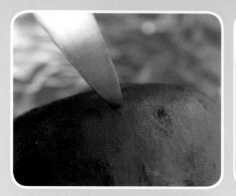
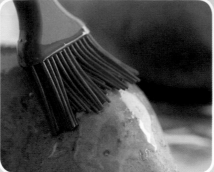
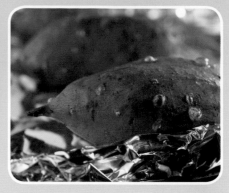
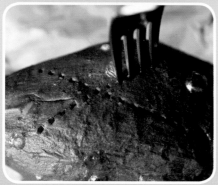
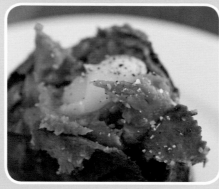
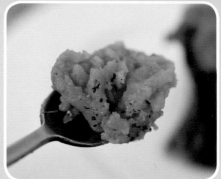

OVEN-BAKED SWEET POTATOES

Plenty of folks eagerly gobble up baked potatoes with butter, so why don't more of us prepare baked sweet potatoes with ghee? Oven-baked sweet potatoes become an impossible-to-resist treat once you dollop on a spoonful of ghee. Bake some up on a cold night, and they'll warm you from the inside out.

Makes 4 servings
Hands-on time: 10 minutes
Total time: 1 hour

4 medium **sweet potatoes**
5 tablespoons **ghee**, divided
Kosher salt
Freshly ground **black pepper**

DO THIS:

1. Preheat the oven to 400°F with the rack in the middle position, and wash, scrub, and dry the sweet potatoes. Prick the sweet potatoes all over with a fork or paring knife, and place them on a foil-lined rimmed baking sheet. Be sure to keep some distance between them.

2. Melt 1 tablespoon of the ghee and brush it onto the sweet potatoes. Bake the sweet potatoes for 45 to 50 minutes, or until they're fragrant and soft to the touch. Remove the tray from the oven, and while the sweet potatoes are still hot, puncture the top of each spud with a fork to form an X. Push the ends of each sweet potato together, and the bright orange flesh will burst out of the seams.

3. Spoon 1 tablespoon of the ghee onto each sweet potato, and season with salt and pepper to taste. Once the ghee melts into the tender sweet potato, it's time to dig in.

CHANGE IT UP:

DON'T BE SHY: ADD MORE TOPPINGS!

SAUSAGE AND PEPPERS ARE A CLASSIC COMBINATION, OR TRY SOME CHOPPED PROSCIUTTO AND COOKED KALE.

BUT HERE'S ONE OF MY FAVORITE MODS: PREHEAT THE OVEN TO 300°F, AND SPREAD ½ CUP OF UNSWEETENED COCONUT FLAKES IN A SINGLE LAYER ON A PARCHMENT-LINED RIMMED BAKING SHEET. TOAST FOR 3 TO 5 MINUTES UNTIL GOLDEN BROWN.

TOP EACH SWEET POTATO WITH TOASTED COCONUT FLAKES, ½ TABLESPOON OF CHOPPED TOASTED ALMONDS, AND A DASH OF GROUND CINNAMON.

PLÁTANOS MADUROS

Hankering for a hunk o' starch? Sweet potatoes aren't the only game in town, you know. Plantains—a staple of Latin American and West African cuisine—can be a fantastic addition to a Paleo eater's menu. I, for one, love *plátanos maduros*—fried plantains. With a pinch of coarse salt and some cinnamon, these sweet and savory plantains make a wonderful side dish. Try them with Peruvian Roast Chicken (page 201)!

Makes 4 servings
Hands-on time: 15 minutes
Total time: 15 minutes

½ cup **ghee** or fat of choice
4 ripe **plantains**, peeled and cut crosswise into ½-inch slices
½ cup **coconut flour**
Fleur de sel or other coarse salt
Ground **cinnamon**

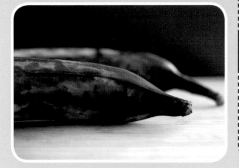

DO THIS:

Heat the ghee in a large skillet over medium-high heat. When it's shimmering, lightly coat the plantain slices in the coconut flour and fry for 2 minutes per side or until golden brown. Transfer to a wire rack and dust on some fleur de sel and cinnamon. Eat 'em hot!

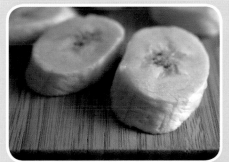

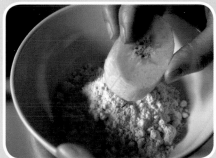

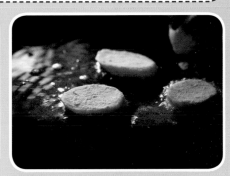

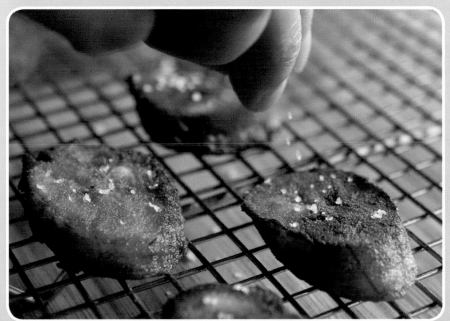

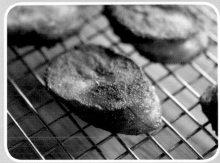

YOU DECIDE!

I prefer ripe, splotchy plantains for their mild sweetness and tender flesh, but feel free to go with green plantains if you like 'em firmer and starchier.

 PSST! FOR A SWEET AND SAVORY TREAT, TRY COATING 'EM WITH MELTED DARK CHOCOLATE.

KABALAGALA (PLANTAIN FRITTERS)

I first learned of this traditional Ugandan fritter from one of our best friends, Sidney. Longtime blog readers will know that we're virtually twins, with identical dispositions and tastes. I'm sure we'd be mistaken for one another more often, except for the fact that Sidney's a foot taller than me. And male. And Ugandan.

Kabalagala is made of just two ingredients: black, super-ripe plantains and cassava flour—also known as tapioca flour. The recipe looks simple enough, but to get it right, you have to put in some practice. Mix the ingredients by hand, and get a feel for the dough. Too little flour will result in a sticky mess; overwork it, and you'll end up with a tray of dense, gummy pucks. But you'll know you got it right when you have puffy fritters that are crunchy on the outside and toothsome in the middle.

I love the chewiness and mild sweetness of these fried, starchy snacks. Just don't expect your *kabalagala* to be airy and spongy like pancakes or beignets. As Sidney explained, "Africans don't do fluffy."

Makes about 24 fritters
Hands-on time: 30 minutes
Total time: 30 minutes

1   large, very ripe black **plantain** (about ¾ pound)
2   cups **tapioca flour** (amount will vary depending on the ripeness of the plantain; you'll need a bit more flour if your plantain is on the riper, moister side)
1   cup **ghee** or fat of choice

DO THIS:

1. Peel the plantain and thoroughly mash it with a fork in a large bowl until smooth.

2. Add 1 cup of the tapioca flour and incorporate into the plantain mash. Slowly add more tapioca flour, but just until the point at which the batter forms a pliable ball of dough that no longer sticks to your hands.

3. Spread some tapioca flour on a smooth, clean surface, and roll out the dough to a thickness of about ¼ inch. Use a round 2-inch cookie cutter or the rim of a cup to form about 20 fritters. Gather the rest of the dough around the cut circles to roll out a few extra fritters.

4. Heat the ghee in a large skillet over medium-high heat until hot and shimmering. Fry the *kabalagala* for 1 to 2 minutes per side or until golden and puffy.

5. Transfer to a wire rack until cool enough to pop into your mouth. Serve immediately.

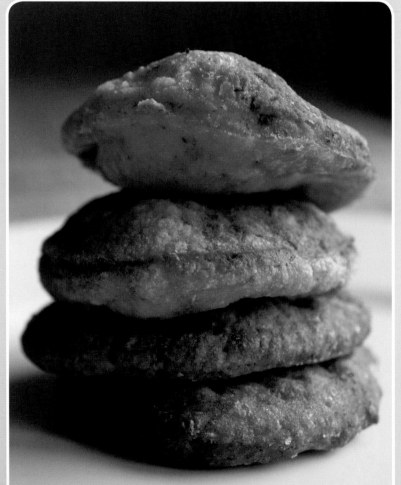

AS A RESULT OF THE STREET VENDORS WHO CALL OUT THE NAME OF THESE FRITTERS TO PASSING MOTORISTS, A POPULAR NEIGHBORHOOD IN KAMPALA, UGANDA'S CAPITAL, IS NOW KNOWN AS KABALAGALA.

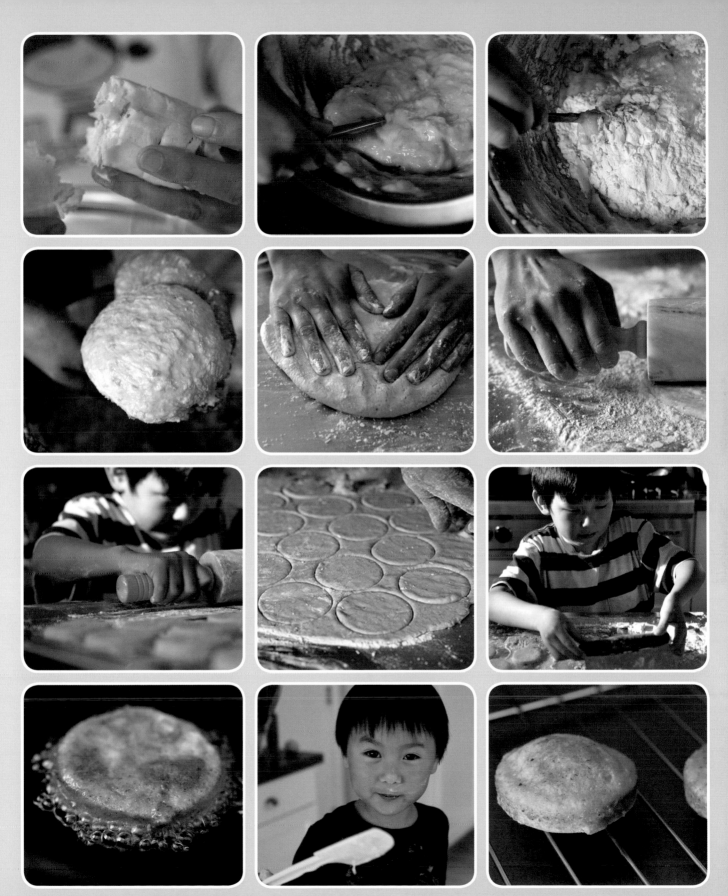

 LITTLE HELPERS MAKE THE PROCESS FUN AND FAST.
AND WHO CARES IF THE KITCHEN GETS TRASHED?

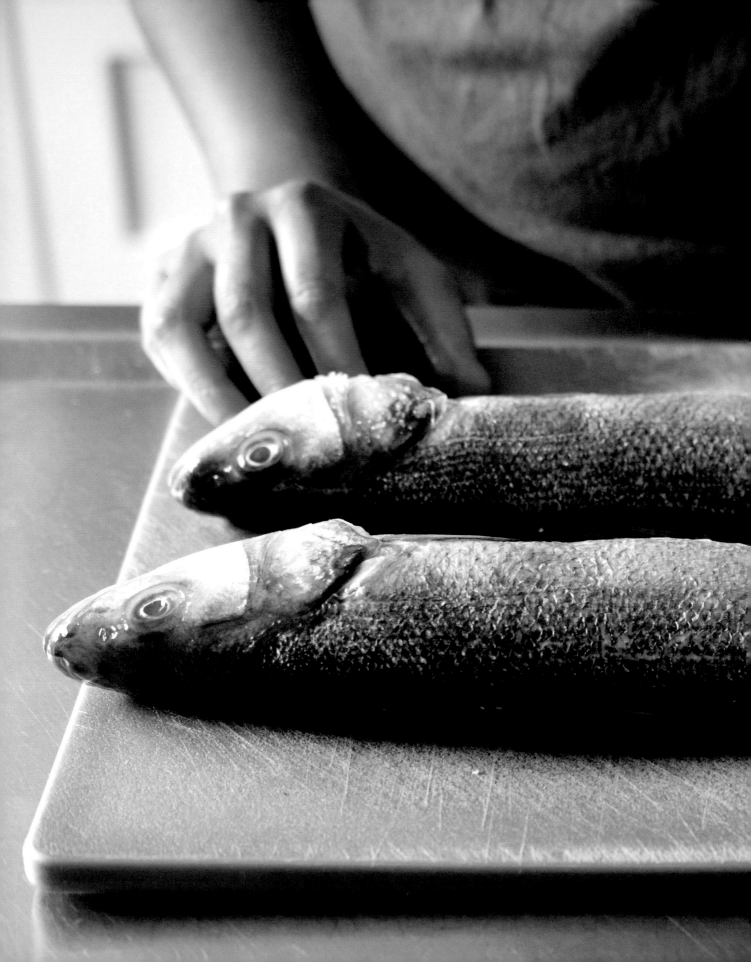

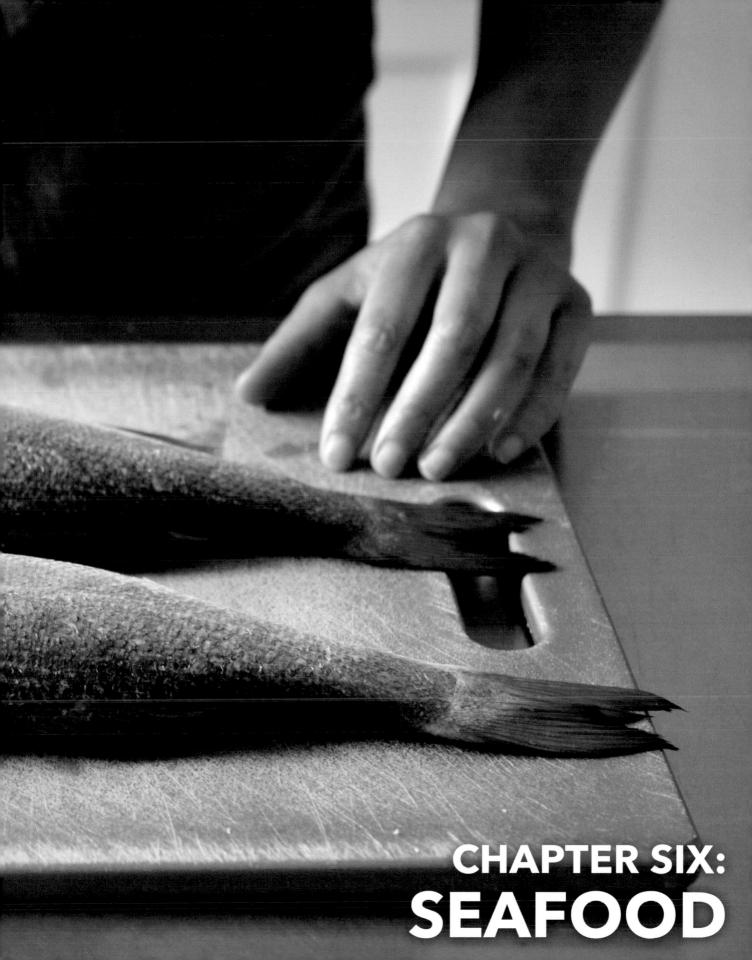

CHAPTER SIX:
SEAFOOD

MUSSELS IN CURRY BROTH

I'm no hunter, but I'm proud to say I've killed my own food. That's right: I've sent scores of bivalves to their quick, painless, and delicious deaths, and I honestly couldn't be happier with the results. Mussels are inexpensive, sustainable, and yummy. Pair 'em with a big, poufy green salad, and slurp away!

Makes 2 servings
Hands-on time: 15 minutes
Total time: 30 minutes

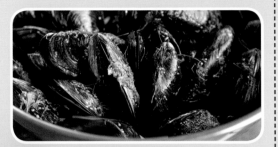

4 **garlic cloves**, minced
¼ cup minced **shallots**
1 cup **chicken broth**
1 small dried **bay leaf**
½ teaspoon **Indian curry powder**
2 pounds fresh, live **mussels**, cleaned
2 tablespoons **ghee** or fat of choice
1 tablespoon chopped fresh **cilantro**
1 tablespoon chopped fresh **mint**
1 tablespoon chopped fresh **basil**
 Kosher salt (optional)

DO THIS:

1. In a stockpot or Dutch oven, combine the garlic, shallots, broth, bay leaf, and curry powder. Bring the liquid to a boil, and then turn down the heat to low and simmer the broth for about 3 minutes.

2. Increase the heat to high, and add the mussels. Give them a good stir before covering the pot. Steam the mussels for 4 to 5 minutes, stirring once at the halfway mark. The mussels are ready when their shells open.

3. Use a slotted spoon to transfer the steamed mussels to a large serving bowl. Toss out the ones that remain closed—those are the ones that died before the cooking process began, and believe me: you *really* don't want to eat them. Cover the mussels with foil.

4. To finish off the sauce, whisk the ghee and herbs into the broth. Taste for seasoning, and add salt only if necessary. Pour the broth over the mussels and serve.

CHEW ON THIS:

- This goes without saying, but always start with super-fresh mussels. Keep them on ice in the fridge, covered with a wet paper towel, until you're ready to cook.

- Fresh mussels are alive, so don't wrap 'em in plastic or they'll die prematurely. Remember: dead mussels = bad mussels.

- To prep mussels for cooking, rinse them off in water, and then yank off their beards—the hairy tendrils that dangle from their insides.

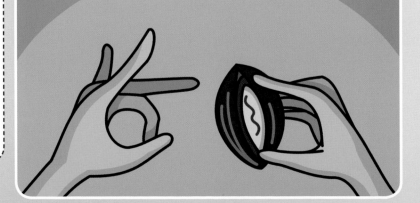

YOU CAN CHECK TO SEE IF A MUSSEL'S ALIVE BY FLICKING YOUR FINGER AGAINST ITS SHELL. IF IT CLOSES, YOU'LL KNOW IT AIN'T DEAD. (YET!)

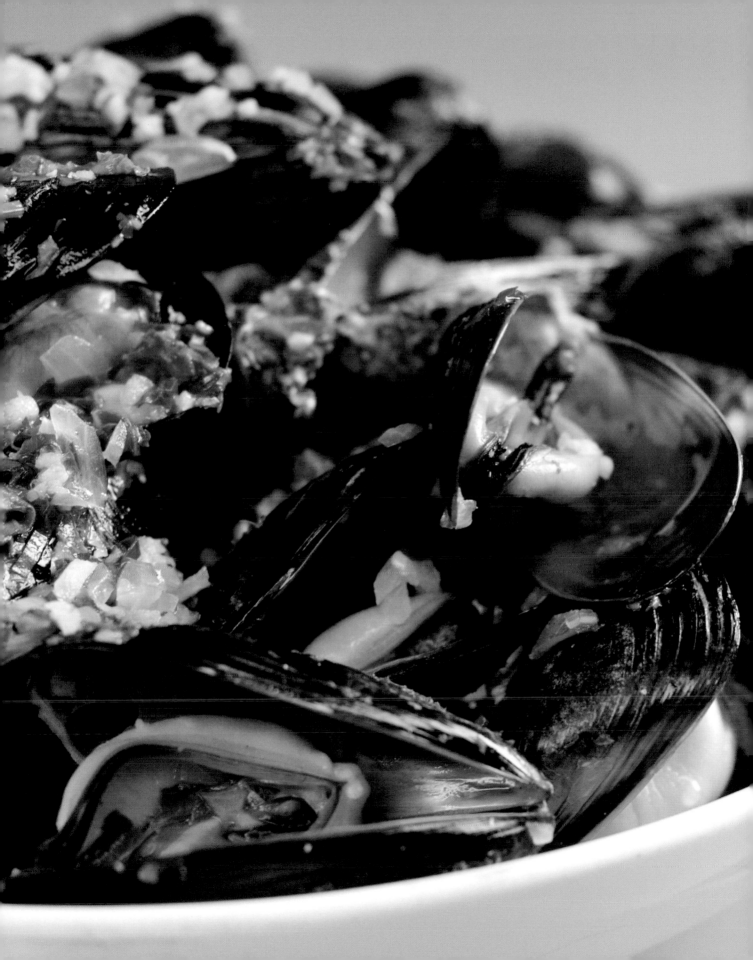

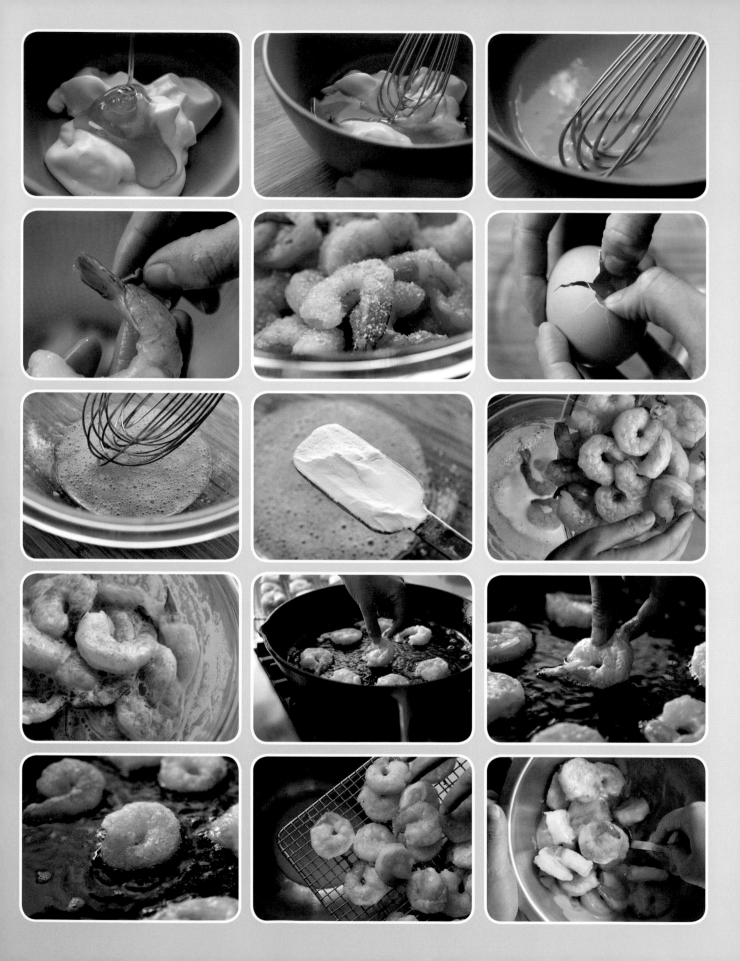

WALNUT PRAWNS

I've always loved walnut prawns. When my parents would take us out for celebratory feasts (in Chinese restaurants, naturally), I could never resist the siren call of crunchy shrimp and candied nuts—all slathered in a creamy, tangy-sweet sauce. When I went Paleo, I resigned myself to a bleak gastronomic future bereft of my favorite childhood dish…until I invented this utterly authentic-tasting real-food version.

Makes 4 servings
Hands-on time: 20 minutes
Total time: 20 minutes

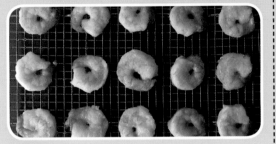

- **3** tablespoons **Paleo Mayonnaise** (page 40)
- **1** tablespoon **honey**
- **1** teaspoon fresh **lemon juice**
- **1** pound (approximately 20 to 25) uncooked large fresh **shrimp**, peeled and deveined
- **¾** teaspoon **kosher salt**
- **1** **egg white**
- **2** tablespoons **tapioca starch**
- **1** cup **ghee** or fat of choice, for frying
- **½** cup **Maple-Spiced Walnuts** (page 67)
- **1** tablespoon **sesame seeds**, toasted

DO THIS:

1. First, make the sauce. In a small bowl, combine the Paleo Mayonnaise, honey, and lemon juice, and whisk to combine into a sweet, creamy dressing. Set it aside.

2. Toss the shrimp in a separate bowl with the salt.

3. In a large bowl, whisk the egg white until frothy, and add the tapioca starch. Mix to form a smooth batter. No clumps, please!

4. Add the shrimp to the batter and mix well, making sure they are completely coated.

5. Melt the ghee in a large cast-iron skillet over medium heat. Once the ghee is shimmering, fry the shrimp in three separate batches. Cook the shrimp for 1 to 2 minutes on each side, or until they're golden on the outside and no longer translucent on the inside. Transfer the cooked shrimp to a wire rack.

6. When all the batches are done, place the shrimp in a bowl with the honey-mayonnaise sauce, and toss gently to coat the prawns before plating. Sprinkle the Maple-Spiced Walnuts and toasted sesame seeds on the prawns, and serve immediately.

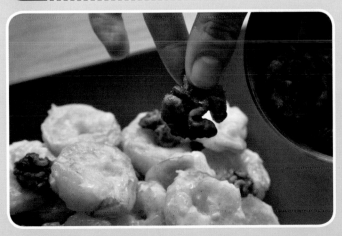
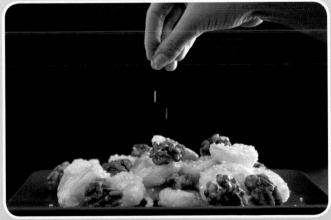

 ENJOY THIS DISH WITH A STEAMING BOWL OF EASY CAULIFLOWER "RICE" (PAGE 156)!

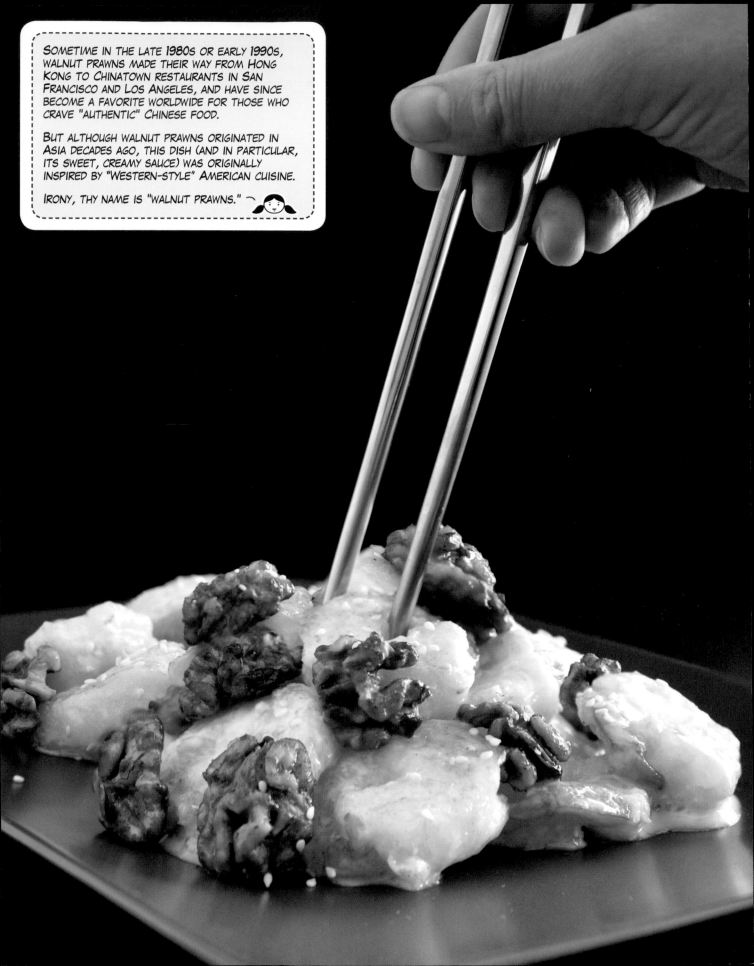

SOMETIME IN THE LATE 1980s OR EARLY 1990s, WALNUT PRAWNS MADE THEIR WAY FROM HONG KONG TO CHINATOWN RESTAURANTS IN SAN FRANCISCO AND LOS ANGELES, AND HAVE SINCE BECOME A FAVORITE WORLDWIDE FOR THOSE WHO CRAVE "AUTHENTIC" CHINESE FOOD.

BUT ALTHOUGH WALNUT PRAWNS ORIGINATED IN ASIA DECADES AGO, THIS DISH (AND IN PARTICULAR, ITS SWEET, CREAMY SAUCE) WAS ORIGINALLY INSPIRED BY "WESTERN-STYLE" AMERICAN CUISINE.

IRONY, THY NAME IS "WALNUT PRAWNS."

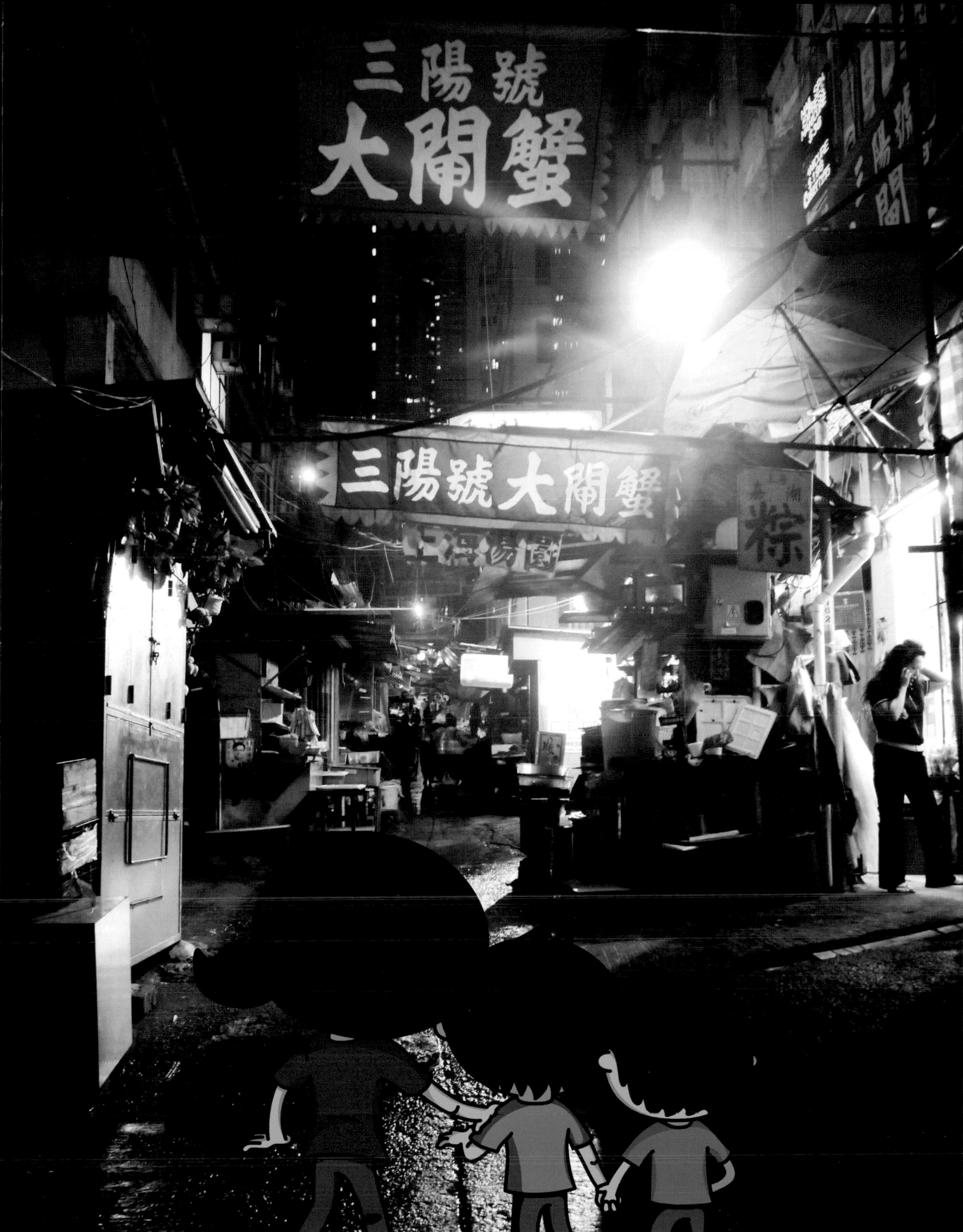
三陽號
大閘蟹
三陽號大閘蟹
粽

SPICY COCONUT SHRIMP

This dish originated in the tropical coasts of Southeast Asia, where both coconuts and crustaceans abound. Coconut shrimp has since spread the world over, but my recipe takes it back to its roots, marrying it with another regional specialty: spicy sriracha. This ain't your momma's coconut shrimp; sink your teeth into the crunchy, golden coconut crust, and you'll discover tender shrimp marinated in a fiery Asian chile sauce.

Makes 4 servings
Hands-on time: 30 minutes
Total time: 1½ hours

TO DEVEIN YOUR SHRIMP, MAKE A SHALLOW SLIT ALONG THE LENGTH OF THE SHRIMP'S BACK, AND PULL OUT THE DARK RIBBON RUNNING FROM HEAD TO TAIL. THE "VEIN" IS NOT ACTUALLY A VEIN, BY THE WAY -- IT'S THE DIGESTIVE TRACT. YOU DON'T HAVE TO REMOVE IT, BUT IT HAS A FLAVOR AND TEXTURE THAT NOT EVERYONE ENJOYS.

1   pound (approximately 20 to 25) uncooked large fresh **shrimp**, peeled and deveined but with tails left intact
¼   cup **Paleo Sriracha** (page 42) or hot sauce of choice
    Finely grated zest from ½ small **orange**
    Melted **ghee**, for greasing
3   **egg whites**, lightly beaten
½   cup **arrowroot powder**
¼   cup **coconut flour**
¼   cup **almond flour**
1   teaspoon **kosher salt**
½   teaspoon **paprika**
¼   teaspoon freshly ground **black pepper**
½   cup shredded unsweetened dried **coconut**

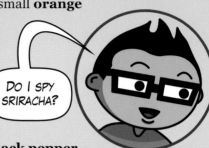

DO I SPY SRIRACHA?

DO THIS:

1. Throw the shrimp in a large bowl or 1-gallon freezer bag, and add the sriracha and orange zest. Mix well, and marinate the shrimp in the fridge for 30 minutes or up to 2 hours.

2. When you're ready to cook, take the marinated shrimp out of the refrigerator and preheat the oven to 400°F with the rack in the middle position. Lightly grease a wire rack with melted ghee, and place it atop a parchment- or foil-lined baking sheet.

3. Put the egg whites in a small bowl.

4. Take out three plates or shallow bowls. Pour the arrowroot powder into the first one. In the second shallow bowl, mix the coconut flour, almond flour, salt, paprika, and pepper. Pour the shredded coconut into the last bowl.

5. Holding each shrimp by the tail, dredge it in the arrowroot powder, shaking off any excess. The arrowroot powder will help keep the batter from falling off the slippery marinated shrimp. Dip the shrimp in the egg white, and then dredge it in the spicy flour mixture. Dip the shrimp in the egg white once more, and then coat it in the shredded coconut.

6. Place the shrimp on the greased wire rack. Bake for 15 to 20 minutes or until the shredded coconut is golden brown and the shrimp is bright pink, flipping the shrimp halfway through the cooking time. Keep an eye on the shrimp, and don't burn the coconut. Serve immediately.

FRY IT!

Prefer pan-fried shrimp? No problem!

Turn the burners on the stove to high, and heat ½ cup of ghee (or enough to reach a depth of ¼ inch) in a cast-iron skillet. Once the oil's hot and shimmering, turn the heat down to medium, and pan-fry the shrimp for 1 to 2 minutes per side, or until golden on the outside and just opaque in the center. Drain on a wire rack before serving.

I KNOW WHAT YOU'RE THINKING: WHAT AM I SUPPOSED TO DO WITH THE **3** LEFTOVER EGG YOLKS? ANSWER: USE THEM TO MAKE PALEO MAYONNAISE (PAGE 40) AND MEXICAN CHOCOLATE POTS DE CRÈME (PAGE 256)!

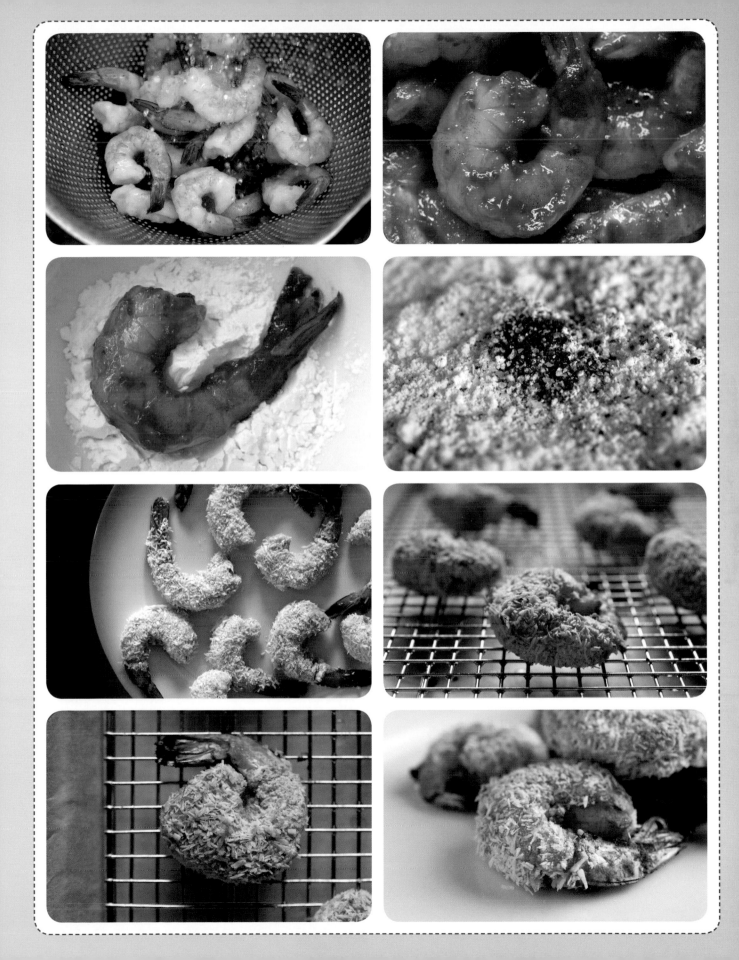

SHRIMP + WATERMELON SKEWERS

These quick and easy skewers are a perfect balance of summery textures and flavors. The snap of briny grilled shrimp pairs surprisingly well with the juicy sweetness of charred watermelon—and a liberal squeeze of lime at the end adds a tangy zing that marries all the components together.

Makes 16 skewers
Hands-on time: 15 minutes
Total time: 15 minutes

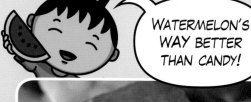

WATERMELON'S WAY BETTER THAN CANDY!

2 pounds (approximately 20 to 25 per pound) uncooked large fresh **shrimp**, peeled and deveined, but with tails intact

2 pounds **watermelon** flesh (from about ½ medium watermelon), cut into 1-inch cubes

3 tablespoons **macadamia nut oil** or melted **ghee**

½ teaspoon **lemon pepper seasoning**

Kosher salt

4 **limes**, quartered

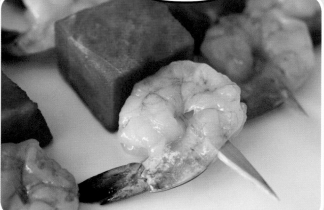

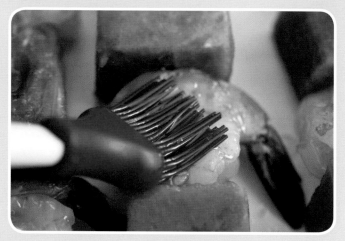

DO THIS:

1. On each skewer, thread 2 to 3 shrimp and 2 to 3 watermelon chunks, alternating each.

2. Brush oil on the prepared skewers and sprinkle with the lemon pepper seasoning and salt.

3. Lay the skewers on a grill over high heat for 4 to 6 minutes, turning once. The skewers are done when the shrimp turn a bright orange and are no longer translucent.

4. Serve with lime wedges (or season to taste with the juice from the limes just prior to serving).

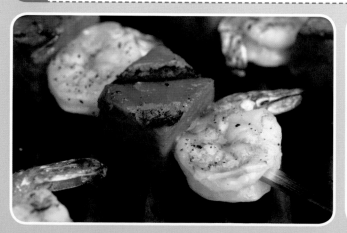

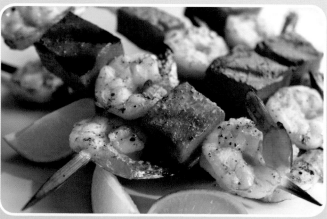

ACCORDING TO THE FOLKS AT AMERICA'S TEST KITCHEN, THERE'S NO NEED TO PRE-SOAK THE WOODEN SKEWERS. THE TIPS WILL ALWAYS BURN NO MATTER WHAT, SO WHY BOTHER?

SLOW-POACHED MAGIC TUNA

If you've got fresh albacore, you must make this dish, which I adapted from a David Tanis recipe. It doesn't get easier than oven-poaching tuna in olive oil, and by adding a generous sprinkle of Magic Mushroom Powder, you exponentially increase the umami in this dish. Bonus: leftovers stored in the braising liquid will keep for up to a week, which means you'll always have a healthy snack at your fingertips.

Makes 4 servings
Hands-on time: 10 minutes
Total time: 30 minutes

2   pounds skinless fresh **albacore fillet**
2   teaspoons **Magic Mushroom Powder** (page 35)
4   **garlic cloves**, minced
⅔   cup **extra-virgin olive oil**

DO THIS:

1. Preheat the oven to 325°F with the rack in the middle position. Cut the fillet crosswise into 1½-inch steaks, and season them with Magic Mushroom Powder.

2. Arrange the tuna steaks in a single layer in a deep-sided oven-safe dish, and evenly distribute the garlic on top of the fish. Pour olive oil into the bottom of the dish, stopping only when it reaches halfway up the tuna steaks. Cover the dish, and poach in the oven for 10 minutes, or until the steaks are cooked halfway through.

3. Gently flip over each tuna steak so that the uncooked sides are now in the olive oil. Cover the dish and continue poaching in the oven for another 10 minutes or until just barely cooked through. Serve with a drizzle of the Magic Mushroom Powder–infused olive oil from the baking dish.

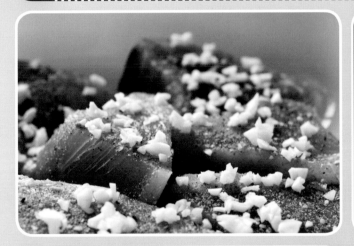
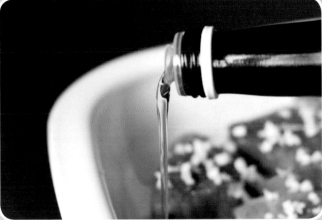
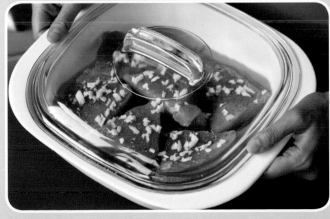
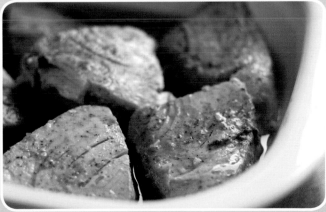

TUNA ITSELF IS ALREADY UMAMI-RICH DUE TO ITS HIGH INOSINATE CONTENT. ADD MAGIC MUSHROOM POWDER TO THE MIX, AND YOUR TASTE BUDS WILL BE GIVING YOU HIGH-FIVES.

FRIED SALMON PATTIES

Fresh, wild-caught salmon is wonderful, but I don't always have the time (or energy) to herd the kids into the car for a drive to the market or fishmonger. Fortunately, I keep a stockpile of canned fish in my pantry; when I'm short on time, I simply whip out my trusty can opener and *voila!* Dinner is served!

What? You're not keen on eating fish straight from the can? Then transform that lowly can of wild salmon into savory, delicate patties. Crisp and golden brown on the outside, tender and moist on the inside, these salmon patties make for a great weeknight meal—and no one'll suspect that you made 'em with canned fish. (Just remember to throw away the open cans. They're a dead giveaway.)

Makes 8 patties | Hands-on time: 30 minutes | Total time: 60 minutes

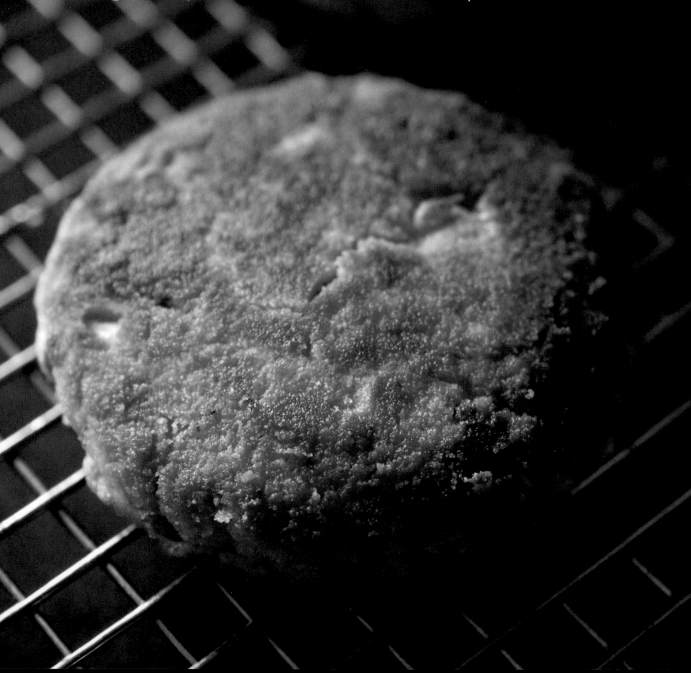

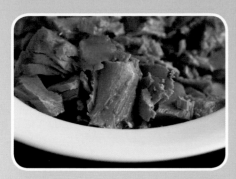

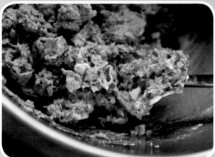

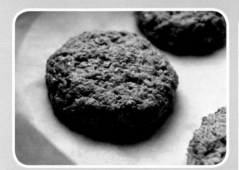

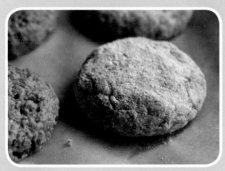

GET:

1½ pounds canned boneless, skinless **wild sockeye salmon** packed in water, drained and broken up into small chunks

¼ cup **Paleo Mayonnaise** (page 40)

2 **scallions**, thinly sliced

2 large **eggs**, lightly beaten

2 tablespoons chopped fresh **Italian parsley**

¼ medium **yellow onion**, minced

¼ cup **coconut flour**, divided

1 teaspoon **paprika**

½ teaspoon dried **dill**

½ teaspoon **kosher salt**

¼ teaspoon dried **mustard**

¼ teaspoon **garlic powder**

¼ teaspoon freshly ground **black pepper**

2 tablespoons **ghee** or fat of choice

2 **lemons**, cut into wedges

¼ cup **Louisiana Rémoulade** (page 63) (optional)

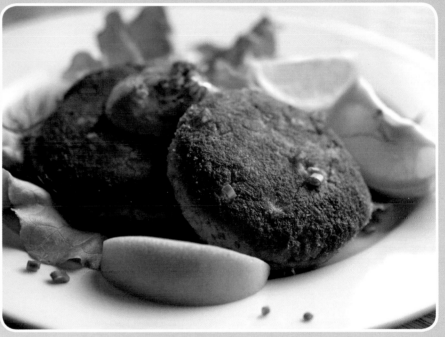

DO THIS:

1. In a large bowl, mix together the salmon, mayonnaise, scallions, eggs, parsley, onion, 1 tablespoon of the coconut flour, the paprika, dill, salt, dried mustard, garlic powder, and pepper.

2. Divide the salmon mixture into 8 equal portions, and use your hands to form each into a patty roughly 3 inches in diameter and ¾ inches in height. Place the cakes on a parchment-lined plate. Cover and chill in the fridge for at least 30 minutes to firm up the cakes.

3. When you're ready to cook, spread the remaining coconut flour in a shallow dish, and lightly coat the cakes, shaking off any excess. Heat the oil over medium heat in a large cast-iron skillet. Once it's shimmering, fry the cakes in the ghee for 2 minutes or until golden brown. Transfer to a wire rack to drain off any excess oil. Serve with lemon wedges (and Louisiana Rémoulade, if desired).

 NOT A SALMON LOVER? SUBSTITUTE TUNA OR LUMP CRAB MEAT INSTEAD!

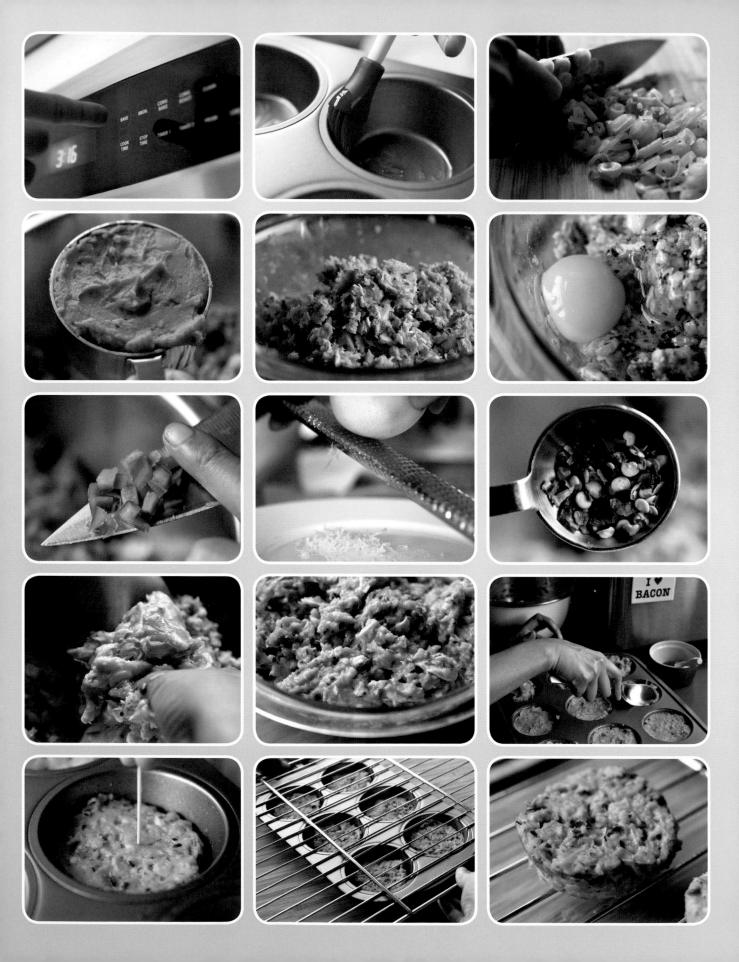

SPICY TUNA CAKES

You may not normally associate canned fish with sweet potatoes and jalapeño peppers, but these hot 'n spicy tuna cakes are a revelation. They're tender and sweet, but with a wickedly peppery bite that sneaks up on you. Eat them for breakfast, lunch, or dinner—or whip up an extra-big batch for your next dinner party.

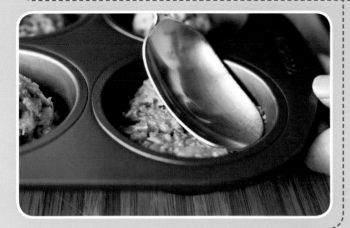

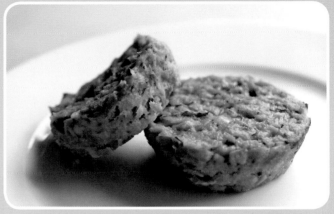

Makes 12 cakes
Hands-on time: 20 minutes
Total time: 45 minutes

YUM!

3	tablespoons melted **ghee**, divided
10	ounces canned **albacore tuna** packed in water, drained
3	**scallions**, thinly sliced (about ⅓ cup)
2	tablespoons finely minced fresh **cilantro**
1⅓	cup mashed **Oven Baked Sweet Potatoes** (page 164)
2	large **eggs**
1	tablespoon minced **jalapeño pepper**
	Finely grated zest from ½ medium **lemon**
½	teaspoon **red pepper flakes**
	Kosher salt
	Freshly ground **black pepper**
3	medium **lemons**, cut into wedges (optional)

DO THIS:

1. Preheat the oven to 350°F with the rack in the middle position, and use a brush or paper towel to grease a 12-cup regular-sized muffin tin with 1 tablespoon of melted ghee.

2. In a large bowl, mix together the tuna, scallions, and cilantro. Add the mashed sweet potato to the tuna mixture, and gently combine. Then, mix in the eggs, remaining 2 tablespoons melted ghee, jalapeño, lemon zest, and red pepper flakes. Don't overwork the ingredients—keep the chunks of fish intact as much as possible. Season with salt and pepper to taste.

3. Scoop a quarter cup of the mixture into each greased muffin tin cup, and flatten with the back of a spoon. Bake the tuna cakes for 20 to 25 minutes or until an inserted toothpick comes out clean.

4. Transfer the cakes to a wire rack to cool. (The easiest way I've found to get them out is to put the wire rack on top of the muffin tin, flip them upside down, and tap them gently on the counter.)

5. Serve with lemon wedges. They're fantastic right out of the oven, but you can also pan-fry them in some melted fat in a skillet over medium heat to crisp the edges and impart some extra crunch.

 WHO NEEDS SANDWICHES? THESE SPICY LITTLE BITES ARE PERFECT FOR PACKED LUNCHES.

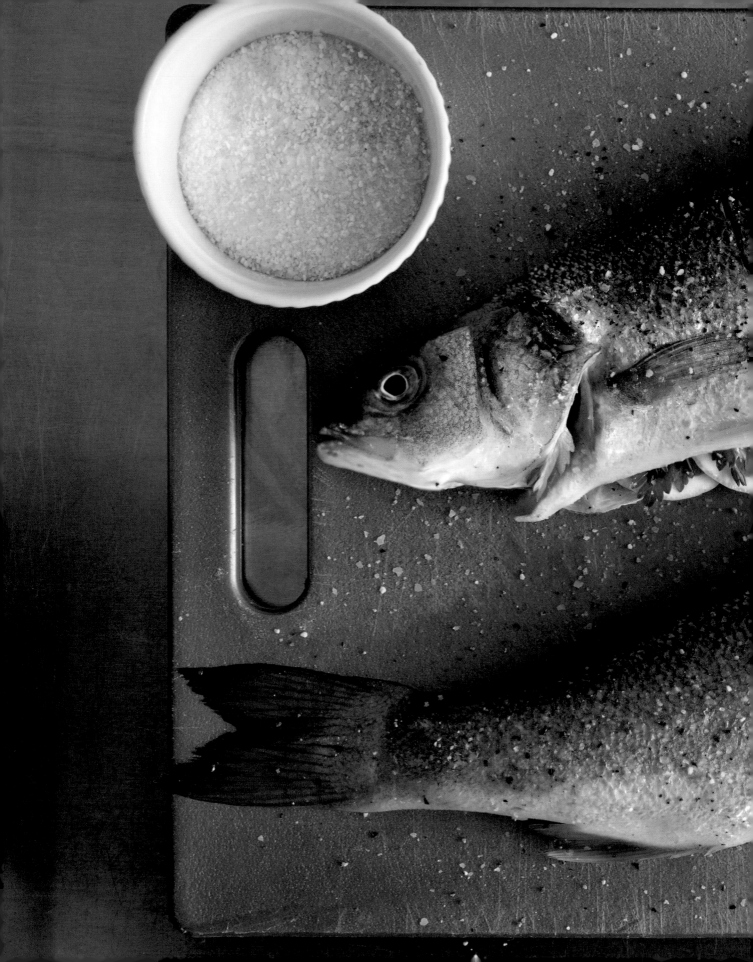

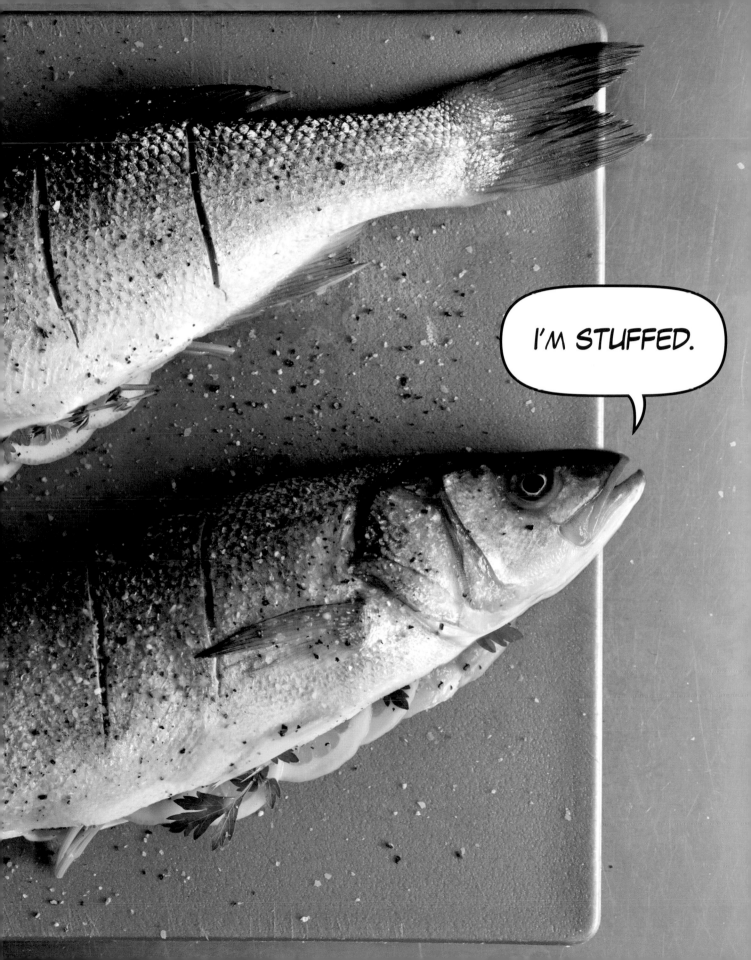

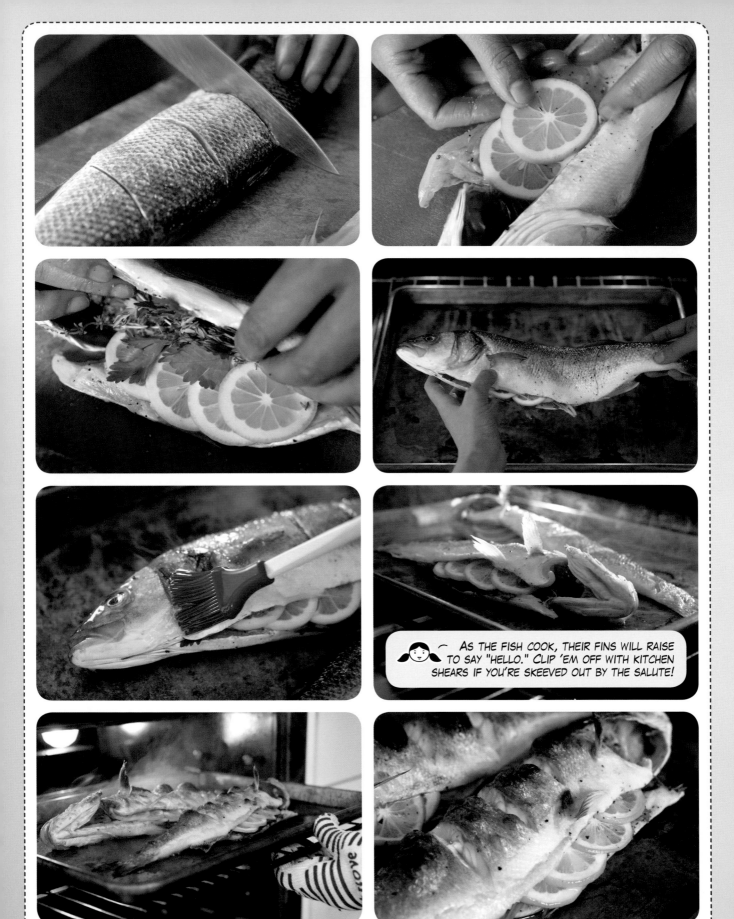

AS THE FISH COOK, THEIR FINS WILL RAISE TO SAY "HELLO." CLIP 'EM OFF WITH KITCHEN SHEARS IF YOU'RE SKEEVED OUT BY THE SALUTE!

WHOLE ROASTED BRANZINI

I had my first bite of branzino over a decade ago, after Henry and I had slowly eaten our way from the Tuscan countryside up to Venice. We lost ourselves for hours each day, exploring every nook and cranny of the vibrant City of Bridges, from the quiet streets of Giudecca to the crowded center of San Marco. No two corners were the same, but at every restaurant we visited, I insisted on ordering whole roasted branzino.

A prized catch in Northern Italy, branzino—also known as Mediterranean seabass or *loup de mer*—is now booming in popularity in restaurants throughout North America, and it's not hard to see why. Branzino isn't expensive, and it's among one of the most eco-friendly seafood choices on the market. Most important (to me, anyway), its flesh is deliciously tender and flavorful, with mildly sweet and nutty notes.

Yes, the prospect of whole-roasting a fish—especially one nicknamed the "wolf of the sea"—can be a bit daunting. But just for you, I've come up with quick, foolproof method that'll dirty just one pan. Ready?

Makes 2 servings
Hands-on time: 10 minutes
Total time: 25 minutes

CAN'T FIND BRANZINI? YOU CAN USE RAINBOW TROUT INSTEAD. JUST SHORTEN THE COOKING TIME IF YOUR FISHIES ARE ON THE SMALLER SIDE!

2 (1-pound) **branzini**, gutted and scaled
Kosher salt
Freshly ground **black pepper**
1 small **lemon**, thinly sliced
4 sprigs fresh **Italian parsley**
6 sprigs fresh **thyme**
2 tablespoons melted **ghee**, divided
1 **lemon**, cut into wedges

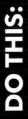

DO THIS:

1. Preheat the broiler with the oven rack 4 to 6 inches from the heating element. Place a non-coated heavy-duty baking sheet on the rack. You want to get the tray red-hot before placing the fish on it.

2. Pat dry the exterior and interior of the fish with a paper towel. Using a sharp knife, cut three evenly spaced slits in the flesh on both sides. Cut deeply—all the way down to the bone. Generously season the fish inside and out with salt and pepper. Shingle the lemon slices so that they slightly overlap, and tuck them into the cavity of the fish along with the herbs.

3. Brush 1 tablespoon of the ghee onto the pan, and place the fish on the hot ghee. The skin should sizzle as soon as it hits the pan. Brush the remaining tablespoon of ghee over the top of the fish, and broil the fish for 3 to 5 minutes or until the skin is blistered on top. Carefully flip the fish with a wide spatula, and continue cooking for another 2 minutes or until they are cooked through. The skin should be browned and crispy, and the tender flesh should flake off the bones easily.

4. Remove the fish from the oven, and rest them for 5 minutes. Discard the herbs and lemon slices, and serve the branzini with fresh lemon wedges.

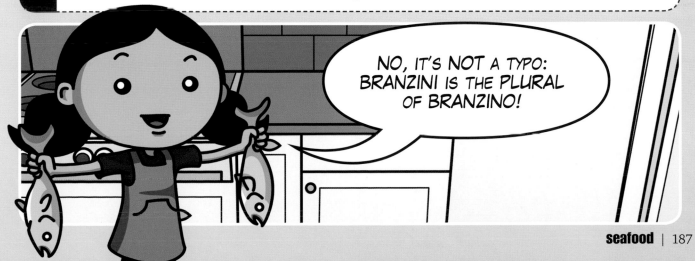

NO, IT'S NOT A TYPO: BRANZINI IS THE PLURAL OF BRANZINO!

CRAB + AVOCADO TEMAKI

We've always been big sushi fans, so temaki (seaweed-wrapped hand rolls) with spicy crab and avocado make regular appearances in our kitchen. I usually have all the ingredients for these creamy, crisp rolls in our fridge and pantry, so it's a breeze to throw together this no-cook recipe. Plus, everyone in the family can assemble their own, which means even less work for me.

Makes 16 hand rolls
Hands-on time: 15 minutes
Total time: 15 minutes

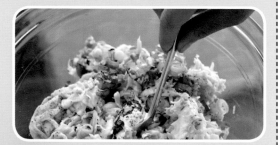

- 2 tablespoons **Paleo Mayonnaise** (page 40)
- 2 **scallions**, thinly sliced
- 1 pound cooked lump **crab meat**
- ½ teaspoon **red pepper flakes** (optional)
- Juice from ½ medium **lime**
- **Kosher salt**
- Freshly ground **black pepper**
- 8 toasted standard-size **nori sheets**, cut in half width-wise
- 1 large **Hass avocado**, pitted, peeled, and thinly sliced
- 2 small Japanese or Persian **cucumbers**, cut into matchsticks
- Handful of **radish sprouts** or **micro greens**

DO THIS:

1. In a large bowl, combine the Paleo Mayonnaise, scallions, crab meat, red pepper flakes (if using), and lime juice. Season with salt and pepper to taste, and mix well.

2. To assemble each roll, hold a piece of nori shiny-side down, and scoop 2 tablespoons of the crab mixture onto the left side of the rectangle. The filling should be at a diagonal, running from the top left corner to the bottom center of the nori.

3. Top the crab with a slice of avocado, some cucumber, and sprouts. Fold the bottom left corner of the nori over the filling before wrapping the long part of the nori around the crab and vegetables to form a cone. Serve immediately—don't let the nori get soft!

HUH?

Nori, the Japanese name for paper-thin sheets of dried seaweed, can be found at most Asian markets.

It's packed with calcium, iron, zinc, and protein, and is used for all kinds of food preparations across Asia. In Japan alone, roughly 9 billion (!) sheets of nori are consumed every year.

I keep nori on hand to roll up sushi or to garnish dishes and clear soups. Keep some toasted nori in your pantry; it can be a culinary lifesaver.

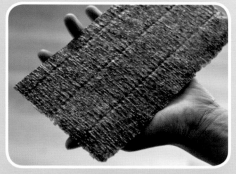
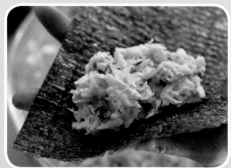
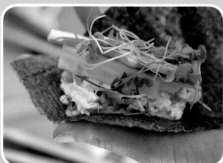
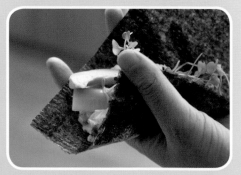

FEELING SPICY? ADD A DASH OF SHICHIMI TOGARASHI (JAPANESE SEVEN-FLAVOR CHILI PEPPER)!

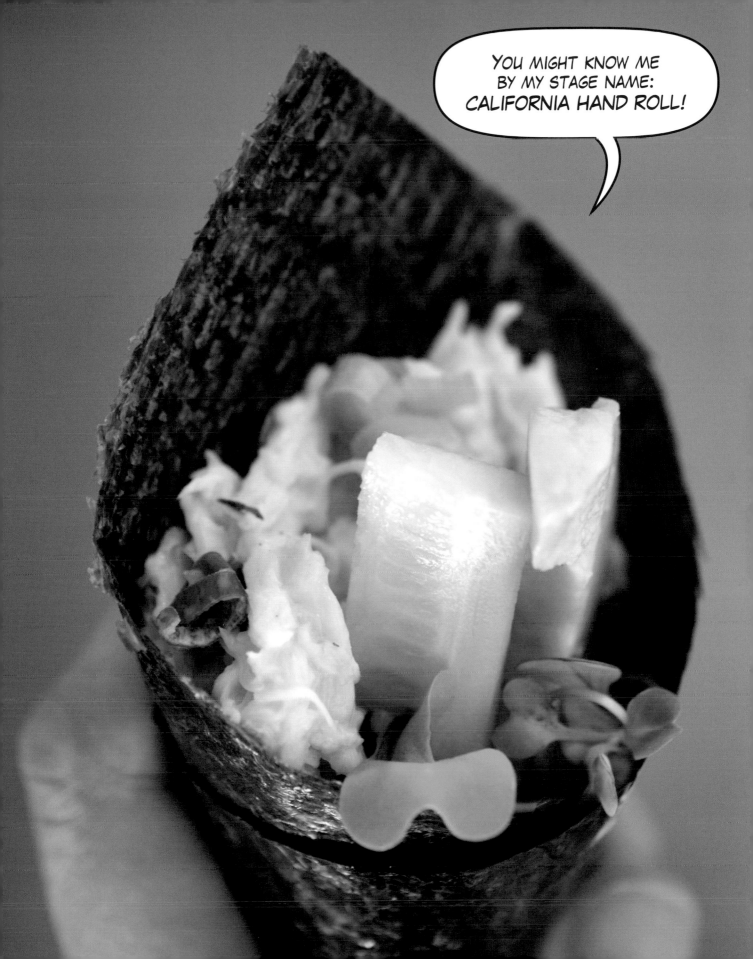

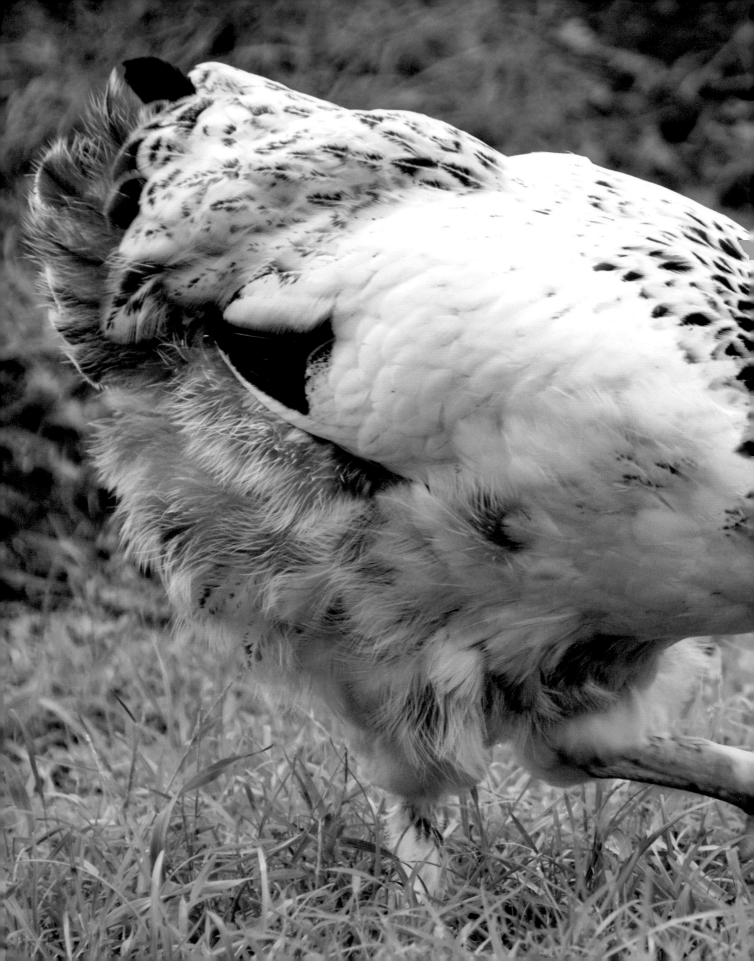

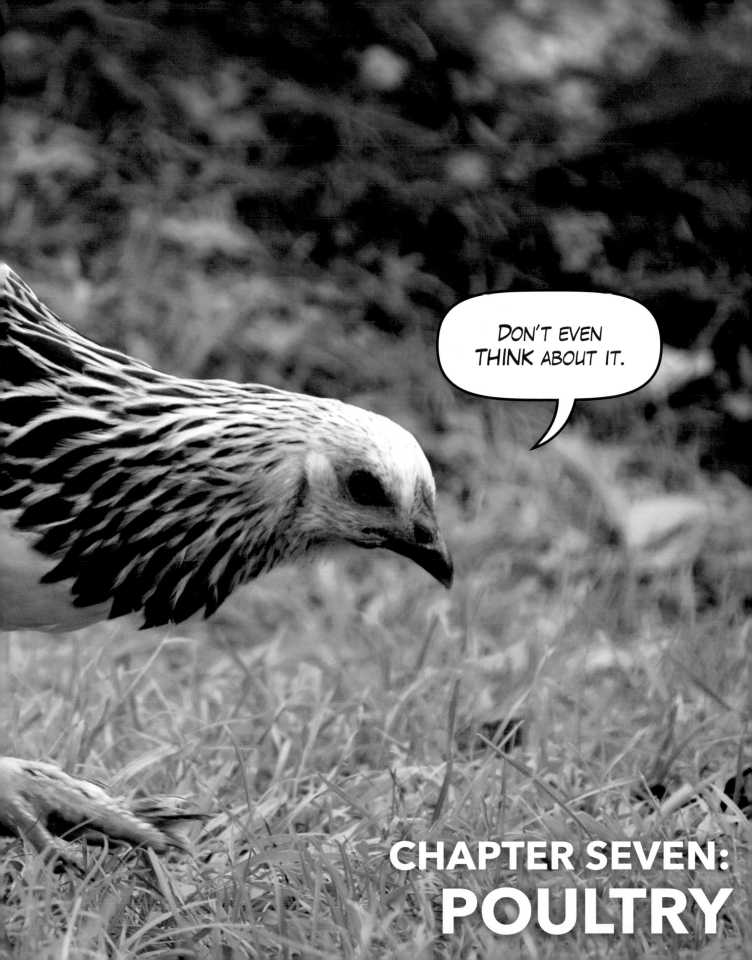

CHAPTER SEVEN:
POULTRY

MY BIG SISTER IS MY GO-TO SOURCE FOR HANDS-ON
COOKING KNOWLEDGE, AND ONE OF MY BIGGEST CULINARY
HEROES AND INFLUENCES. PLUS, SHE'S A SUPER READER.

SEE?

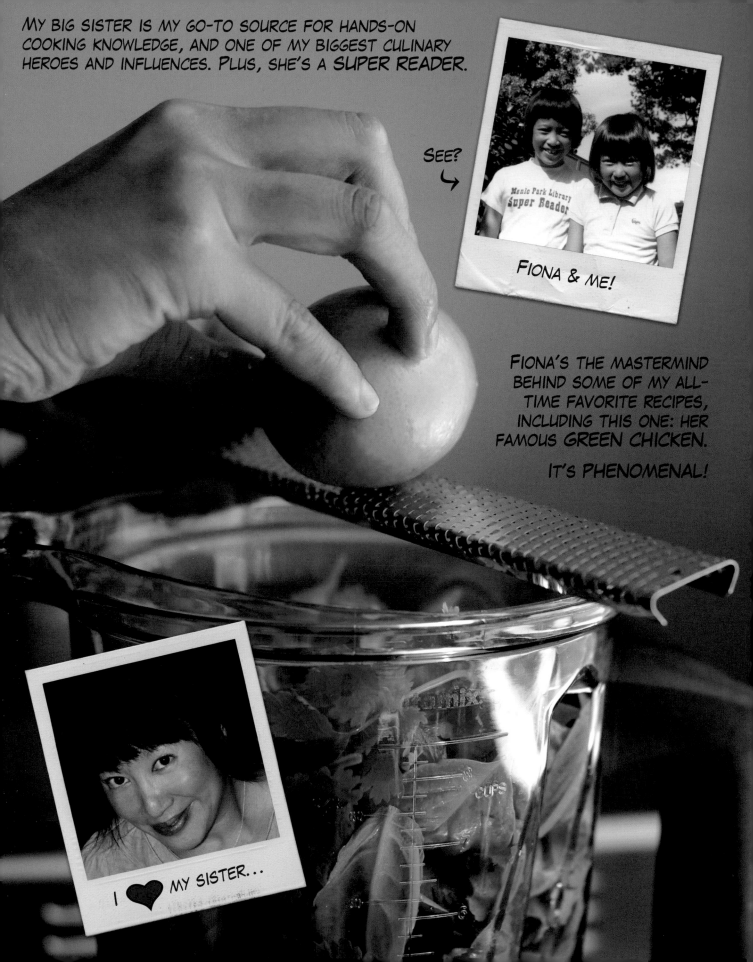

FIONA & ME!

FIONA'S THE MASTERMIND
BEHIND SOME OF MY ALL-
TIME FAVORITE RECIPES,
INCLUDING THIS ONE: HER
FAMOUS GREEN CHICKEN.

IT'S PHENOMENAL!

I ♥ MY SISTER...

FIONA'S GREEN CHICKEN

Makes 6 servings
Hands-on time: 15 minutes
Total time: 2 hours

After pestering my crazy-awesome chef sister for a Paleo marinade recipe, she finally relented and sent me the secret formula for her go-to, Thai-inspired, green herb marinade. This stuff is truly phenomenal—and not just on chicken.

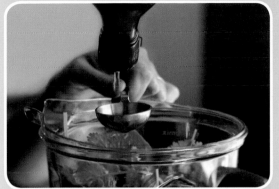

1   medium sweet **onion**, coarsely chopped (about 1 cup)
1¼ cups packed fresh **basil**
1   cup packed fresh **cilantro** (leaves and stems)
¼   cup packed fresh **mint**
3   **garlic cloves**, peeled
¼   cup Paleo-friendly **fish sauce**
2   tablespoons **apple juice**
1   teaspoon **Aleppo pepper** or **red pepper flakes**
½   teaspoon freshly ground **black pepper**
    Finely grated zest from 1 medium **lime**
3   pounds skin-on **chicken drumsticks** or **thighs**
2   **limes**, cut into wedges

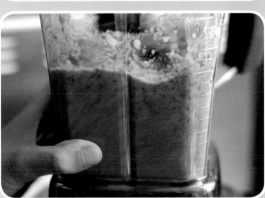

DO THIS:

1. In a blender, purée the onion, basil, cilantro, mint, garlic, fish sauce, apple juice, Aleppo pepper, black pepper, and lime zest. The mixture should be thick and smooth, with no chunks. Taste and adjust for seasoning.

2. Place the chicken in a gallon-size zip-top bag. Pour in the marinade and squeeze out the air in the bag before sealing. Marinate the chicken in the refrigerator for at least 1 hour and up to a day.

3. Take the chicken out of the fridge at least 30 minutes before cooking so it can come up to room temperature. Remove the chicken from the bag.

4. If oven-roasting: Preheat the oven to 400°F with the rack in the middle position. Then, place a wire rack atop a foil-lined rimmed baking tray. Arrange the chicken in a single layer on the rack, and roast for 35 to 40 minutes, flipping the bird (ha!) at the midpoint.

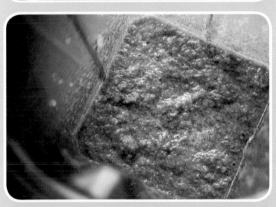

5. If grilling: Arrange the marinated chicken on a medium-hot grill and cook for about 25 minutes, turning every 5 to 7 minutes.

6. The chicken's ready when the internal temperature reaches 170°F or when the juices run clear. Serve with lime wedges.

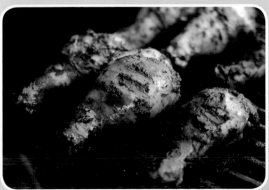

INSTEAD OF USING THE GREEN STUFF AS A MARINADE, TRY DRIZZLING IT IN SOUPS OR ON GRILLED MEATS!

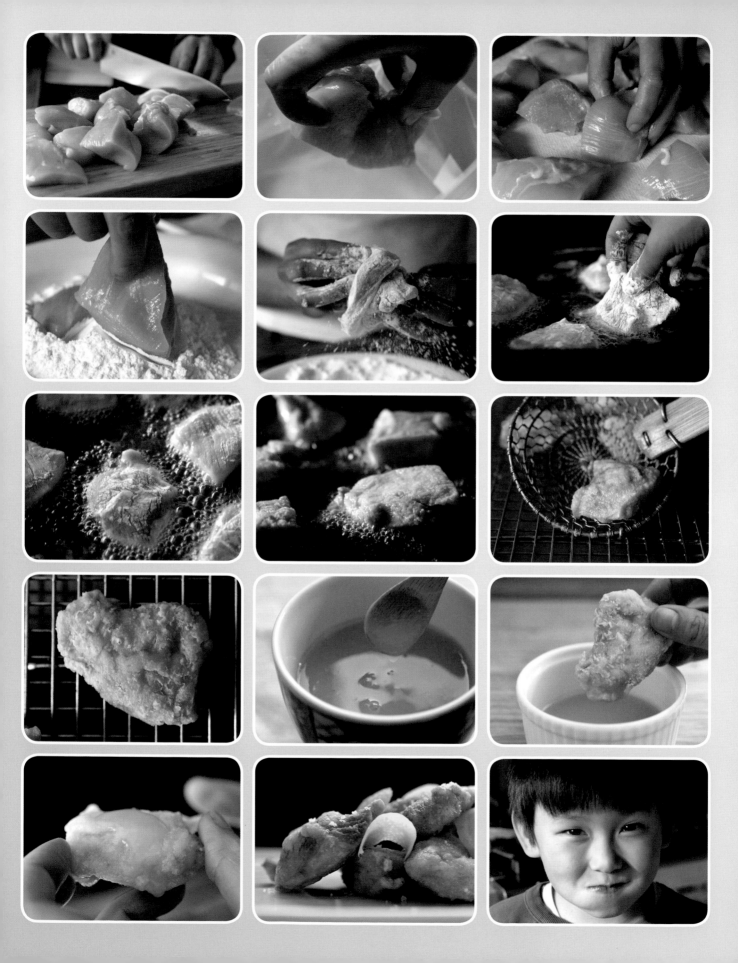

CHICKEN NUGGETS

No, I'm not talking about processed hunks of fried pink slime served up in fast food containers. Instead, we're making nuggets from pieces of whole breast meat, brined for maximum juiciness and fried in healthy fats. These crispy chicken pieces are the perfect finger food for anyone who loves eating with their hands.

Makes 6 servings
Hands-on time: 20 minutes
Total time: 1 hour

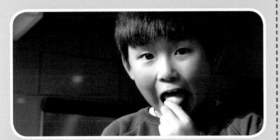

6 cups **water**
½ cup **kosher salt**
1 cup **ghee** or fat of choice, for frying
1 cup **tapioca powder** or **arrowroot powder**
4 large skinless, boneless **chicken breasts** (about 2½ pounds), cut into ½-inch-thick nuggets
Fleur de sel or other coarse sea salt (optional)
½ cup **Sriracha Mayonnaise** (page 45), **Lemon Honey Sauce** (page 57), **Honey Mustard Dressing** (page 58), **Avocado + Basil Dressing** (page 61), **Paleo Ranch Dressing** (page 62), or **Louisiana Rémoulade** (page 63)

DO THIS:

1. Mix the water and salt in a gallon-sized zip-top bag. Seal and agitate it to dissolve the salt. Add the chicken to the brine and refrigerate for 30 minutes to an hour.

2. When you're ready to cook, melt the ghee in a large skillet over medium-high heat. Make sure there's enough oil to reach halfway up the chicken pieces.

3. Remove the chicken from the brine and blot dry with paper towels. Put the tapioca or arrowroot powder in a shallow bowl, and coat each piece of chicken in the powder, shaking off any excess.

4. Once the oil's hot and shimmering, fry the chicken until crispy, about 2 minutes per side. Transfer to a wire rack to drain off any extra oil. If desired, sprinkle on some fleur de sel while hot, and serve with your favorite dipping sauce(s).

JUICY LEAN MEATS: NOT AN OXYMORON!

All too often, chicken breast and other lean cuts can turn out dry and powdery. The key to firm, juicy, savory chicken? Brining. Soaking lean poultry or pork in a salt water solution reshapes the protein molecules in the meat, keeping it plump and moist throughout the cooking process. Brining also breaks down the structural integrity of the meat, resulting in greater tenderness. Try it!

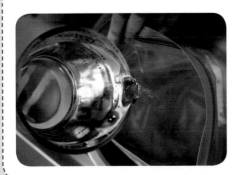
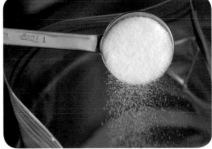
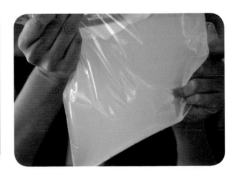

THE BEST WAY TO REHEAT COLD NUGGETS IS TO FRY 'EM AGAIN. THEY MAY CRISP UP EVEN CRUNCHIER THAN THE FIRST TIME!

MAGIC WINGS

Hosting a party? Want to serve finger food that's easy to prepare yet packed with umami? This recipe fits the bill. If you have time, marinate the chicken for a few hours in advance of cooking—but if you're expecting guests within the hour, these wings will taste magical even if you're making them to order.

Makes 6 servings
Hands-on time: 10 minutes
Total time: 1 hour

4 pounds **chicken wings**
2 tablespoons **Magic Mushroom Powder** (page 35)
½ teaspoon Paleo-friendly **fish sauce** (optional)
Melted **ghee**
2 small **limes**, cut into wedges

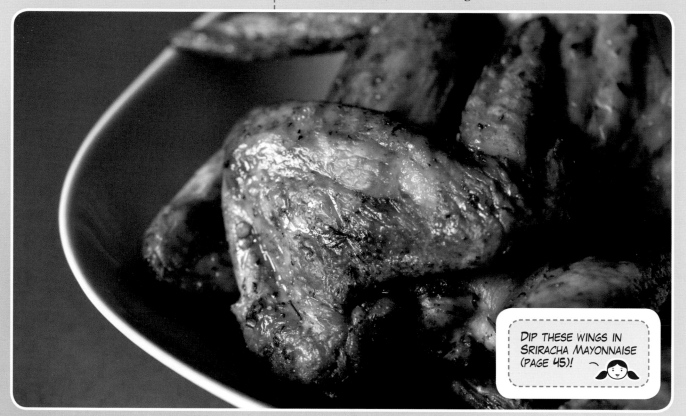

DIP THESE WINGS IN SRIRACHA MAYONNAISE (PAGE 45)!

DO THIS:

1. Toss the chicken wings with Magic Mushroom Powder (and if desired, fish sauce) in a large bowl, making sure to evenly distribute the seasoning. Cover and marinate the wings in the refrigerator for up to 24 hours.

2. A half-hour before serving, take the wings out of the refrigerator and preheat the oven to 425°F with the rack in the middle position. (Got a convection bake setting on your oven? You can set it to 400°F on convection bake for this recipe.) Place a wire rack on top of a foil-lined rimmed baking sheet. You'll likely need to cook the wings in two batches, so if you have two trays, use 'em.

3. Grease the rack with melted ghee, and arrange the wings in a single layer on the wire rack. Be careful not to overcrowd the wings. Bake for 15 minutes, and then flip the wings and rotate the tray. Bake for another 10 to 15 minutes or until the skins are crisp, taut, and golden brown.

4. Plate and serve with lime wedges.

PREPARE THIS DISH WITH THIGHS FOR AN EASY WEEKNIGHT MEAL! JUST COOK FOR 15 MINUTES MORE, OR UNTIL THE INTERNAL TEMPERATURE OF THE BIRD REACHES 170°F.

CRISPY SMASHED CHICKEN

So you've had a long, stressful day, and no clue what to make for dinner. But you have chicken breasts in the fridge, right? Believe it or not, you can easily transform that cold poultry into hot, crispy paillards in 30 minutes or less. Plus, you can release your pent-up rage by going medieval on the chicken. Win-win!

Makes 4 servings
Hands-on time: 30 minutes
Total time: 30 minutes

"PAILLARD" IS A FANCY FRENCH CULINARY TERM THAT DESCRIBES A PIECE OF MEAT THAT'S BEEN THINLY SLICED OR POUNDED TO FACILITATE QUICK COOKING. IT'S FUN TO THROW BIG WORDS AROUND!

- **4** skinless, boneless **chicken breasts** (about 6 ounces each)
- **½** cup **coconut flour**
- **1** tablespoon **kosher salt**
- **½** teaspoon **garlic powder**
  Freshly ground **black pepper**
- **2** tablespoons **ghee** or fat of choice, plus more as needed
- **2** **limes**, cut into wedges (optional)
- **2** cups **Spicy Pineapple Salsa** (page 55) or **Salsa Roja Asada** (page 54) (optional)

DO THIS:

1. Sprinkle a few drops of water on the chicken and place it between two pieces of plastic wrap or parchment. Then, hulk out and smash the breasts with a meat pounder, rolling pin, or small cast-iron skillet until the chicken is uniformly flattened into ½-inch-thick paillards.

2. In a large bowl, mix the coconut flour, salt, garlic powder, and a few grinds of pepper. Dredge the chicken in the flour mixture, and pat off any excess.

3. Heat the ghee over medium-high heat in a large cast-iron skillet until it's shimmering.

4. Once at a time, fry each chicken breast in the skillet, letting it cook undisturbed for 3 to 4 minutes before flipping. Then, cook the other side for another 3 to 4 minutes, or until the exterior is crisp and golden brown. Transfer the chicken to a wire rack, and tent it with foil while you fry up the remaining pieces.

5. Slice up the paillards, and serve with lime wedges and your favorite salsa.

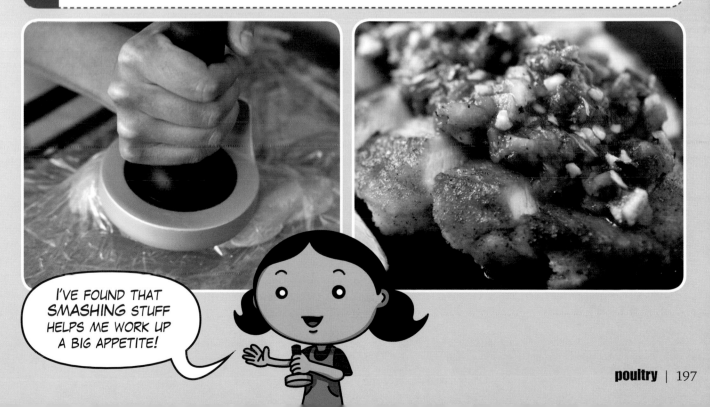

I'VE FOUND THAT SMASHING STUFF HELPS ME WORK UP A BIG APPETITE!

SLOW COOKER CHICKEN + GRAVY

Ever try to prepare a whole chicken in the slow cooker? With most recipes, the bird winds up overcooked, stringy, and dry. Super icky—but not with this recipe. This preparation will yield a moist, tender chicken and a thick, savory gravy. Serve it for supper, and everyone will lick their plates clean. Plus, you'll finally get to show off that awesome gravy boat that your mom gave you.

By the way, the fish sauce is optional, but trust me: it adds a ton of umami to this dish. Omit it at your peril!

Makes 4 servings
Hands-on time: 30 minutes
Total time: 6 hours

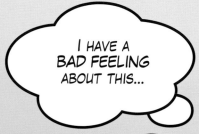

I HAVE A BAD FEELING ABOUT THIS...

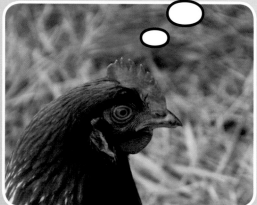

2	tablespoons **ghee** or fat of choice
3	large **leeks**, white parts only, chopped medium
6	**garlic cloves**, smashed and peeled
1	teaspoon **tomato paste**
	Kosher salt
	Freshly ground **black pepper**
½	cup **chicken stock**
1	(4-pound) whole **chicken**
1	tablespoon dried **poultry seasoning** or dried herb blend of choice
1	teaspoon Paleo-friendly **fish sauce** (optional)

DO THIS:

1. Melt the ghee in a large skillet over medium heat. Once the fat starts to shimmer, add the leeks and garlic and cook for a few minutes or until fragrant. Add the tomato paste and stir to incorporate. Season with salt and pepper to taste.

2. Cook until the aromatics are softened and lightly browned, 8 to 10 minutes. Deglaze the pan with chicken stock and transfer the cooked vegetables to a slow cooker.

3. Pat the chicken dry, and season well—both inside and out—with salt, pepper, and poultry seasoning. Place the chicken breast-down in the slow cooker, and if desired, add the fish sauce. Place the cover on the slow cooker, and cook on low for 4 to 6 hours, depending on the size of the bird. The smaller the chicken, the less time is required.

4. When the chicken's done cooking, transfer it to a platter and tent it with a piece of foil. Rest it for 20 minutes.

5. In the meantime, defat the cooking liquid. Taste and adjust for seasoning. Transfer the liquid and vegetables to a large measuring cup, and use an immersion blender to purée the contents. The result? A thick, rich gravy.

6. Once the chicken's rested, place it on a cutting board and break it down. (Better yet, just rip it all up with your hands like a true caveperson.) Pile all the juicy, tender chicken pieces on a platter and serve it with the gravy.

CHEW ON THIS:

- Don't leave the bird in the slow cooker for more than 6 hours unless you enjoy eating powdery, dessicated chicken. And don't set the slow cooker to "high" in an effort to save time, either.

- Save some gravy and store it in a sealed container in the fridge for a week (or in the freezer for a few months). It'll come in handy for everything from Loco Moco (page 228) to Thanksgiving dinner.

WASTE NOT, WANT NOT: SAVE THE CHICKEN BONES TO MAKE BONE BROTH (PAGE 104)!

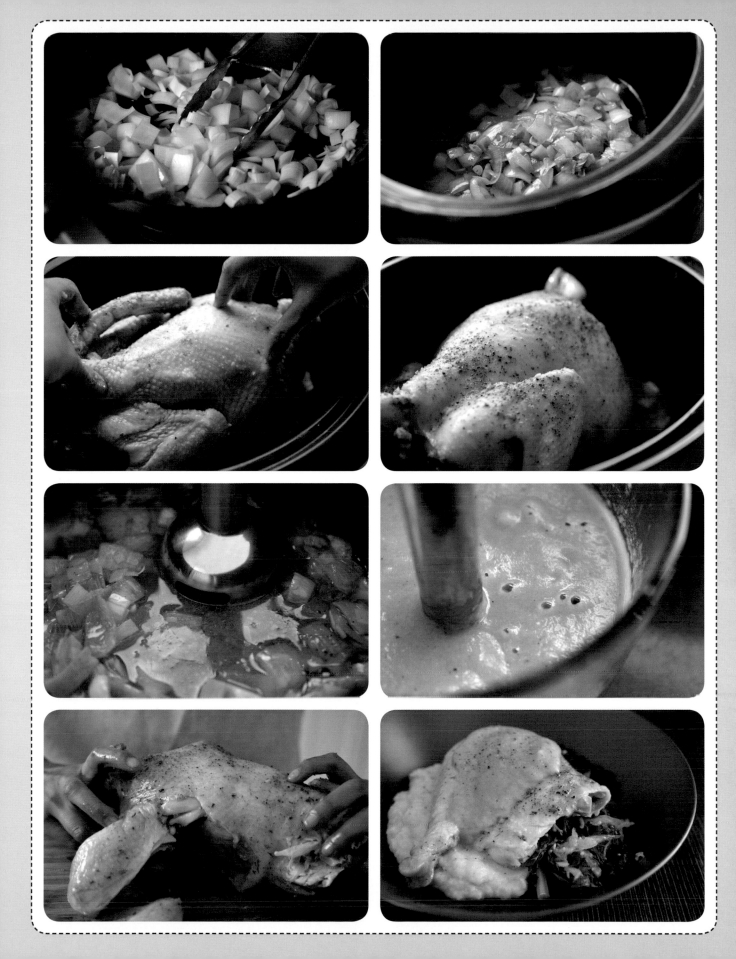

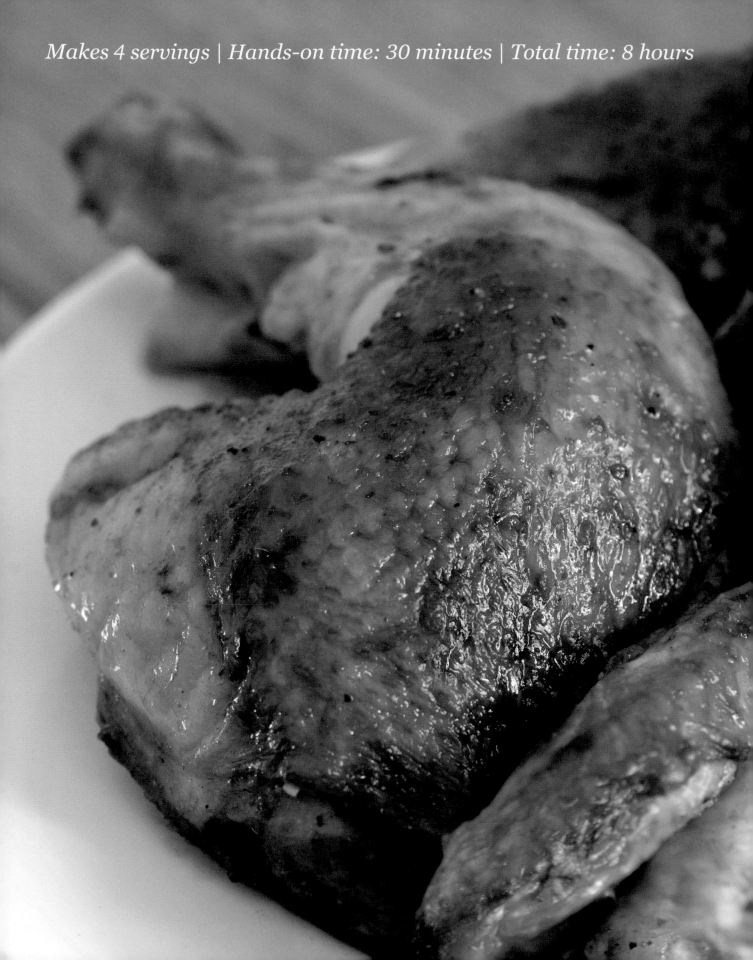

PERUVIAN ROAST CHICKEN + AJI VERDE CHILI SAUCE

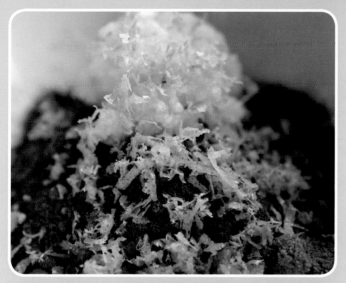

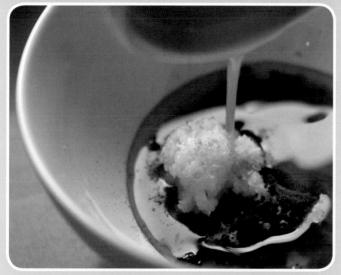

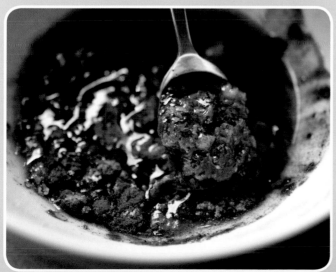

My childhood best friend, Evelyn, was born in Peru—but as kids, we were much more interested in the craptacular contents of our school's vending machines than the South American dishes her mom would make. So it wasn't until decades later that I finally had a taste of Peruvian-style roast chicken at a San Francisco restaurant. A paste of garlic and spices had been rubbed both under and over the crisp, golden-brown skin of the chicken, giving the tender meat a hint of tartness and smoke. I was hooked.

Making authentic Peruvian chicken at home, however, posed a few challenges. First of all, I don't have a rotisserie. (My kitchen's already overflowing with gadgets; one more appliance and my neat-freak husband will keel over.) Secondly, I don't have easy access to the Peruvian black mint known as *huacatay*—a distinctively flavored Andean herb used to make the luscious green aji verde chili sauce that traditionally accompanies the roast chicken.

But I can never resist a challenge.

The solution to the rotisserie problem was simple: I'd spatchcock the bird before oven-roasting it. Spatchcocking sounds dirty, but it simply means removing the backbone and butterflying the bird to ensure that the breasts and thighs will cook to juicy perfection at the same time.

Finding common ingredients to replace the *huacatay* was tougher, but after some research and taste-testing, I found that a mix of fresh basil, cilantro, and mint produces a remarkably similar perfume and herby notes.

My recipe for homemade Peruvian chicken takes a bit of pre-planning and patience, but it's a cinch to prepare and yields a juicy and intensely flavorful meal. Paired with the cool, tangy contrast of the aji verde chili sauce, this dish will be one that you'll want to make—and devour—again and again.

Besides, it sure beats soda and chips from my high school's vending machines.

 EVERYTHING TASTES BETTER WITH AJI VERDE CHILI SAUCE: FROM MEAT AND FISH TO SALADS AND SOUPS!

GET:

Aji Verde Chili Sauce

2	tablespoons **extra-virgin olive oil**
2	**garlic cloves**, minced
3	**jalapeño** peppers, stemmed, seeded, and roughly chopped
1	**scallion**, roughly chopped
½	cup **Paleo Mayonnaise** (page 40)
⅓	cup fresh **basil**
⅓	cup fresh **cilantro**
⅓	cup fresh **mint**
2	teaspoons fresh **lime juice**
1	teaspoon **white vinegar**

Peruvian Marinade

4	**garlic cloves**, minced
3	tablespoons melted **ghee** or fat of choice
1	tablespoon **kosher salt**
1	tablespoon freshly ground **black pepper**
1	tablespoon ground **cumin**
1	tablespoon **smoked paprika**
1	teaspoon dried **oregano**
	Finely grated zest and juice from 1 small **lime**

1	(4-pound) whole **chicken**

DO THIS:

1. To make the aji verde chili sauce, gently heat the olive oil and garlic in a small cast-iron skillet over low heat for 2 to 3 minutes. Once the garlic is fragrant and the oil bubbles, take the skillet off the heat and turn off the stove.

2. Blitz the remaining aji verde chili sauce ingredients in a food processor or blender until well combined, scraping down the sides as necessary. Then, add the garlicky oil and blend until smooth. The sauce can be made ahead of time and kept in a covered container in the refrigerator for a few days.

3. To make the marinade for the chicken, mix together all the marinade ingredients in a small bowl. (This probably goes without saying, but always zest before you juice.) As the ghee in the mixture cools, the marinade will firm up and form a thick paste (unless you're cooking someplace really warm, where ghee never solidifies—in which case I hope you have something cool to drink.)

4. Next, spatchcock the bird. Using kitchen shears, cut out the backbone of the chicken by making parallel cuts along each side of the spine. (Save the backbone to make Bone Broth later.) Open up the bird like a book, and lay it breast-side down. With a sharp knife, make a ½-inch incision in the cartilage of the breast bone, and firmly press down with your hands to flatten the chicken. The splayed-open chicken should now look like the facehugger from *Aliens*.

5. Flip the bird (tee hee!) over, and use your fingers to gently separate the skin of the chicken from the breast and thigh meat to create pockets, making sure not to tear any holes. Spread the marinade under the skin, and rub it all over the outside of the chicken, too.

6. Marinate the chicken in a covered container in the refrigerator for 6 to 24 hours.

7. About an hour before you cook the bird, take it out of the refrigerator and bring it up to room temperature. Preheat your oven to 400°F and place the rack in the upper-middle position. Set a wire rack on top of a foil-lined rimmed baking sheet, and place the chicken skin-side up on the wire rack. Tuck the wing tips behind the breasts.

8. Roast the chicken for 45 minutes or until the breast meat reaches 150°F and the thigh meat hits 170°F as measured by an instant-read thermometer. Take the chicken out of the oven and rest it for 10 minutes before carving.

9. Serve with the aji verde chili sauce on the side.

SPATCHCOCK, SPATCHCOCK, SPATCHCOCK! I LOVE THAT WORD.

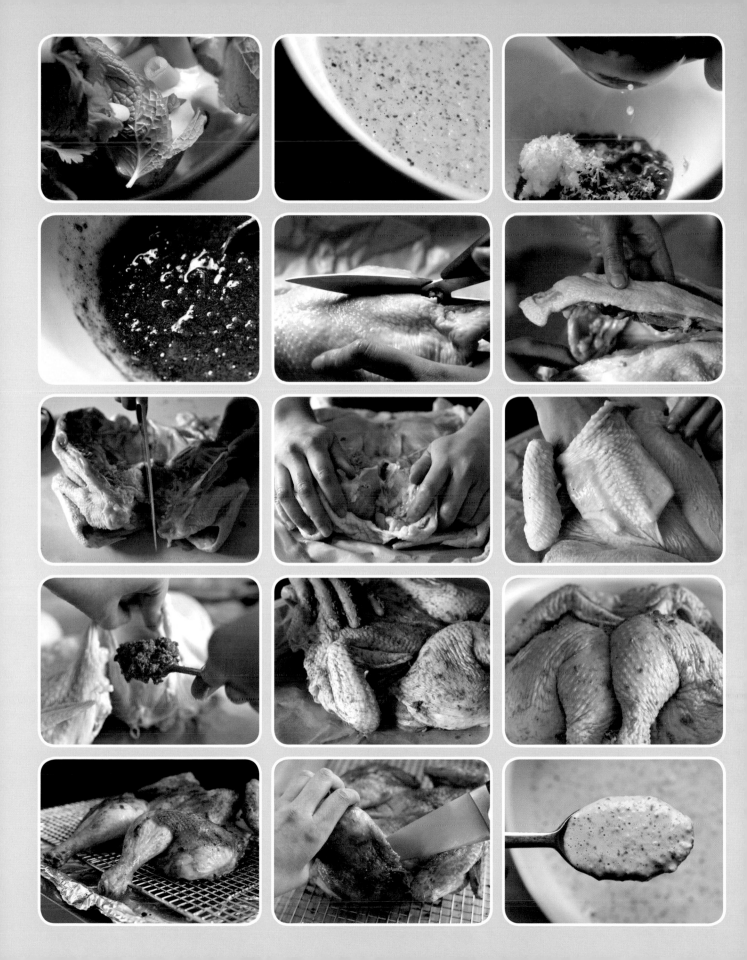

SLOW-ROASTED DUCK LEGS

When it's cooked properly, roast duck is sublime, with thin, crackling-crisp skin and moist, fork-tender meat. This slow-roasted duck is infused with bright, peppery aromatics, and it's a cinch to prepare. Just give the marinade ingredients some time to intensify the flavors of the meat, and pop these duck legs in the oven for a comforting seasonal dish. Serve it up with an autumn salad, and you won't be disappointed.

Makes 4 servings
Hands-on time: 20 minutes
Total time: 2 days

I'M ADDICTED TO DUCK. DOES THAT MAKE ME A QUACKHEAD?

4	**duck legs**
1½	teaspoons **kosher salt**
2	strips **lemon peel**, each approximately ½ inch by 2 inches (use a vegetable peeler!)
10	whole black **peppercorns**
6	**garlic cloves**, smashed and peeled
4	fresh **thyme** sprigs
½	teaspoon **red pepper flakes**
1	tablespoon **duck fat** or fat of choice

DO THIS:

1. Rub the duck legs with salt, and place them skin-side down in a shallow dish. Place the other ingredients except for the duck fat on top of the duck. Cover and marinate the legs for 1 to 2 days in the refrigerator.

2. When you're ready to cook, preheat the oven to 300°F with the rack in the middle position. Melt the duck fat, and use it to grease a baking dish.

3. Place the duck skin-side up in the dish, with the aromatics from the marinade tucked underneath the duck. Don't worry about crowding the duck—it should be a fairly snug fit.

4. Roast the duck legs in the oven for 2 to 3 hours, or until the fat under the skin has rendered, the legs are golden brown, and the meat is tender.

5. Discard all the aromatics except for the garlic cloves, which can be served with the duck. If the legs aren't browned to your liking, melt some more duck fat in a cast-iron skillet over medium heat, and fry the legs for a few minutes until the skin's golden and crisp. Serve immediately.

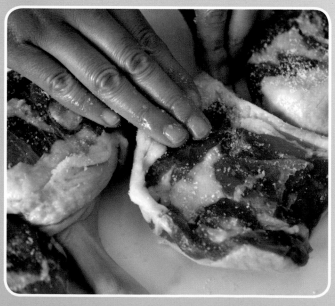
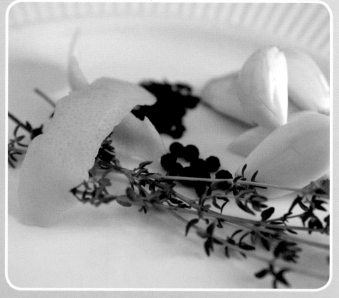

SERVE THIS WITH A SIMPLE SALAD OF WATERCRESS AND FRISÉE, SEASONED WITH SALT AND PEPPER, AND TOSSED WITH CITRUS VINAIGRETTE (PAGE 59)!

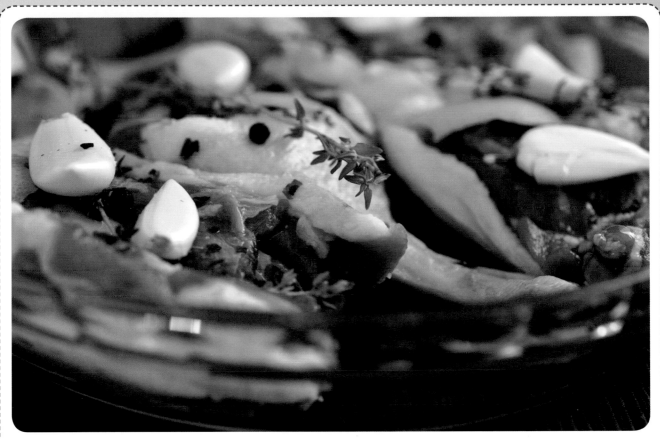

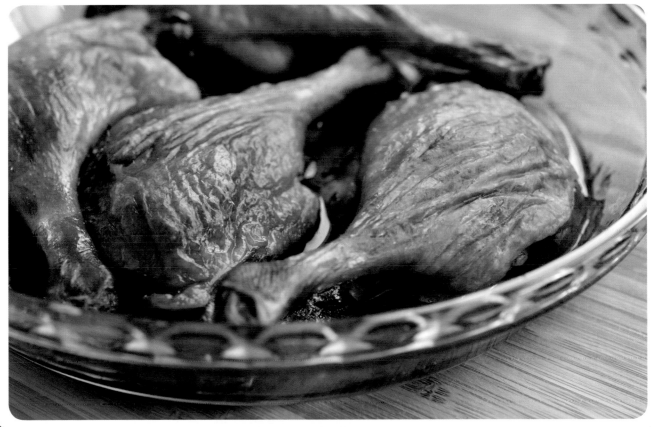

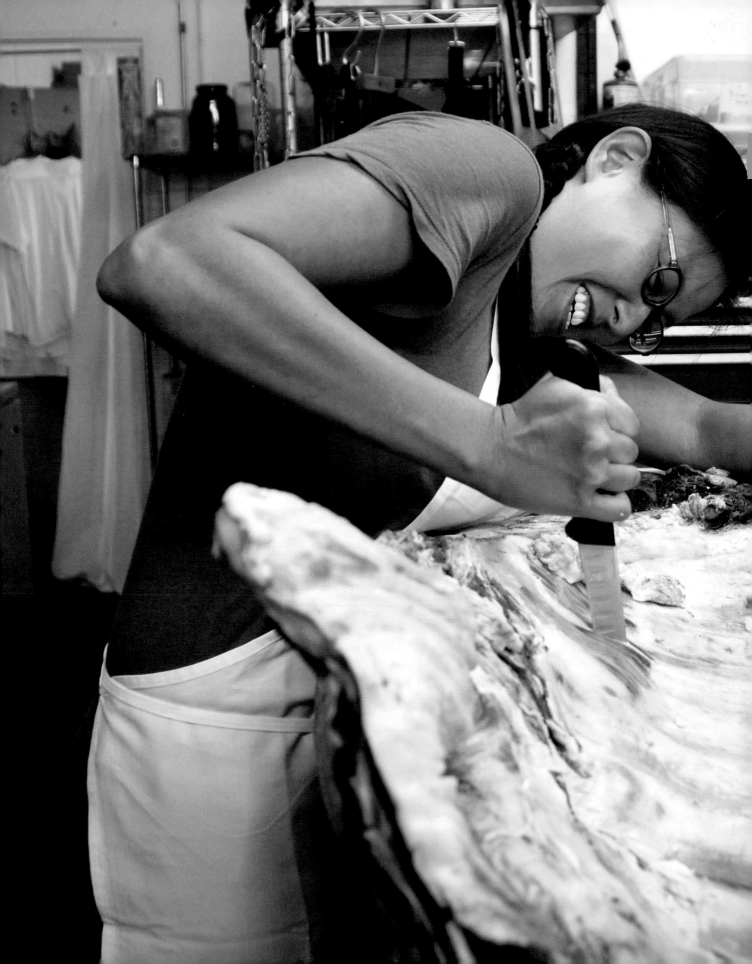

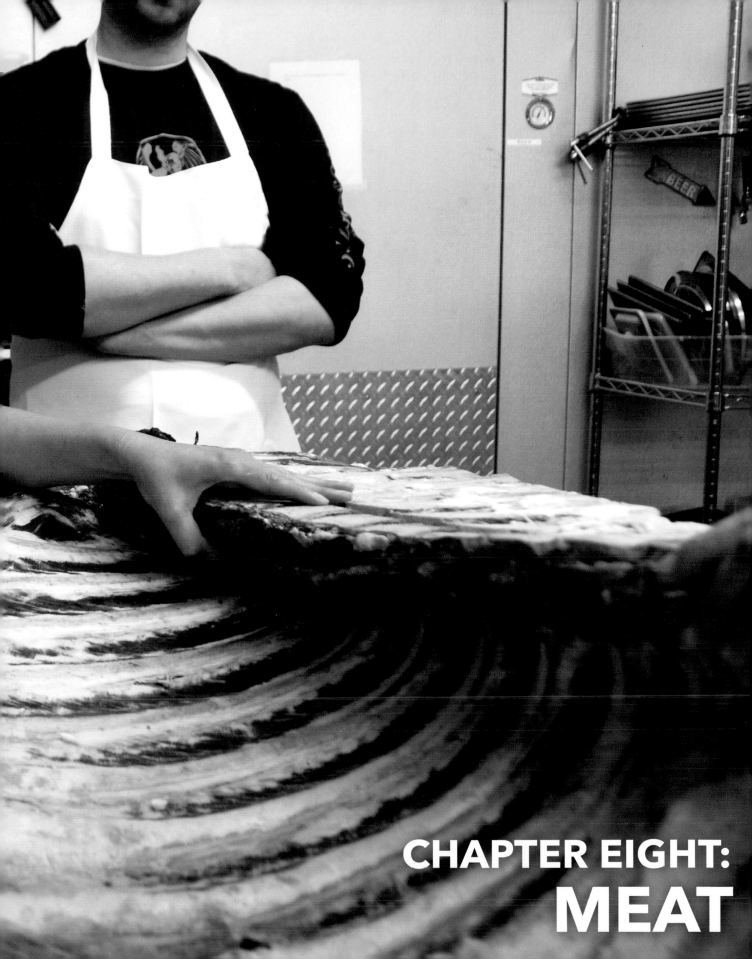

CHAPTER EIGHT:
MEAT

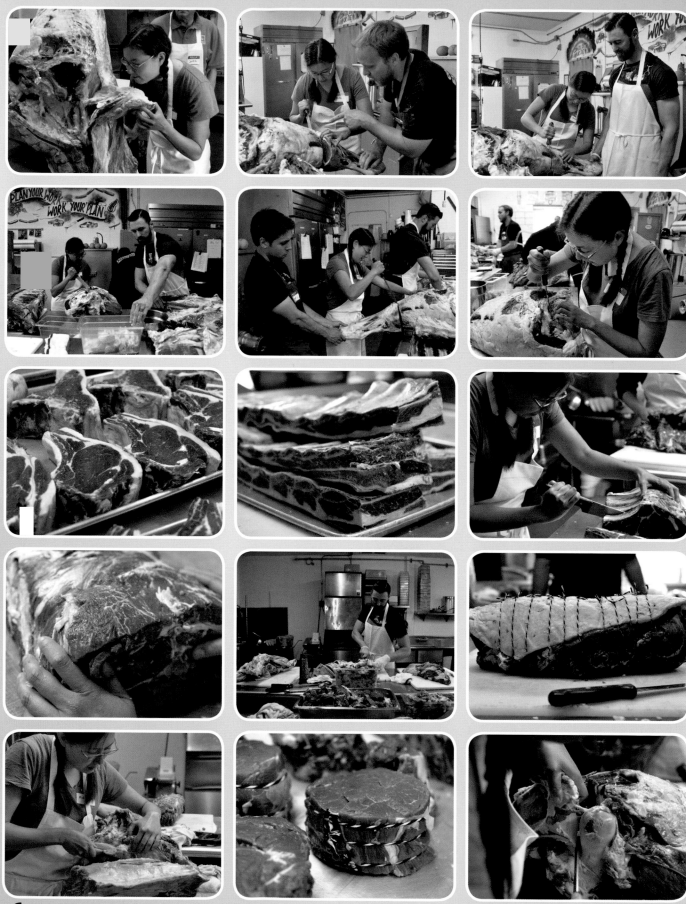

RYAN FARR AND KENT SCHOBERLE OF SAN FRANCISCO'S 4505 MEATS TAUGHT ME AND MY PAL DALLAS HOW TO BUTCHER A STEER!

I LOVE ANIMALS.
THEY'RE DELICIOUS.

Scientists agree: humans evolved to eat meat. So for optimal health, I include a healthy amount of it in my diet.

Eating meat isn't just good for you; it can be ethical and sustainable, too. Just try to stick to the highest possible standards that your pocketbook can accommodate. Buy your meat from local farms and farmer's markets, or join a cowshare or a Community Supported Agriculture (CSA) program that offers farm-fresh pick-ups or deliveries. After all, the food we put in our bodies has a huge impact not just on our health, but on our environment as well.

If you're prioritizing your protein purchases, put grass-fed, sustainably raised beef, lamb, goat, and venison at the top of your list. Whenever possible, make sure your grass-fed meat is grass-finished, too; otherwise, "grass-fed" could just mean that the animal was fed the unholy triumvirate of soy, wheat, and corn as soon as it was old enough to be crammed into a feedlot at a factory farm.

The meat of grass-fed ruminants can be pricy, so when you spot a sale or discount, stock up on as many different cuts as you can haul away in the trunk of your car: steaks, ribs, roasts—you name it. Tougher cuts are cheaper, and can be slow-cooked or pressure-cooked to tender perfection. Make sure you have plenty of ground beef, too. It can come in handy when you need to whip up a quick dinner.

Pigs aren't "grass-fed" because they aren't vegetarians, but with a bit of extra effort, you can find pasture-raised pork. Avoid pigs that are raised on garbage and chemical injections, and get the ones that eat what nature intended.

Do your best to get the good stuff, but if you're stuck with conventionally-raised, grain-fed meat, don't freak out. Just choose lean cuts and trim off the excess fat. (The fat profile of factory-farmed animals is less than optimal.)

One final tip: get yourself an extra freezer. A big one.

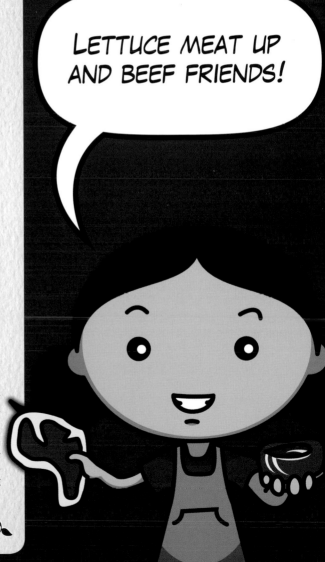

LETTUCE MEAT UP AND BEEF FRIENDS!

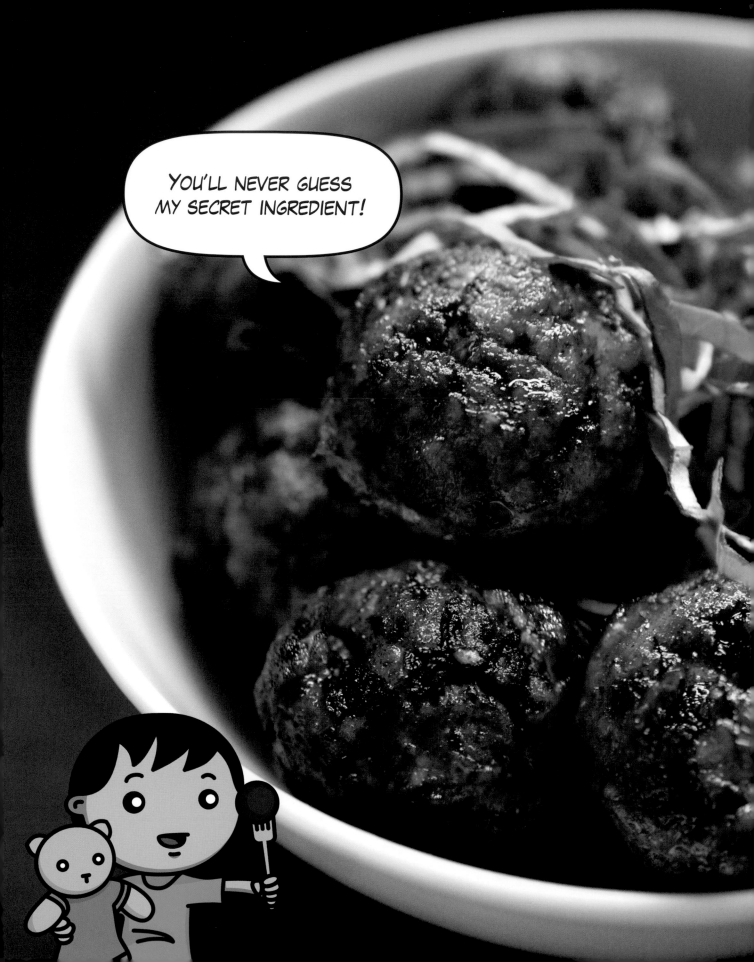

POLPETTE DI VITELLO

Makes 48 meatballs
Hands-on time: 30 minutes
Total time: 30 minutes

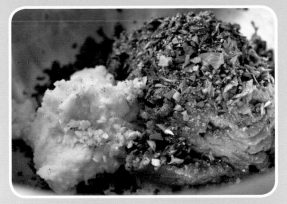

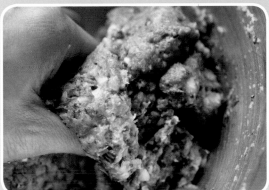

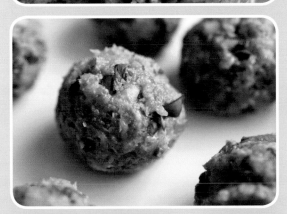

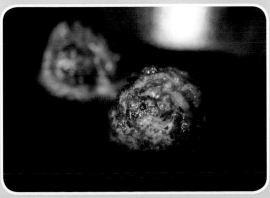

Close your eyes and imagine a meatball. Are you picturing a humongous orb of "imbreaded" meat drowning in spaghetti sauce? Well, don't. Classic Italian *polpette* are typically enjoyed as-is—no toppings required. Rather than relying on tomato sauce to punch up the flavor, these veal meatballs are seasoned with fragrant spices and subtle herbs. Sure, you can still enjoy *polpette* with some marinara sauce on the side, but the meatballs themselves are the main attraction.

Unfortunately, traditional *polpette* recipes call for adding milk-soaked bread crumbs as a moist, spongy binding agent. What are gluten-free, dairy-free cooks to do? Many turn to almond flour or coconut flour as a substitute for the bread crumbs, but more often than not, they wind up with dry, dense, overcooked lumps of meat.

Luckily, I've uncovered the secret to making tender meatballs without bread: mashed cauliflower. A bit of mash binds the ingredients together while adding just the right amount of lightness. But don't tell anyone, or I'll track you down.

2	pounds **ground veal**
½	cup minced fresh **basil**
½	cup minced fresh **Italian parsley**
2	teaspoons **kosher salt**
1	teaspoon freshly ground **black pepper**
1	cup **Garlic Mashed Cauliflower** (page 155)
½	medium **yellow onion**, finely minced
2	**garlic cloves**, minced
1	cup **ghee**, for frying
½	cup **marinara sauce**, warmed (optional)

DO THIS:

1. Using your hands, gently combine the veal, basil, parsley, salt, pepper, mashed cauliflower, onion, and garlic in a large bowl. Form the meat mixture into 1½-inch balls.

2. Heat the ghee in a large skillet over medium-high heat. Make sure there's enough oil to reach halfway up the meatballs. Once the oil's hot and shimmering, fry the meatballs, turning occasionally, for 2 minutes or until cooked through.

3. Transfer to a wire rack to drain off any extra oil, and serve with marinara sauce, if desired.

IN ABRUZZO, MEATBALLS ARE ROLLED OUT TO THE SIZE OF MARBLES, ABOUT ½ INCH IN DIAMETER. THEY'RE CALLED POLPETTINE (NOT TO BE CONFUSED WITH PALPATINE, THE EVIL EMPEROR FROM STAR WARS).

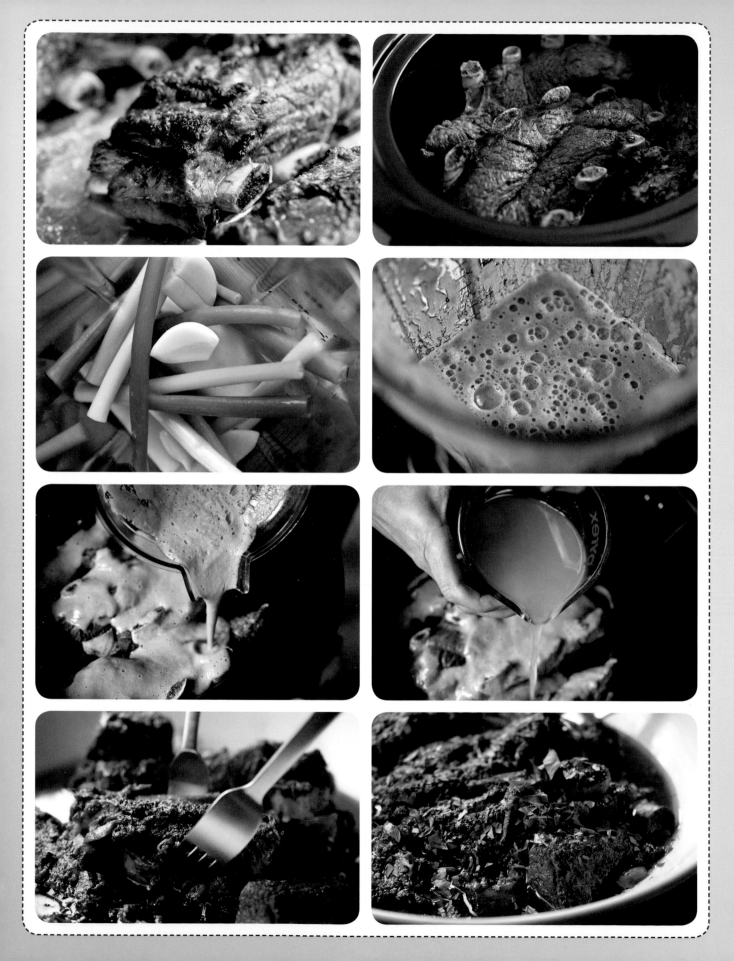

SLOW COOKER KOREAN SHORT RIBS

After stumbling home in the too-bright morning sunshine from another graveyard shift at the hospital, I just want to spend time with my little guys and then face-plant into my pillow. Prepping for dinner is the last thing on my mind. Fortunately, I can quickly toss some ingredients into my slow cooker and pass out, confident that I'll wake up to the smell of a simmering pot of slow-cooked, Asian-spiced short ribs.

This recipe was inspired by the smarty-pants over at America's Test Kitchen, who—in the course of making a similar dish—found that searing the meat in advance isn't strictly necessary. The flavors will develop and intensify on their own in the slow cooker, so if you're short on time, skip the browning and just throw everything into your slow cooker.

Makes 4 servings
Hands-on time: 15 minutes
Total time: 10 hours

6	pounds bone-in English-style **beef short ribs**
	Kosher salt
	Freshly ground **black pepper**
1	medium **pear** or **Asian pear**, peeled, cored, and chopped medium
½	cup **coconut aminos**
6	**garlic cloves**, smashed and peeled
3	**scallions**, chopped medium
1	(1-inch) piece fresh **ginger**, peeled and cut into coins
2	teaspoons Paleo-friendly **fish sauce**
1	tablespoon **apple cider vinegar**
1	cup **Bone Broth** (page 104) or stock of choice
¼	cup minced fresh **cilantro**

YOU MAY WANT TO MAKE THIS DISH AHEAD OF TIME AND STORE IT IN YOUR FRIDGE. DURING THE COOKING PROCESS, THE SHORT RIBS WILL RELEASE A TON OF FAT INTO THE GRAVY, WHICH YOU CAN EASILY REMOVE WHEN THE CHILLED FAT HARDENS.

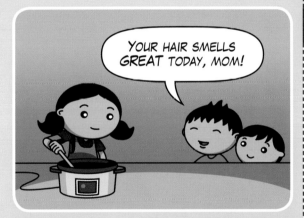

YOUR HAIR SMELLS GREAT TODAY, MOM!

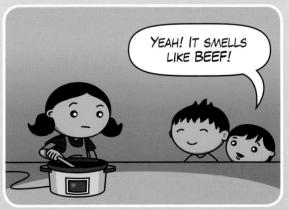

YEAH! IT SMELLS LIKE BEEF!

DO THIS:

1. Arrange an oven rack 4 to 6 inches from the heating element, and preheat the broiler.

2. Generously season the short ribs with salt and pepper, and lay the ribs bone-side up on a foil-lined baking sheet. Broil the ribs for 5 minutes, and then flip and broil for an additional 5 minutes or until browned on both sides.

3. Stack the ribs in a single layer in the slow cooker. You may need to lay them on their sides to fit 'em all in.

4. Toss the pear, coconut aminos, garlic, scallions, ginger, fish sauce, and vinegar in a blender and purée until smooth. Pour the sauce evenly over the ribs, and add the broth to the pot. Cover the slow cooker and set it to low. Cook the ribs for 9 to 11 hours.

5. When you're ready to eat, transfer the meat from the slow cooker to a serving platter. After 5 minutes, you can ladle the fat off the surface of the braising liquid if you wish. Adjust the seasoning with salt and pepper to taste, and pour a cup of the sauce over the ribs. Garnish with cilantro and serve the remaining sauce on the side.

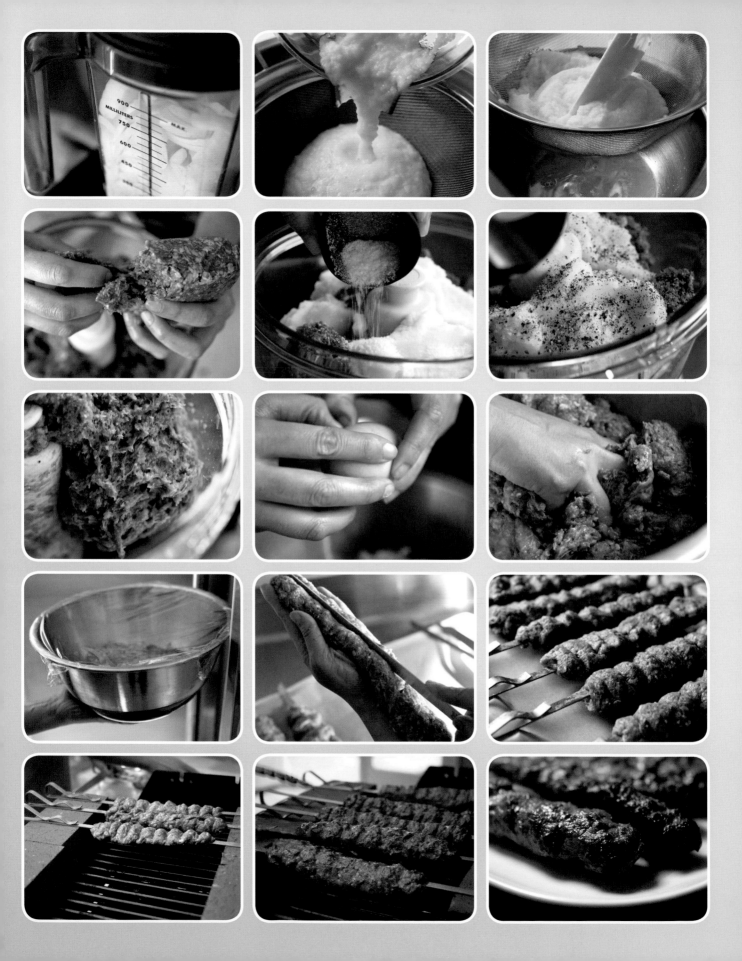

KABOB KOOBIDEH

Persian in origin, *kabob koobideh* was originally prepared by using a wooden mallet to hammer seasoned meat on a flat stone and cooking it on skewers. Modern versions are a tad less smash-tastic, but just as juicy, tender, and delicious. If you've got some ground beef or lamb in the fridge, these meat sticks are a fantastic change of pace. Just be sure to thoroughly knead the mixture of meat and finely minced onions, and use flat metal skewers (at least ⅜ inch wide) so these delicate kabobs will hold together and cook evenly.

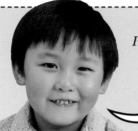

Makes 6 kabobs
Hands-on time: 30 minutes
Total time: 4½ hours

MEAT ON A STICK!

- 2 medium **yellow onions**, roughly chopped
- 2 pounds **ground beef**
- 2 teaspoons **kosher salt**
-    Freshly ground **black pepper**
- 1 large **egg**
- 1 teaspoon ground **sumac** (optional)

DO THIS:

1. Purée the onions in a blender until it resembles an onion slushy. Spoon the onions into a fine-mesh sieve set over a bowl to drain off the liquid. Reserve the liquid in a bowl.

2. Add the beef, drained onions, salt, and several grinds of pepper to the work bowl of a large food processor fitted with a chopping blade. Pulse until the ingredients are well incorporated.

3. Transfer the meat to a large bowl and mix in the egg. Squeeze the mixture between your fingers and knead until the texture is tacky. Refrigerate the meat for at least 4 hours and up to 12 hours.

4. When you're ready to cook the kabobs, preheat your grill to high. Line a rimmed baking sheet with parchment paper.

5. Divide the meat into 6 portions. Wetting your hands with the reserved onion water or tap water will keep the raw meat from sticking to your hands. Grab a portion of meat and wrap it around the skewer. Squeeze the meat around the skewer to form a long tube. "Scissor" the meat with your fingers to form rippled bite-size segments.

6. Lay the finished kabobs on the baking sheet. With the ends of the skewers resting on the rims of the baking sheet, the meat should stay suspended. You can cover and refrigerate the kabobs ahead of time until you're ready to cook.

7. Place two (or more) bricks on the grill so that you can suspend the kabobs between them. Don't rest the meat directly on the grates; otherwise, it'll stick, and you'll be sad. *Waaah.*

8. Flip the kabobs every couple of minutes to ensure even cooking. Be careful not to cook them too long on one side, or the kabobs may sag, split, and fall. (Which, once again, will make you want to weep.) The kabobs'll be done cooking in 8 to 10 minutes, depending on the heat of the grill.

9. Carefully slide the kabobs off the skewers and dust with sumac (if desired) before serving. By the way, *kabob koobideh* pairs wonderfully with Slow-Roasted Tomatoes (page 38), Caramelized Onions (page 38), and Easy Cauliflower "Rice" (page 156).

NO SKEWERS? NO GRILL? NO PROBLEM.

Fancy tools are fun, but these kabobs are just as tasty when broiled in the oven. Here's how you can do it:

Instead of using skewers, carefully place the kabobs on a greased wire rack atop a foil-lined baking sheet. Broil the kabobs 6 inches from the heat source for 3 to 4 minutes on each side. Easy, right?

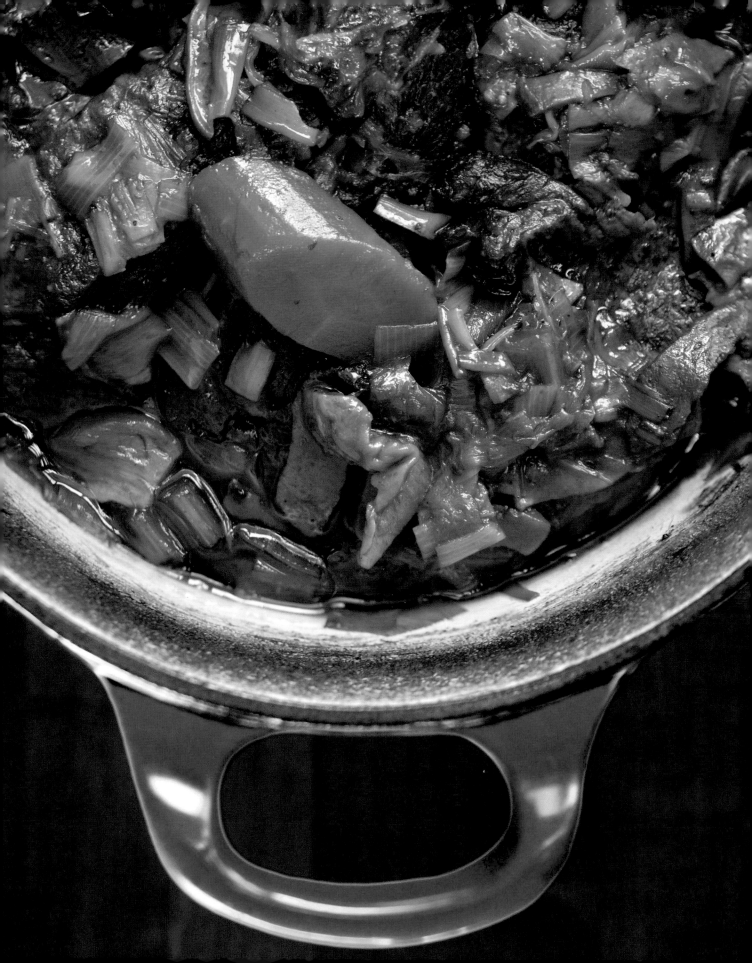

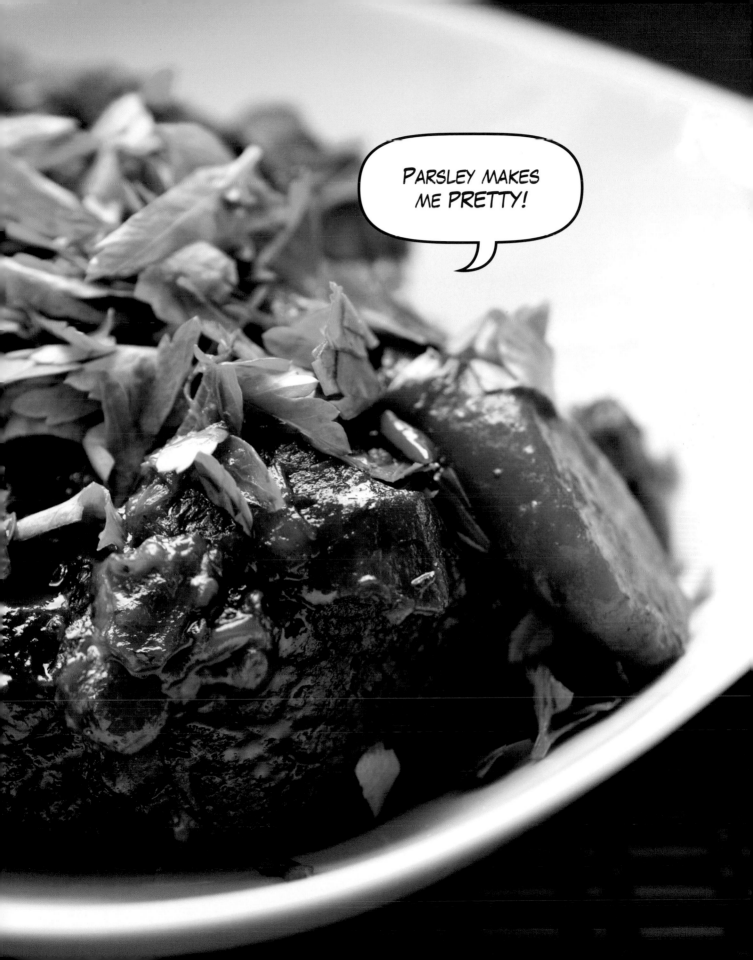

YANKEE POT ROAST

I love that there's nothing fussy about Yankee pot roast. With roots in nineteenth-century New England, this one-pot comfort meal has never gone out of style. The basic formula has remained unchanged since the 1880s: sear off a cheap, tough cut of meat, and then slowly braise it with aromatics and broth until the roast is succulent and tender. Of course, that doesn't mean our palates have to be stuck in the past. My version adds modern flair to this timeless classic, with a sweet balsamic reduction and bursts of umami that transcend eras and tastes. Mark my words: this ain't your great-great-great-great-grandmother's pot roast.

Makes 6 servings
Hands-on time: 30 minutes
Total time: 4 hours

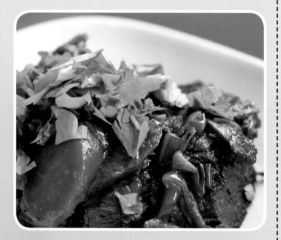

- **1** (3½-pound) boneless **beef chuck-eye roast**
- **Kosher salt**
- Freshly ground **black pepper**
- **2** tablespoons **ghee** or fat of choice, divided
- **3** **leeks**, white and light green ends only, cleaned, trimmed, and thinly sliced
- **2** **celery stalks**, chopped medium
- **2** medium **carrots**, chopped medium
- **2** **garlic cloves**, smashed and peeled
- **1** tablespoon **tomato paste**
- **¼** cup **balsamic vinegar**
- **½** ounce dried **porcini mushrooms**, soaked in hot water for 30 minutes, drained, and chopped medium
- **2** sprigs fresh **thyme**
- **2½** cups **Bone Broth** (page 104) or stock of choice
- **¼** cup chopped fresh **Italian parsley**

DO THIS:

1. Adjust an oven rack to the lower middle position and heat the oven to 275°F. Pat the roast dry with paper towels, and season it with ¾ tablespoon of salt and a few generous grinds of pepper.

2. Melt 1 tablespoon of the ghee in a large Dutch oven over high heat. Once it's sizzling hot, sear the roast until evenly browned, about 3 minutes per side. Transfer the beef to a platter.

3. Lower the heat to medium, and add the remaining tablespoon of ghee. Toss in the leeks, celery, and carrots, and a pinch of salt. Sauté the vegetables until softened, about 5 minutes.

4. Add the garlic and tomato paste, and stir for 30 seconds or until fragrant. Pour in the vinegar and deglaze. (Kitchen newbies: "deglaze" means to scrape the browned goodness—known in French as the *fond*—from the sides and bottom of the pot so that it dissolves in the liquid.)

5. Nestle the roast atop the bed of vegetables on the bottom of the pot. Throw in the mushrooms, tuck in the thyme, and pour in the broth. The liquid should reach at least halfway up the sides of the roast. Bring the contents of the pot up to a simmer, and then remove it from the heat.

6. Place a piece of parchment paper on top of the stew and carefully push down until it touches the surface of the roast. Try not to burn your fingers. Cover the pot and place it in the oven.

7. Roast for 3 to 4 hours or until the meat easily comes apart with a fork. Remove the roast and the vegetables from the pot and tent it with a piece of foil. Boil the remaining liquid over high heat until it's reduced by half. (In other words, make a reduction.) Taste and adjust for seasoning.

8. Slice the beef against the grain and serve with the sauce. Garnish with the Italian parsley.

YOU'LL LOVE THIS WITH GARLIC MASHED CAULIFLOWER (PAGE 155)!

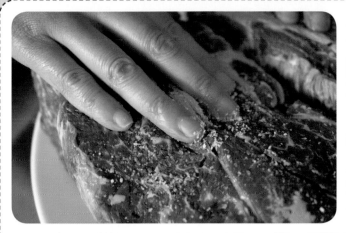

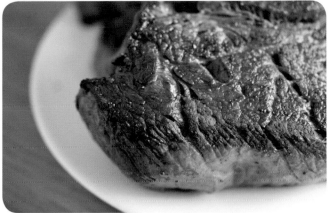

NO-FUSS, NO-MUSS LEEK CLEANING!

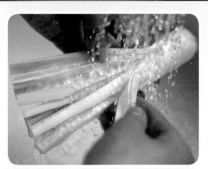

Your leeks may look clean, but there's still plenty of dirt hidden in the folds. Here's how you can quickly and easily clean a leek:

1. Keeping the root end intact, cut the rest of the leek in half lengthwise.

2. Give the leek a quarter-turn, and then slice it lengthwise again (at a right angle from the initial cut)—again, keeping the root end intact.

3. Fan the leaves under running water to release the sand and mud. Finally, flick off the excess water and slice away!

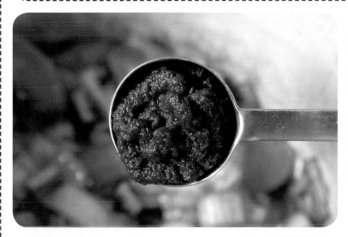

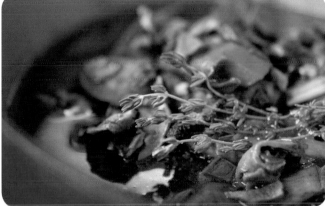

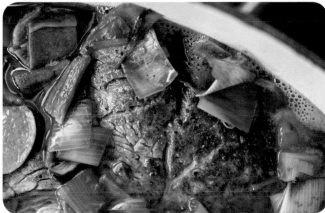

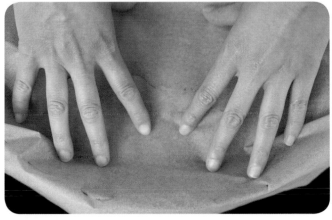

SMASHED STEAK SKEWERS + CHERRY BARBECUE SAUCE

Makes 16 skewers | Hands-on time: 45 minutes | Total time: 45 minutes

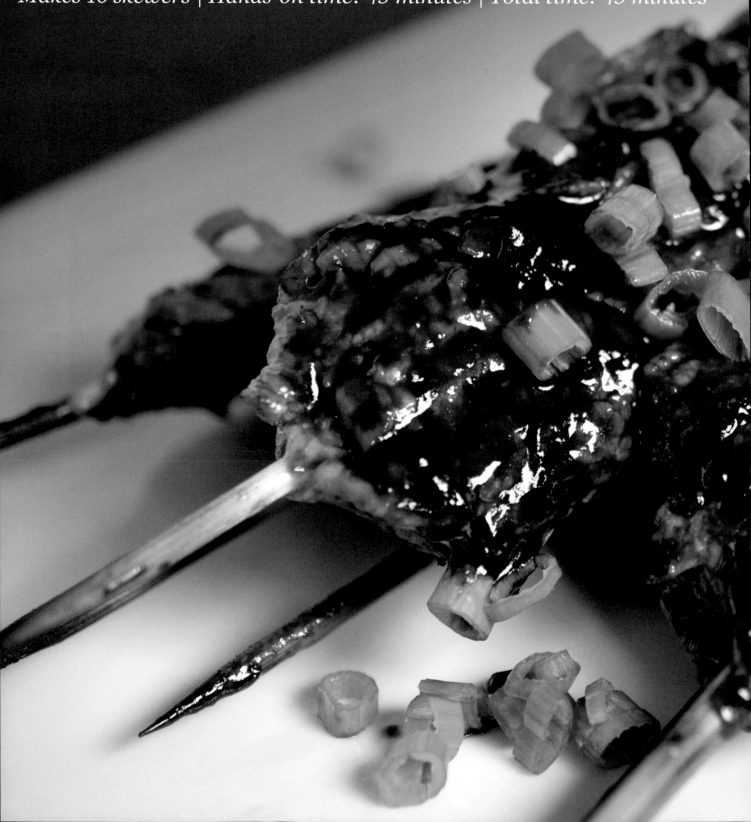

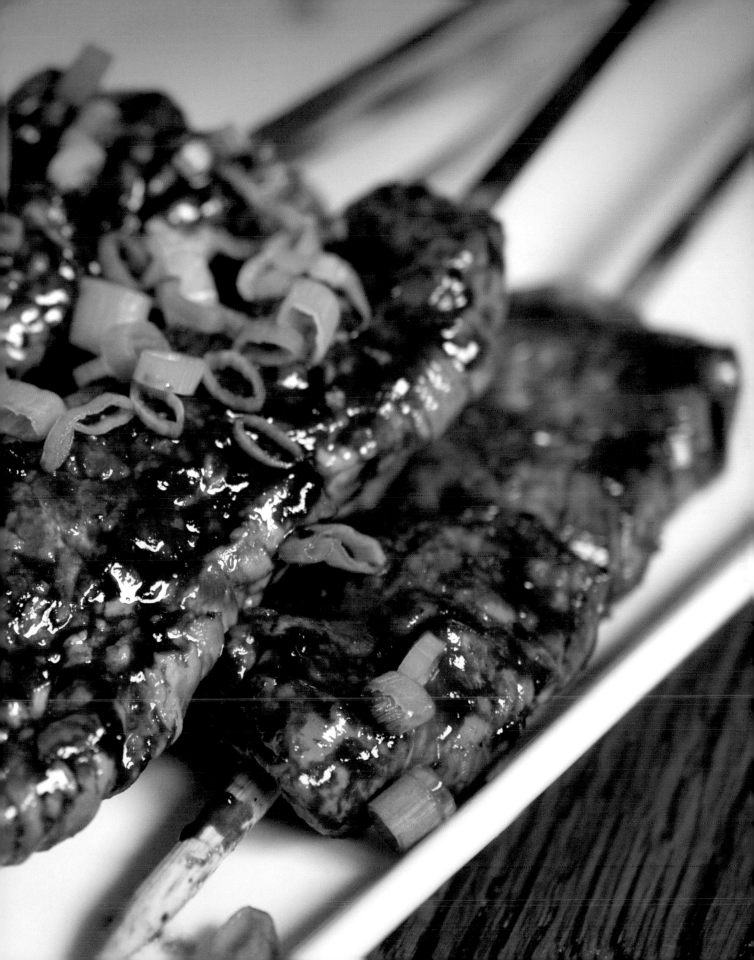

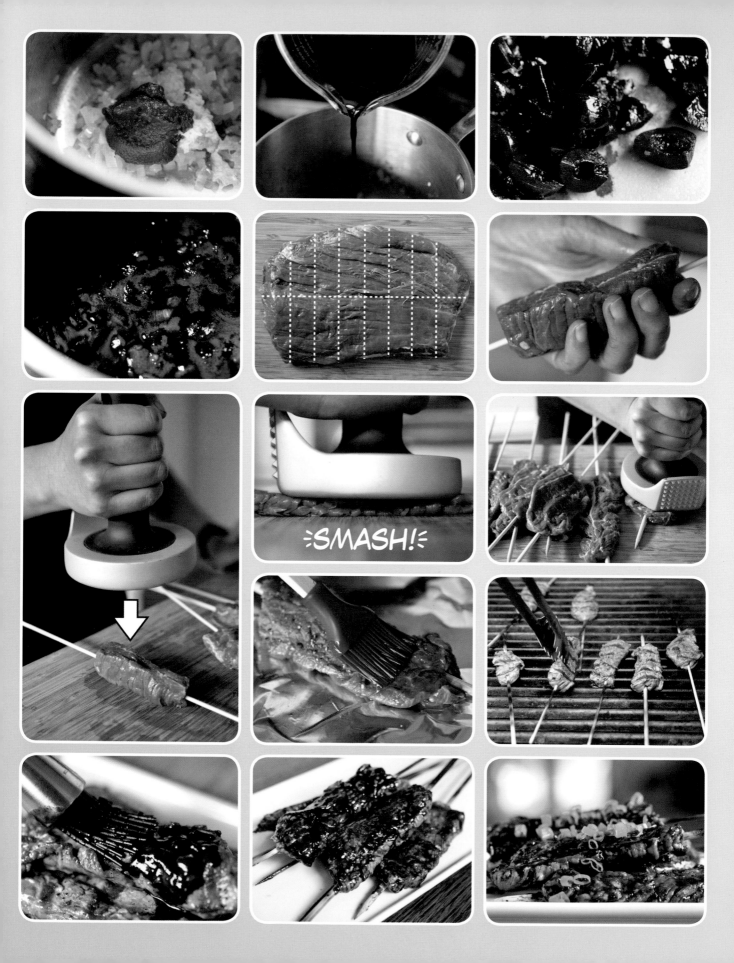

:SMASH!:

I rarely throw around the term "caveman diet." As I mentioned earlier, in our house, we simply try to prioritize whole, nutrient-dense ingredients, and steer clear of foods that tend to be more harmful than healthful. Sadly, I've found that when the word "caveman" is associated with the way we eat, people tend to stare at us like we're absolutely bonkers. (Which we are, but that's beside the point.)

Still, embracing the "caveman" label can be a fun way to get the whole family into the spirit of Paleo chow. Take these smashed steak skewers: they're simple, tasty, and kid-approved. I can't think of anything more primal than speared hunks of meat, flattened with a heavy object and grilled over an open fire—can you?

GET:

Cherry Barbecue Sauce

- 2 teaspoons **ghee** or fat of choice
- ½ cup minced **shallots**
  Kosher salt
- 1 **garlic clove**, minced
- 1 (1-inch) piece fresh **ginger**, peeled and finely grated (about 1 tablespoon)
- 1 tablespoon **tomato paste**
- ¼ cup **coconut aminos**
- ¼ cup **balsamic vinegar**
- ¼ cup **apple juice**
- 10 ounces pitted fresh or frozen dark sweet **cherries**, roughly chopped
  Freshly ground **black pepper**

Smashed Steak Skewers

- 1 (1½-pound) **flank steak**
  Kosher salt
  Freshly ground **black pepper**
- 2 tablespoons melted **ghee** or fat of choice
- ¼ cup **scallions**, thinly sliced (optional)

DO THIS:

1. First, make the barbecue sauce. Melt the ghee over medium heat in a small saucepan. Add the shallots and a pinch of salt and sauté until translucent, about 5 minutes. Stir in the garlic, ginger, and tomato paste, and sauté for 30 seconds until fragrant. Add the coconut aminos, vinegar, apple juice, and cherries, and bring the ingredients to a boil.

2. Lower the heat and simmer for 10 minutes or until the cherry mixture is thickened. While the sauce is simmering, stir occasionally and smush the cherries against the side of the pot.

3. Season the sauce with salt and pepper to taste. Transfer the sauce to a bowl and set aside.

4. Cut the steak in half lengthwise (along the grain). Then, slice the steak in half across the grain, then in fourths, and finally in eighths. You should end up with 16 rectangular pieces of meat. Carefully stab each chunk of meat through the center with a skewer.

5. Now comes the fun part: grab a hefty meat pounder or small cast-iron skillet, and smash each steak skewer until it's about ½ inch thick. Season the beef with salt and pepper, and brush both sides with melted ghee.

6. Fire up your backyard grill, and cook over high heat for 1 to 2 minutes on each side.

7. Rest the meat skewers for 5 to 10 minutes before brushing on the cherry barbecue sauce. A garnish of fresh green scallions is optional, but it can instantly transform this rugged plate of skewers into a more refined dish. Serve immediately.

GRAB SOME NAPKINS 'CAUSE THIS IS GONNA GET MESSY!

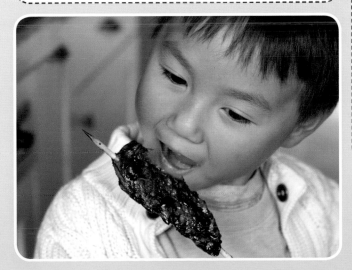

SOUTHWEST COWBOY CHILI

GET:

1	(4-pound) **beef chuck roast**, cut into 2-inch cubes
2	teaspoons **kosher salt**
4	slices **bacon**, cut into ¼-inch pieces
1	medium **yellow onion**, cut into ½-inch dice
2	tablespoons **tomato paste**
¼	cup **ancho chile powder**
2	tablespoons ground **cumin**
1	tablespoon dried **oregano**
2	teaspoons **smoked paprika**
6	cups **Bone Broth** (page 104) or chicken stock, divided
1	ounce **unsweetened chocolate**, shaved
4	**garlic cloves**, minced
	Juice from 1 small **lime**
	Freshly ground **black pepper**
½	medium **white onion**, cut into ¼-inch pieces (optional)
½	cup minced fresh **cilantro** (optional)
½	cup julienned **radishes** (optional)
2	small **limes**, quartered (optional)

Makes 6 servings
Hands-on time: 45 minutes
Total time: 4 hours

During college, Henry and I worked at the same research institute on campus, and every summer, the staff organized a friendly chili cook-off. Most of the participants approached the contest with casual good humor, thinking only of kicking back with bowls of chili and cold bottles of beer in the California sunshine.

But not us. We were in it to win it.

My future husband and I spent days tinkering with our chili, adding and subtracting ingredients until we landed on what we thought was a sure winner: a spicy mélange of meat and peppers…and beans and corn.

And just to be sure that we'd emerge victorious, we badgered some friends into brazenly stuffing the ballot box in our favor. Our chili won by a hair, but it was a hollow victory—and not just because everyone was already on to our vote-rigging scheme. We knew our chili wasn't the best submission.

The true winner was a pot of rich, meaty, no-bean stew, with fork-tender pieces of flavorful chuck roast and just the right balance of salt and heat. It's been twenty years since the contest, but I still dream about that chili. After countless hours in the kitchen, this recipe is the closest I've come to replicating the dish that should've rightfully won that cook-off all those summers ago. If you're anything like me, you won't soon forget this Southwestern-style chili, with its smoky spices and tender chunks of beef.

DO THIS:

1. Preheat the oven to 275°F. In a large bowl, toss the beef with the salt and set aside. Cook the bacon in a large Dutch oven over medium heat. Stir occasionally to ensure even browning. Once it's crisp, transfer the crunchy bacon to a platter with a slotted spoon.

2. Increase the heat to medium-high. In batches, add the beef in a single layer to the bacon drippings in the Dutch oven, and brown the meat on two sides, about 2 minutes per side. Transfer the beef to a plate.

3. Lower the heat to medium, and add the yellow onion and tomato paste. Sauté until the onion is tender and translucent, about 5 minutes. In the meantime, combine the chile powder, cumin, oregano, paprika, and ½ cup of the stock in a small bowl. Mix until smooth, and then stir in the chocolate shavings.

4. When the onion is soft, stir in the garlic and chili-chocolate mixture, and cook for 1 minute or until fragrant. Add the seared beef, cooked bacon, the remaining 5½ cups broth, and the lime juice. Stir well. Increase the heat to high and bring the contents of the Dutch oven up to a boil. Cover, but leave the lid slightly ajar. Place the pot in the oven, and cook for 3 hours or until the meat is fork-tender.

5. Season with salt and pepper, and place the chili in the refrigerator overnight or up to 5 days to enable the flavors to meld. Reheat on the stove, and if desired, top with chopped white onion, cilantro, radishes, and limes.

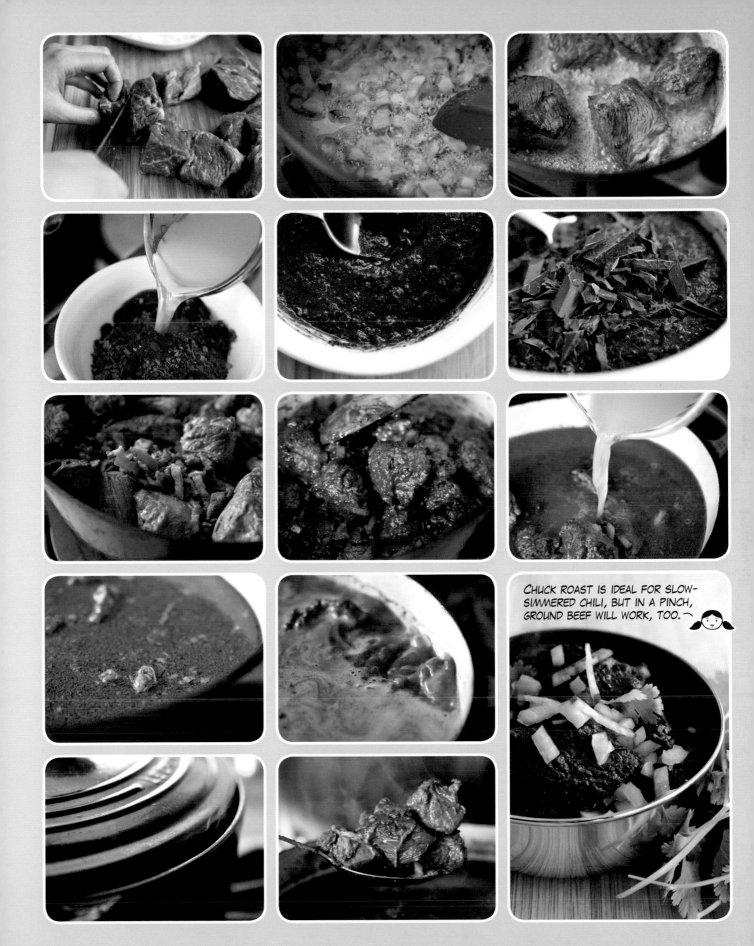

CHUCK ROAST IS IDEAL FOR SLOW-SIMMERED CHILI, BUT IN A PINCH, GROUND BEEF WILL WORK, TOO.

BIG-O BACON BURGERS

Makes 4 burgers | Hands-on time: 30 minutes | Total time: 30 minutes

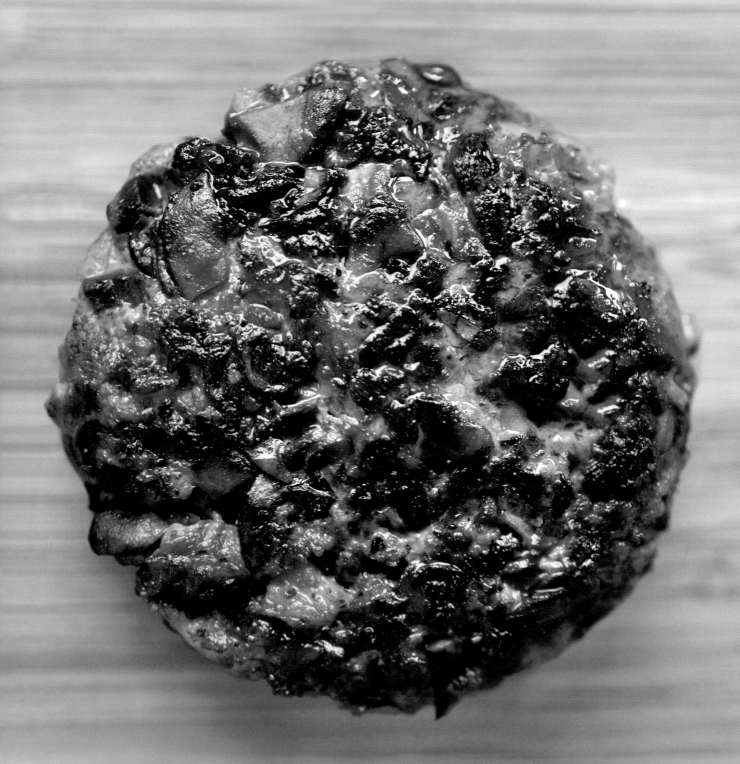

Bacon. Mushrooms. Beef. Dangerously good.

GET:

2	tablespoons **lard** or fat of choice, divided
½	pound **cremini mushrooms,** minced
4	ounces **bacon**, frozen and cross-cut into small pieces
1	pound **ground beef**
1½	teaspoons **kosher salt**
	Freshly ground **black pepper**
1	ripe heirloom **tomato**, sliced
4	**butter lettuce leaves**, rinsed and dried
8	whole **Roasted Portobello Mushrooms** (page 144) (optional)

OPTIONAL TOPPINGS:

- **Slow-Roasted Tomatoes** (page 38)
- **Caramelized Onions** (page 38)
- **Roasted Bell Peppers** (page 39)
- **Paleo Mayonnaise** (page 40)
- **Paleo Sriracha** (page 42)
- **Sriracha Mayonnaise** (page 45)
- **Quick-Pickled Carrot Strings** (page 50)
- **Spicy Pineapple Salsa** (page 55)
- **Holy 'Moly (Easy Guacamole)** (page 51)
- **Paleo Ranch Dressing** (page 62)
- **Louisiana Rémoulade** (page 63)

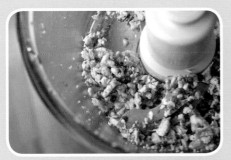 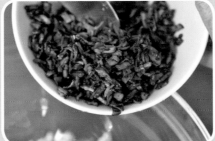 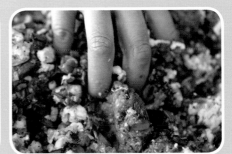

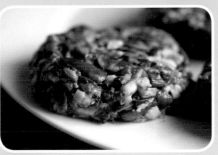 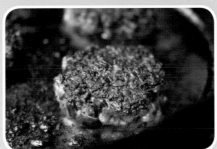 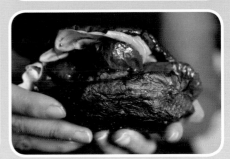

DO THIS:

1. Heat 1 tablespoon of the lard in a cast-iron skillet over medium heat, and sauté the cremini mushrooms until the liquid they release has cooked off. Set aside the cooked mushrooms.

2. Pulse the frozen bacon pieces in a food processor to the consistency of ground meat.

3. In a large bowl, combine the ground beef, bacon, and cremini mushrooms, and season with salt and pepper. Using your hands, gently combine the ingredients. Be careful not to overwork the meat. Divide the mixture into 4 portions (or more, if you're making sliders), and use your hands to flatten each into ¾-inch-thick patties.

4. Melt the remaining tablespoon of lard in a cast-iron skillet over medium heat, and fry up the patties in the hot fat, turning once. Regular-sized (6-ounce) burgers should take about 3 minutes per side; slider burgers should take about 2 minutes per side. The meat inside should be perfectly pink all the way through, and studded with pretty little pieces of smoky bacon and mushrooms.

5. Transfer the patties to a wire rack so that any excess cooking fat can drain off. Wrap each patty in sturdy butter lettuce leaves and serve with tomato slices.

6. Looking for an alternative to hamburger buns? Use Roasted Portobello Mushrooms instead. Oh, and don't forget to load up your burgers with any or all of the suggested toppings above, people.

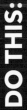 *A WORD TO THE WISE: MAKE MORE THAN YOU THINK YOU'LL NEED!*

LOCO MOCO

As you peer into your fridge, wondering what to make for dinner, your gaze lands on a carton of eggs and some leftovers: Easy Cauliflower "Rice," Big-O Bacon Burgers, gravy from your Slow Cooker Chicken. Jackpot—the stars have aligned. Aloha, loco moco.

Loco moco combines hamburger patties, rice, brown gravy, and fried eggs to create a singularly rib-sticking plate of Hawaiian comfort food. Invented in the 1940s by a Hilo restaurant owner in response to requests from famished teenage customers, loco moco can now be found at virtually every roadside joint on the islands. And with any luck, the Paleo version of this ono grind will soon grace your table, too.

Makes 2 servings
Hands-on time: 15 minutes
Total time: 15 minutes

2   large **eggs**
1   tablespoon **ghee** or fat of choice
     Kosher salt
     Freshly ground **black pepper**
2   cups **Easy Cauliflower "Rice"** (page 156) or **Coconut Pineapple "Rice"** (page 157)
½   cup **Caramelized Onions** (page 38) (optional)
2   **Big-O Bacon Burger** patties (page 226), hot
½   cup gravy from **Slow Cooker Chicken + Gravy** (page 198)

 A FUN GARNISH: CHOPPED NORI AND A PINCH OF CRUSHED RED PEPPER FLAKES!

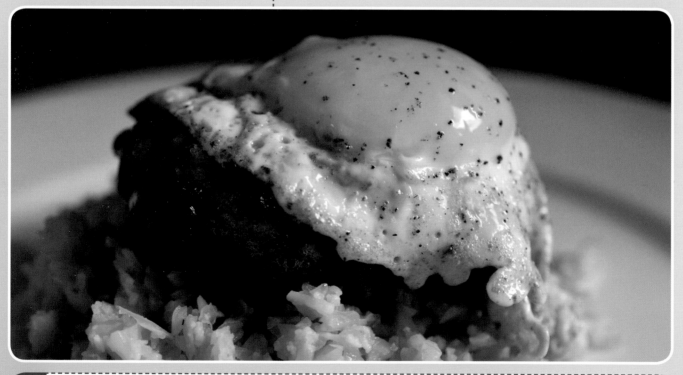

DO THIS:

1. Break the eggs into a bowl. Heat the ghee in a skillet over medium heat. Once it's sizzling hot, gently pour in the eggs. As the eggs cook, season them with salt and pepper.

2. Fry the eggs to your desired doneness. I prefer firm whites and runny yolks, so I like to cook my eggs for 1 minute before flipping and cooking them for about 2 minutes more.

3. Divide the reheated "rice" onto 2 plates, and if desired, top with a mound of warm caramelized onions. Place a hot burger patty atop each plate of rice, and spoon on some gravy. Top with a fried egg before serving.

ROAST BEAST

When it comes to properly cooking meats, I have notoriously high standards. I want my steaks and roasts to be perfectly pink and medium-rare from stem to stern—a result that's difficult to accomplish without a sous-vide cooker. (This, of course, explains my obsession with my temperature-regulated water oven.)

But sous vide isn't the only game in town. Ryan Farr of San Francisco's 4505 Meats—who once spent an entire day patiently teaching me how to butcher a steer—is an advocate of slow, low-temperature roasting. There's no need to purchase any counter-hogging equipment; with an oven and an in-oven thermometer, anyone can transform any big cut of meat into juicy, perfectly cooked protein.

Don't believe me? Check out how easy it is to make roast beef (or *beast*, if you prefer) using Ryan's method.

Makes 6 servings
Hands-on time: 15 minutes
Total time: 12 hours

1   (3-pound) **beef eye of round roast**
    Kosher salt
¼   cup **Dukkah** (page 34)
    Freshly ground **black pepper**

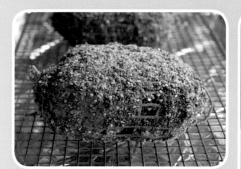

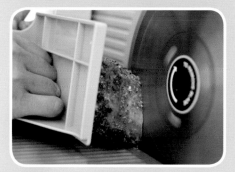

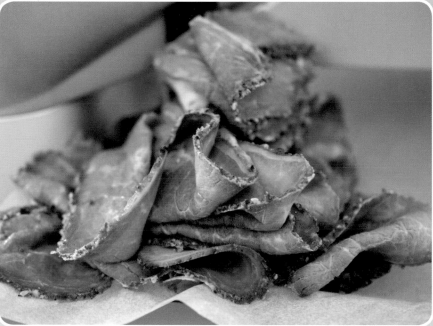

DO THIS:

1. Liberally season the roast with salt, and then refrigerate in a large uncovered bowl overnight. Take the roast out of the fridge 1 hour before you start cooking to bring it up to room temperature.

2. Preheat the oven to 250°F with the rack in the middle position, and place a wire rack atop a foil-lined baking tray. Using paper towels, pat the roast dry. Rub the dukkah onto the surface of the roast, and season liberally with pepper.

3. Place the roast on the wire rack, and put it in the oven. Stick an instant-read, in-oven thermometer probe into the thickest part of the meat, and slow-roast for approximately 1½ hours or until the internal temperature reaches 130 to 132°F for medium-rare (or 140°F for medium).

4. Set the oven to broil, and adjust the rack so that the meat is about 4 inches from the heating element. Broil for 1 minute, and then flip the roast over and broil the other side for 1 more minute.

5. Transfer the roast to a plate, and tent with foil. Rest the meat for 15 minutes before slicing.

I'M OBSESSED WITH MY DELI SLICER, BUT A SHARP KNIFE AND A STEADY HAND ARE JUST AS GOOD!

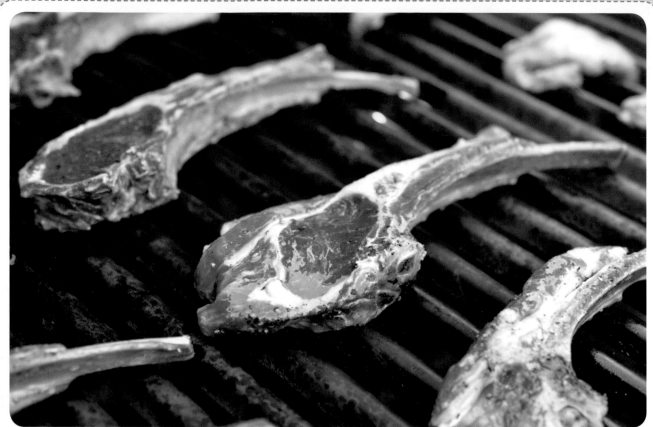

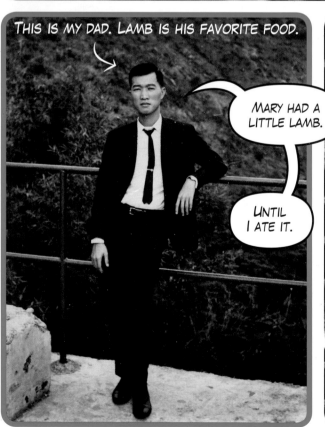

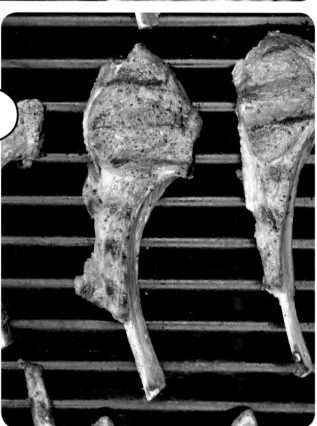

GRILLED LAMB CHOPS
+ MINT CHIMICHURRI

Makes 4 servings | Hands-on time: 30 minutes | Total time: 1 hour

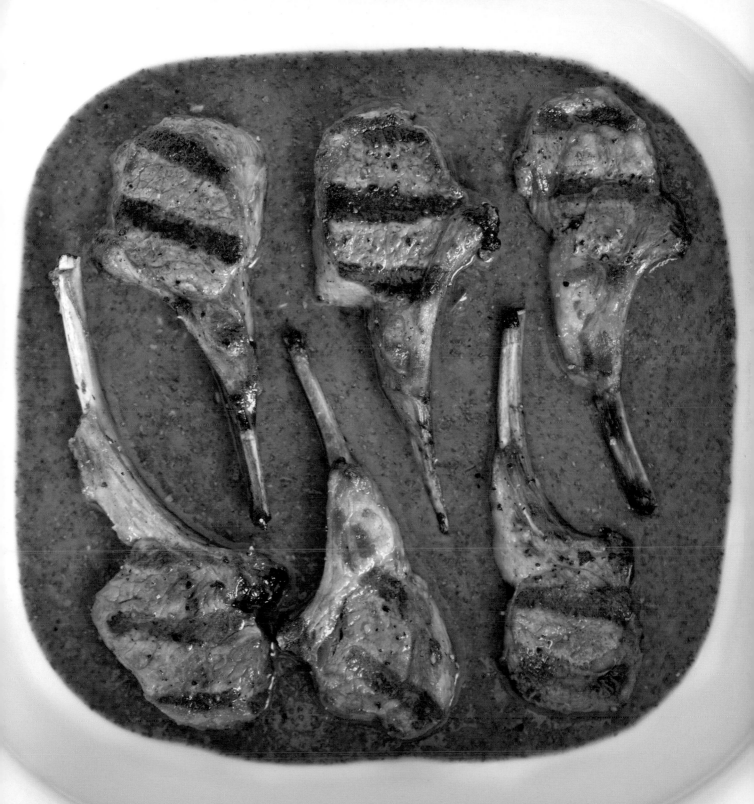

The beauty of this recipe is that you don't have to waste precious hours of your life marinating these lamb chops before it's time to cook. Just pick up a couple of racks of lamb on your way home from work, and in about an hour, you'll have a platter of zesty chops ready for your hungry clan. The secret? By resting your grilled lamb in a pool of minty chimichurri, the meat'll soak up all the finger-lickin' flavors in no time at all.

GET:

Grilled Lamb Chops

Kosher salt
16 **lamb rib chops**, frenched
Freshly ground **black pepper**
2 tablespoons **ghee** or fat of choice, melted

Mint Chimichurri

1 cup fresh **parsley**, chopped
½ cup fresh **mint**, chopped
¼ cup minced **shallots**
¼ cup **balsamic vinegar**
1 tablespoon salt-packed **capers**, soaked, rinsed, drained, and minced
1 teaspoon minced **garlic cloves**
¼ teaspoon crushed **red chile flakes**
Freshly ground **black pepper**
½ cup **extra-virgin olive oil**

DO THIS:

1. Salt the chops on both sides and bring them up to room temperature on the counter while you're making the chimichurri.

2. Put all the chimichurri ingredients except the olive oil into a food processor or blender, and pulse until the contents are roughly chopped. Then, resume pulsing while adding the olive oil in a steady stream. Once a smooth chimichurri forms, pour it into a large, deep dish than can fit all of the lamb chops.

3. Pat the chops dry with a paper towel and season with pepper. Brush with melted ghee.

4. Set a gas grill to medium-high or build a medium-hot fire in a charcoal grill. (No grill? Use a cast-iron skillet over medium heat.) Cook the chops for 2 to 3 minutes on each side or until the lamb reaches your desired doneness. Place the chops directly into the chimichurri, and toss to coat well. Rest the chops for 10 minutes before serving.

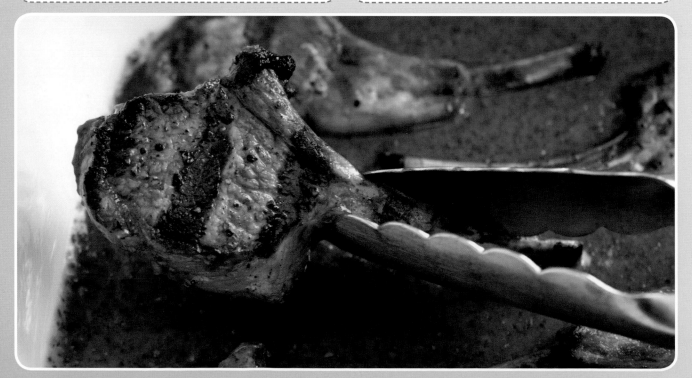

MY KIDDOS CALL 'EM LAMB LOLLIPOPS!

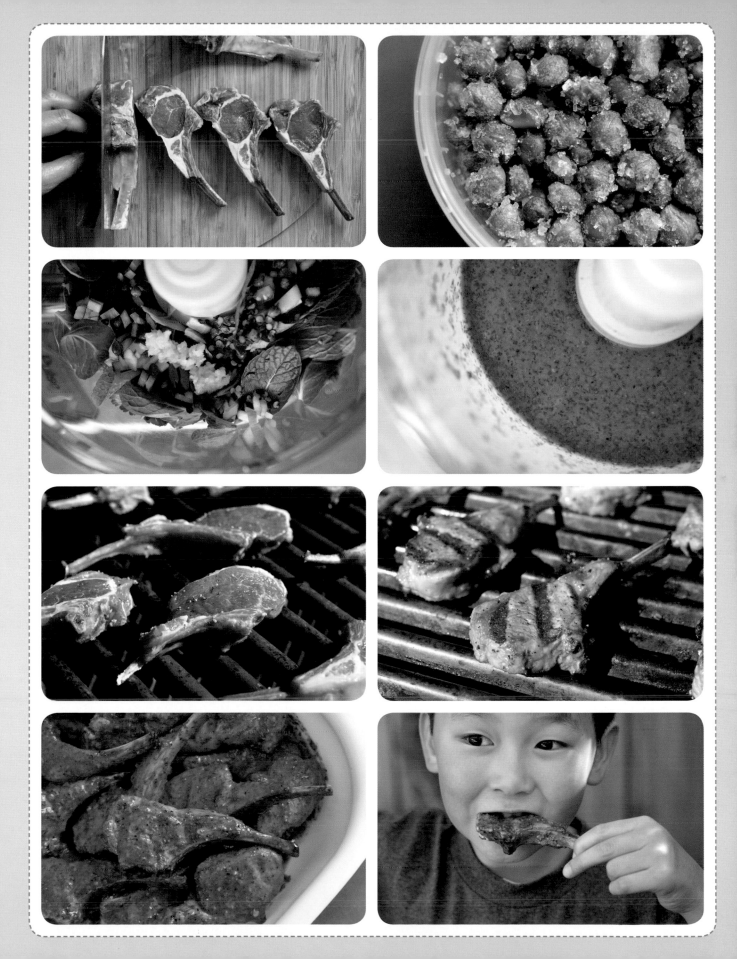

SLOW COOKER KALUA PIG

Makes 8 servings | Hands-on time: 10 minutes | Total time: 16 hours

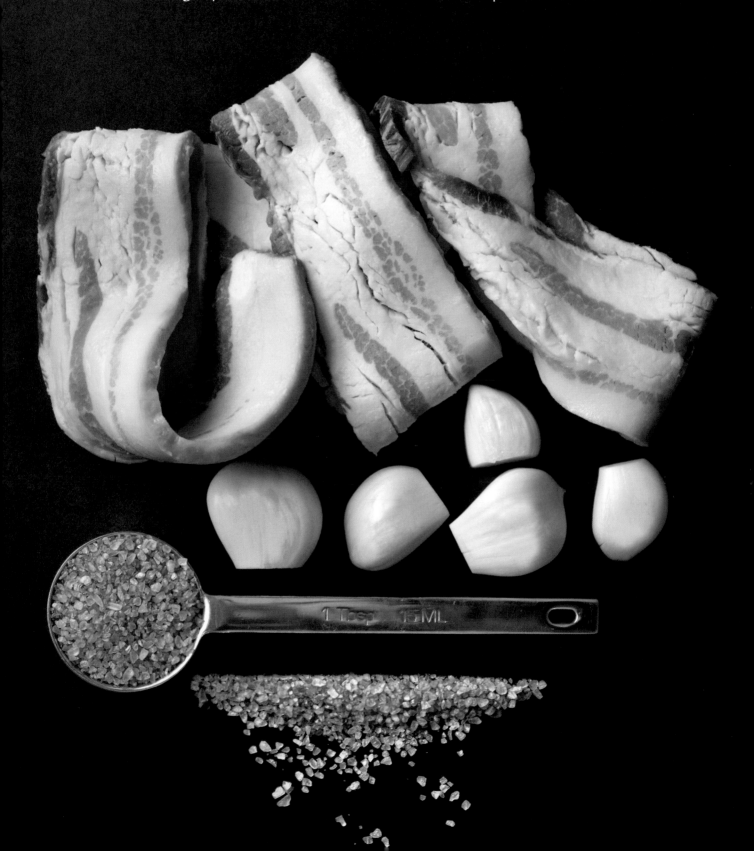

Once or twice a year, our family decamps to Hawaii—our home away from home. I love everything about the islands: the people, the pace, the climate, the beaches, the sunsets, the food.

Foremost among the Hawaiian dishes I crave? Kalua pig.

Often the headlining dish in a lu'au, kalua pig is the epitome of slow-roasted porky goodness. And I do mean *slooow*.

To make kalua pig the old school way, you first have to dig an *imu*—a big underground pit oven—and build a fire in it. Into the imu goes a whole pig, stuffed with hot volcanic rocks and wrapped in ti and banana leaves. The pig (*pua'a* in Hawaiian) is usually enveloped by chicken wire, too, so that once the pork is cooked and ready for removal, the fall-apart-tender meat stays together. The pua'a is then covered by burlap, a tarp, and a mound of dirt. Eight to ten hours of slow roasting (and a good amount of shoveling) later, dinner is served.

But something tells me that your local fire marshal is less than enthusiastic about you excavating part of your backyard so you can bury and cook a pig in it. So to keep you out of trouble, here's a much less labor-intensive recipe for succulent, Hawaiian-style kalua pig. All you need are a few strips of bacon, a pork roast, Hawaiian sea salt, a slow cooker, and a little patience. The slow cooker helps retain all the juices of the meat, producing a roast pork that's ridiculously tender and flavorful.

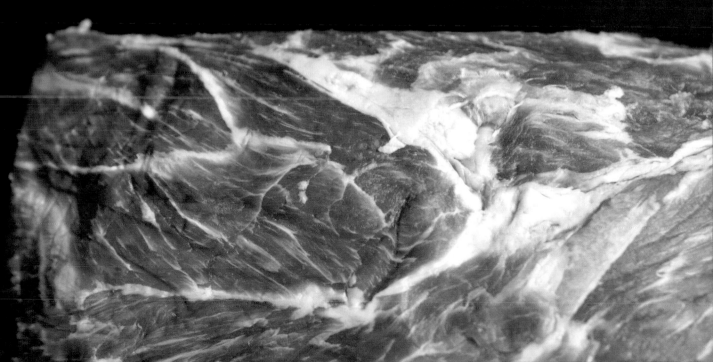

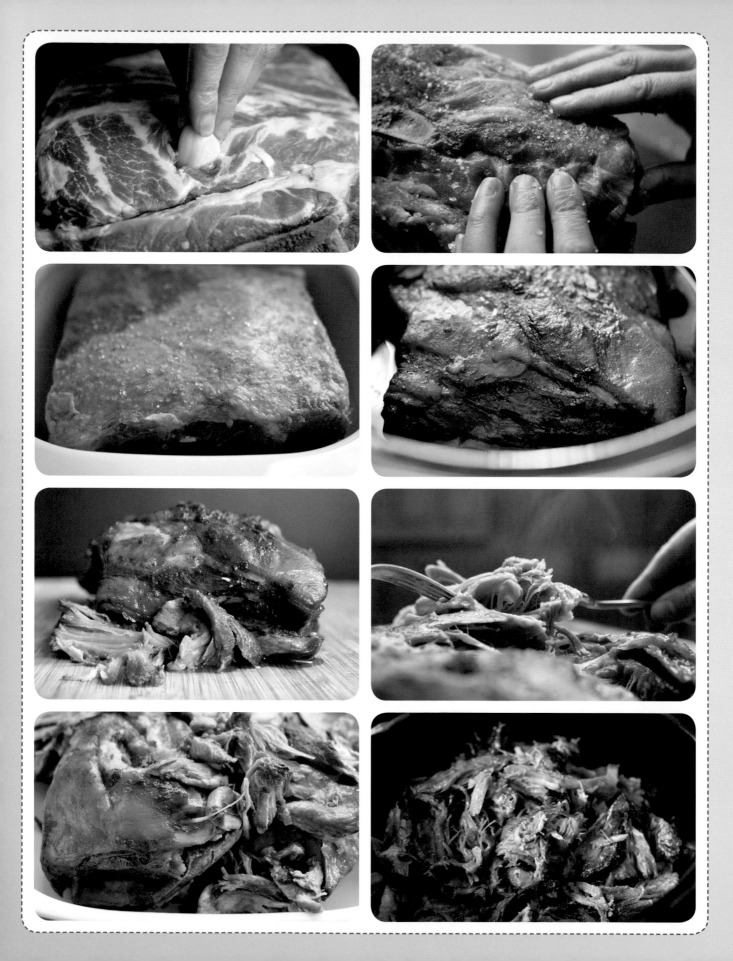

GET:

- **3** slices **bacon**
- **1** (5-pound) **pork shoulder roast**, bone-in or out (it doesn't matter)
- **5** **garlic cloves** (optional)
- **1½** tablespoons coarse **Alaea Hawaiian sea salt**

ALAEA WHAT?

Coarse and unrefined, Alaea sea salt gets its deep terra-cotta hue from *alae*, a purified red volcanic clay that originated on the island of Kauai. The red clay is more mineral-rich than most salts, and imparts a subtle earthiness to dishes.

I stock up on Alaea salt whenever I visit Hawaii, but you don't need to fly to paradise to get your hands on this wondrous ingredient—it's widely available for purchase online.

Even if you don't have any Alaea salt on hand, don't fret. There's nothing quite like the real thing, but in a pinch, any coarse salt will work.

DO THIS:

1. Line the bottom of a slow cooker with bacon slices. (No bacon? No worries. You can replicate the smoky flavor with 2 teaspoons of smoked paprika rubbed over the surface of the pork. Bacon does make it better, though.)

2. If desired, make 5 small incisions in the pork roast and tuck the garlic cloves inside.

3. Season the pork with the sea salt, making sure to get it in all the nooks and crannies.

4. Place the roast in the slow cooker on top of the bacon, skin-side up.

5. Cover and cook on low for 16 hours or until the meat is tender and easily shreds with a fork.

6. When the pork's done, transfer the roast to a separate platter before shredding. Don't shred the pork directly in the slow cooker; the cooking liquid can render the meat too salty.

7. Season to taste with some of the remaining cooking liquid before serving.

PUT THAT PIG TO WORK!

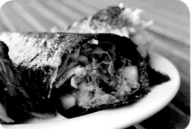
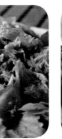
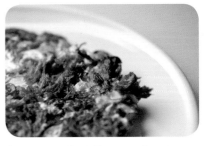

JUICY, TENDER SLOW COOKER KALUA PIG IS FANTASTIC WHEN SERVED AS-IS, BUT IT ALSO MAKES FOR AN INCREDIBLY VERSATILE FILLING. I'M NOT KIDDING, FOLKS: YOU CAN STICK IT IN JUST ABOUT ANYTHING, AND IT'LL BE DELICIOUS.

ENTERTAINING VISITORS FOR BRUNCH? MAKE PORKY BREAKFAST SCRAMBLES, OMELETS, OR FRITTATAS. HOSTING A MEXICAN FIESTA? FILL CRISP LETTUCE TACOS WITH SAVORY KALUA PIG AND TOP IT WITH HOMEMADE GUACAMOLE AND TOMATOES. (CALL IT CARNITAS, AND YOUR GUESTS WON'T BE THE WISER.)

AND ON THOSE BUSY NIGHTS WHEN YOU'RE DESPERATELY IN NEED OF EMERGENCY PROTEIN (AND WISHING YOU WERE MAGICALLY WHISKED AWAY TO HAWAII), JUST GRAB YOUR LEFTOVER PORK AND TOSS IT ON A SUMMER SALAD OR WRAP IT IN TOASTED SHEETS OF NORI. DINNER'LL BE ON THE TABLE IN NO TIME AT ALL!

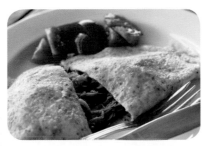
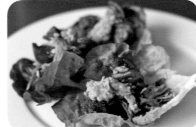
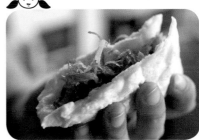

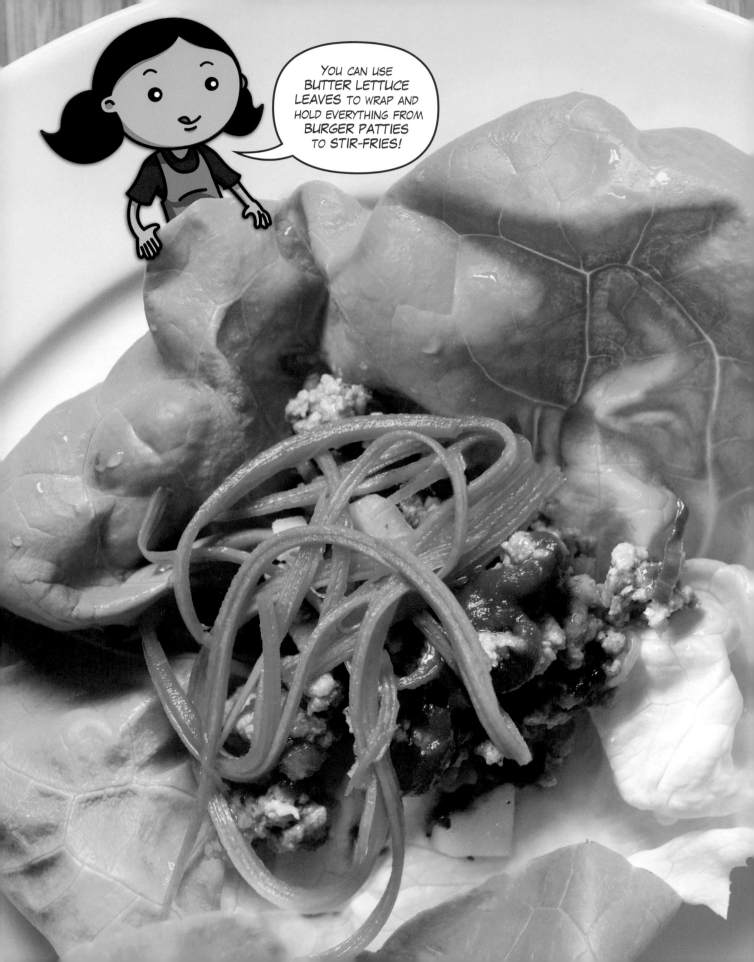

VIETNAMESE LETTUCE CUPS

Makes 4 servings
Hands-on time: 30 minutes
Total time: 30 minutes

Blending Chinese and French influences, Vietnamese cuisine is pure alchemy; it balances and mixes flavors, textures, and temperatures to create unique, surprising dishes that pop.

This easy weeknight meal is a fantastic example. Scoop the steaming-hot filling into cool, crisp lettuce cups, add sweet-tart pickled carrot strings and a squirt of spicy sriracha, and get ready to be transported. Sure, this recipe requires some basic knife skills, but once your *mise en place* is set, it'll take just minutes to get these wraps from wok to table.

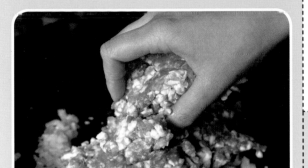

1   tablespoon **coconut oil** or fat of choice
1   small **shallot**, minced
    Kosher salt
1   pound ground **pork**
1   teaspoon minced fresh **ginger**
1   **garlic clove**, minced
1   teaspoon Paleo-friendly **fish sauce**
2   teaspoons fresh **lime juice**
    Freshly ground **black pepper**
½   medium Golden Delicious **apple**, cut into ¼-inch dice
2   **scallions**, thinly sliced
¼   cup minced fresh **cilantro**
1   teaspoon minced fresh **mint**
2   tablespoons minced fresh **basil**
1   head **butter lettuce**, leaves separated
    Quick-Pickled Carrot Strings (page 50)
    Paleo Sriracha (page 42)

DO THIS:

In a large skillet or wok, melt the fat over medium heat. When it's shimmering, add the shallot and a pinch of salt and sauté for about 3 minutes or until translucent. Toss in the ground pork and cook, stirring, until no longer pink. Add the ginger and garlic, and stir-fry until fragrant. Season with fish sauce, lime juice, and pepper. Remove from heat, add the apple and minced herbs, and stir to combine. Serve in individual butter lettuce leaves with a garnish of pickled carrot and sriracha.

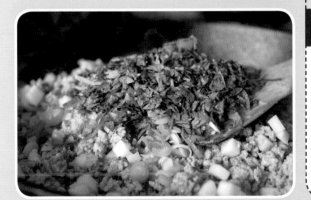

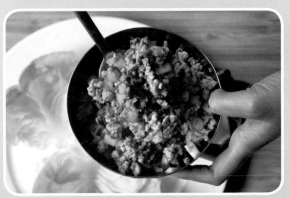

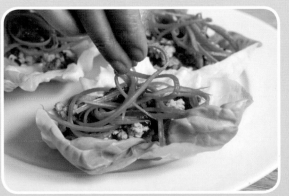

NO SRIRACHA ON HAND? TOP WITH THIN SLICES OF JALAPEÑO PEPPER INSTEAD!

MAPLE SAUSAGE PATTIES

Don't you think it's time to throw away that box of chemically enhanced, frostbitten sausage pucks buried in the back of your icebox? It's not hard to make your own, you know. Seasoned with fresh herbs and a dash of maple syrup, these hearty homemade breakfast patties are the perfect way to start your day.

Makes 16 patties
Hands-on time: 30 minutes
Total time: 30 minutes

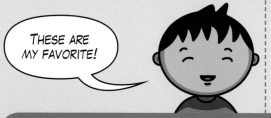

THESE ARE MY FAVORITE!

2	pounds **ground pork**
2	tablespoons **maple syrup**
1	tablespoon **kosher salt**
1	teaspoon freshly ground **black pepper**
2	teaspoons minced fresh **sage**
1	teaspoon minced fresh **thyme**
½	teaspoon minced fresh **rosemary**
½	teaspoon **ancho chile powder**
2	tablespoons **ghee** or fat of choice

DO THIS:

1. In a large bowl, mix all the ingredients together except the ghee. Be careful not to overwork the meat—you don't want your patties to be dense and tough.

2. Use your hands to form the meat into sixteen 2-inch rounds. The patties should be roughly ¾ inch in height.

3. Melt the ghee in a large (12-inch) cast-iron skillet over medium heat. In two batches, cook the patties in the hot ghee for 4 minutes on each side, or until they're cooked through and golden brown.

CHEW ON THIS:

- Don't use lean or extra-lean pork, or you'll end up with dry, crumbly, flavorless patties. Instead, shoot for pork that's at least 20 percent fat. And remember: pastured is best!

- Wondering about ancho chile powder? It's made from dried poblano peppers, and imparts a smoky, fruity heat to your food.

- If you're avoiding sweeteners, feel free to replace the maple syrup with apple. Grate a peeled and cored apple and drain off the excess liquid before mixing it into the meat. Apple plus pork always equals yum.

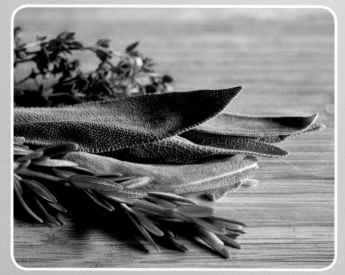

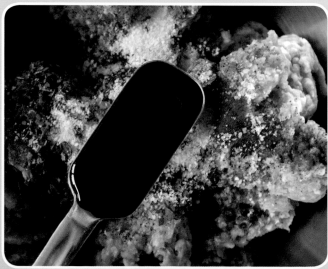

 WANNA MAKE PALEO SAUSAGE EGG MUFFIN SANDWICHES FOR BREAKFAST? VISIT ME AT NOMNOMPALEO.COM FOR THE RECIPE!

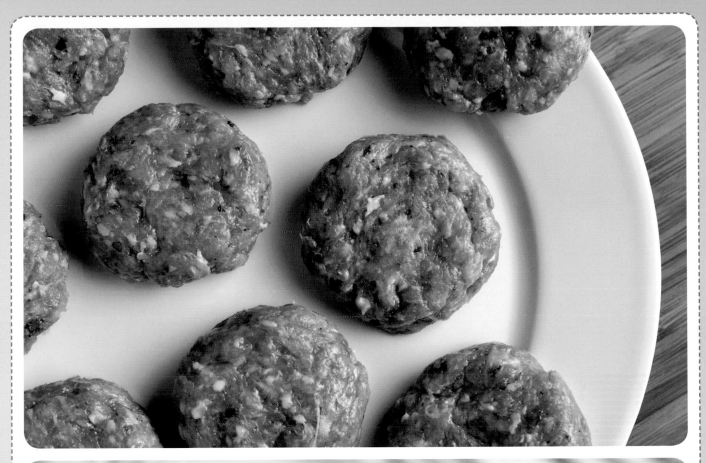

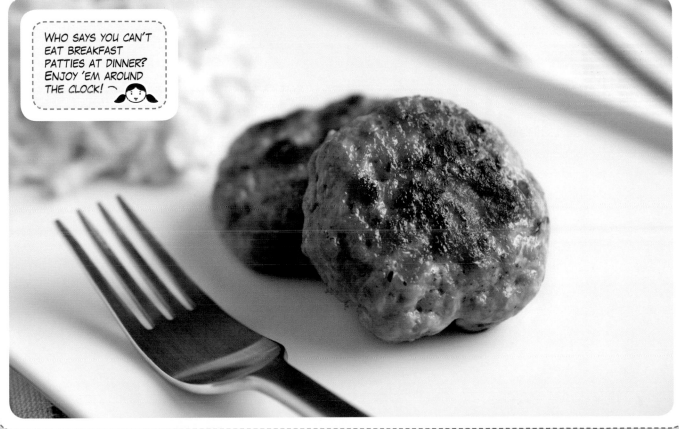

WHO SAYS YOU CAN'T EAT BREAKFAST PATTIES AT DINNER? ENJOY 'EM AROUND THE CLOCK! ⌐

BRINNER IS BREAKFAST FOR DINNER! SCRAMBLE SOME EGGS WITH A GENEROUS PINCH OF MAGIC MUSHROOM POWDER (PAGE 35), AND THROW SOME MAPLE SAUSAGE PATTIES ON THE SIDE!

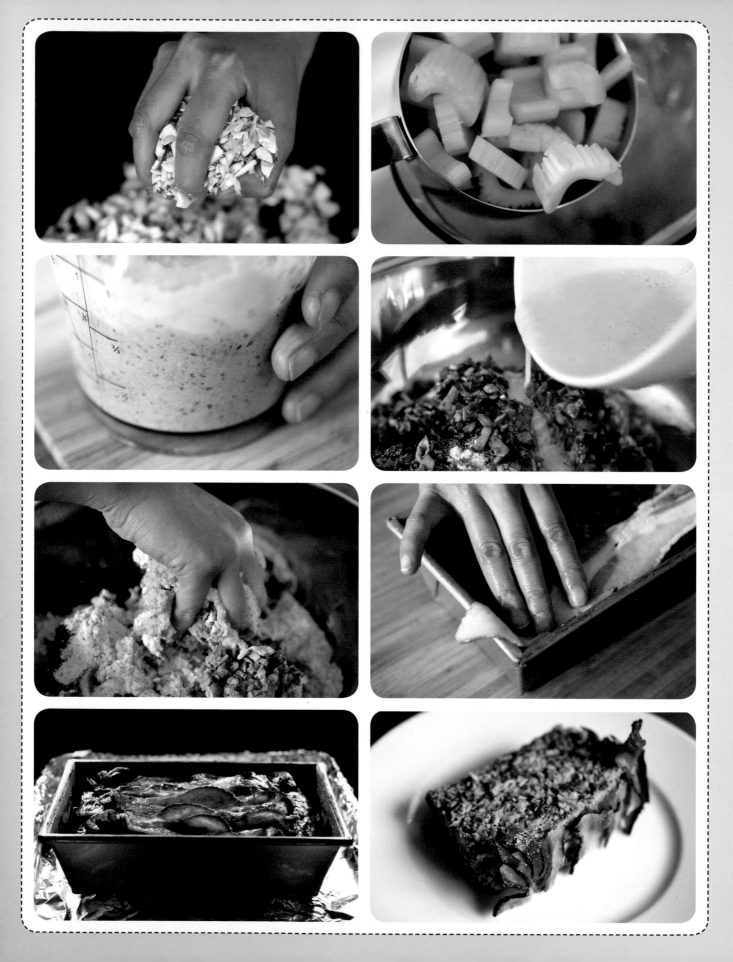

SUPER-PORKTASTIC MEATLOAF

This tender, flavorful, porky loaf was a clear-cut winner the very first time I made it. Don't believe me? My (then) six-year-old declared that this dish merited "FIVE STARS!" and demanded seconds. But then again, just like all of us, he has a special place in his heart for just about anything topped with bacon.

Makes 6 servings
Hands-on time: 30 minutes
Total time: 2 hours

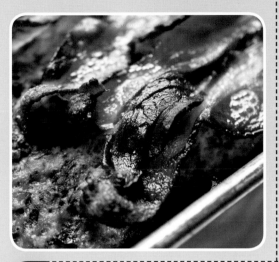

- 1 tablespoon **ghee** or fat of choice
- 1 small **yellow onion**, cut into ½-inch dice
- ½ pound **cremini mushrooms**, minced
- 2 medium **celery** stalks, chopped medium
- ½ cup loosely packed fresh **Italian parsley**
- ¼ cup **coconut cream**
- 1 pound **ground pork**
- 1 pound frozen chopped **spinach**, thawed and squeezed dry
- ¼ cup **coconut flour**
- 1 teaspoon **kosher salt**
- 1½ teaspoons freshly ground **black pepper**
- ¼ teaspoon freshly grated **nutmeg**
- 1 **garlic clove**, minced
- 2 large **eggs**, lightly beaten
- 5 **bacon** slices
- **Marinara sauce**, warmed, for serving (optional)

DO THIS:

1. Preheat the oven to 350°F with the rack in the middle position.

2. Heat the ghee over medium heat in a large cast-iron skillet. Add the chopped onion and mushrooms, and sauté until all the liquid evaporates and the onions are softened.

3. Toss the celery, parsley, and coconut cream into a blender or an immersion blender cup, and blend the ingredients until smooth.

4. In a large bowl, combine the ground pork, chopped spinach, coconut flour, salt, pepper, nutmeg, garlic, and cooked mushrooms and onions. Add the eggs to the rest of the ingredients. Pour the blended green mixture into the bowl, and use your hands to gently combine all of the ingredients.

5. Transfer the mixture to an ungreased 9-inch-by-5-inch loaf pan, and use your hands to form a smooth, flat top.

6. Layer the bacon slices on top, making sure to overlap them a bit. Don't worry if the bacon slices dangle off the ends of the loaf pan—they'll shrink as they cook. (The thicker the bacon, the less the shrinkage.)

7. You can cover and refrigerate the uncooked loaf for up to a day in advance of baking, but if you're cooking it immediately, put the loaf pan on a foil-lined baking sheet before sticking it in the oven.

8. Bake for 70 minutes, rotating the loaf pan at the halfway point. Then, stick it under the broiler for 3 minutes to crisp up the bacon.

9. Rest the loaf for 20 minutes, and then slice it up. If you're feeling particularly saucy, spoon some warmed marinara sauce on top before serving.

 DO YOU PREFER A MOISTER, LIGHTER-TEXTURED MEATLOAF? TRY SUBSTITUTING A QUARTER-CUP OF GARLIC MASHED CAULIFLOWER (PAGE 155) IN PLACE OF THE COCONUT FLOUR!

SIU YOKE
(CRISPY ROAST PORK BELLY)

Whenever I spy a slab of crisp roast pork belly hanging in the window of a Chinese barbecue joint, I start salivating. With a crackling-crisp golden-orange exterior and a lusciously succulent and juicy interior, Chinese *siu yoke* is every bit as smashing as it looks. Best of all, with just a bit of time and effort, you won't even need to brave the Chinatown crowds to enjoy this utterly authentic version at home.

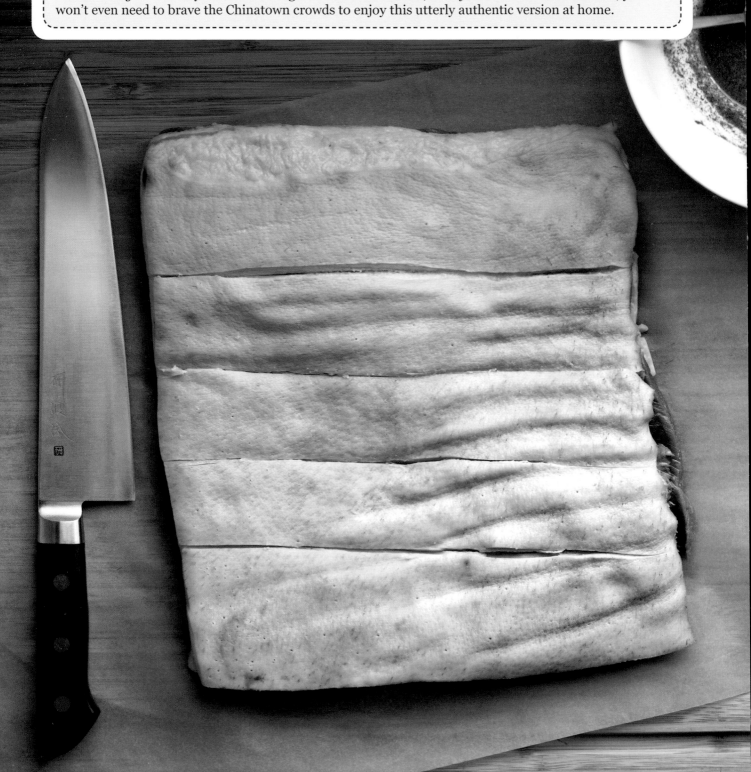

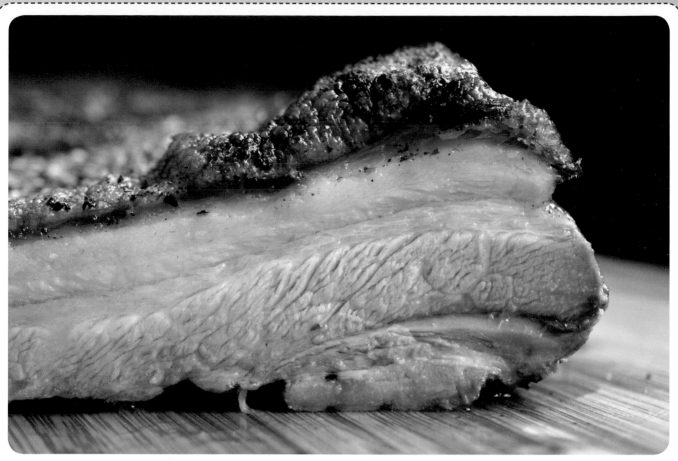

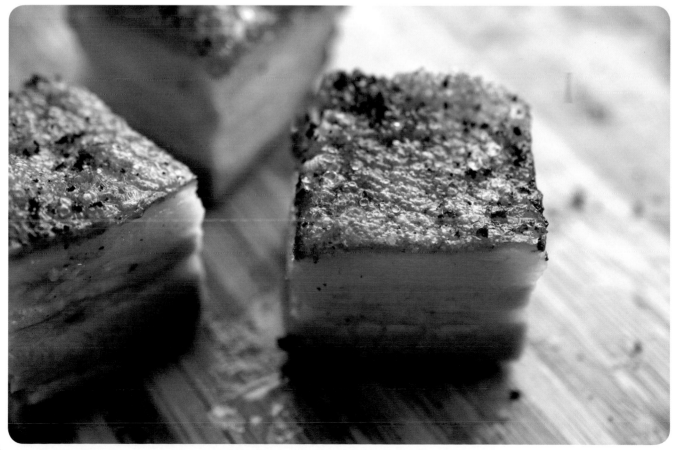

GET:

Roast Pork

1   (4-pound) **pork belly**
1½ tablespoon **baking soda**
1   quart boiling **water**, plus more for roasting
½   teaspoon **kosher salt**

Siu Yoke Marinade

2   teaspoons **five spice powder**
2   tablespoons **kosher salt**
2   tablespoons **apple cider vinegar**
1   tablespoon Paleo-friendly **fish sauce**
1   tablespoon **honey**

Makes 8 servings
Hands-on time: 45 minutes
Total time: 12 hours

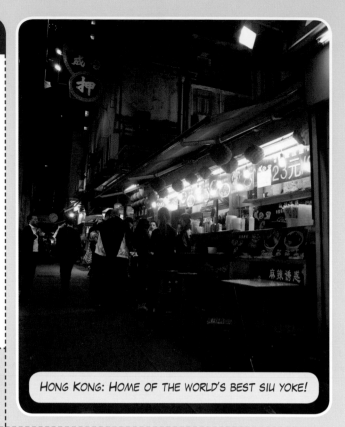

HONG KONG: HOME OF THE WORLD'S BEST SIU YOKE!

DO THIS:

1. Using a sharp, multi-pronged blade tenderizer or thumbtack (or, frankly, anything sharp, pointy, and clean), prick the pork skin all over. Make sure to pierce the skin, but don't poke into the meat.

2. With a sharp knife, score the skin with parallel lines running along the width of the pork, about 1 to 2 inches apart. Again, cut through the skin, but not into the meat.

3. Place the pork skin-side up on a tilted wire rack in the sink. Dissolve the baking soda in the boiling water, and pour the scalding-hot alkaline solution over the skin of the belly. Pat the skin very dry with a clean cloth or paper towels.

4. In a bowl, combine the marinade ingredients and stir thoroughly to form a uniform mixture.

5. Place the pork belly skin-side down on a flat surface. Rub the marinade onto the surface of the exposed meat (but don't spread it on the skin side).

6. Flip the belly over and place it skin-side up in a baking dish. Refrigerate it overnight, uncovered.

7. One hour before you plan to cook the pork belly, remove it from the refrigerator so it can come up to room temperature. In the meantime, preheat the oven to 375°F with the rack placed in the middle position. Fill a foil-lined roasting tray with at least a half-inch of boiling water.

8. Pat the pork belly skin dry (yes, again), and sprinkle ½ teaspoon kosher salt over the skin. Place the pork skin-side up on a wire rack, and set the rack atop the prepared roasting tray.

9. Roast in the oven for 60 to 80 minutes or until the internal temperature of the pork belly reaches 160°F. (Use an instant-read thermometer to be sure.)

10. Increase the heat to broil, and cook the pork belly until the skin is crispy and a char develops, 5 to 10 minutes. Rest the pork for 15 minutes, and then use a serrated knife to scrape off the salt and any charred bits. Cut into 1½-inch pieces before serving.

AS A BOY, HENRY CALLED THE SIU YOKE SKIN "BOK-BOK" DUE TO ITS AUDIBLY CRUNCHY POP WHEN YOU TAKE A BITE. WE TEASE HIM MERCILESSLY ABOUT IT.

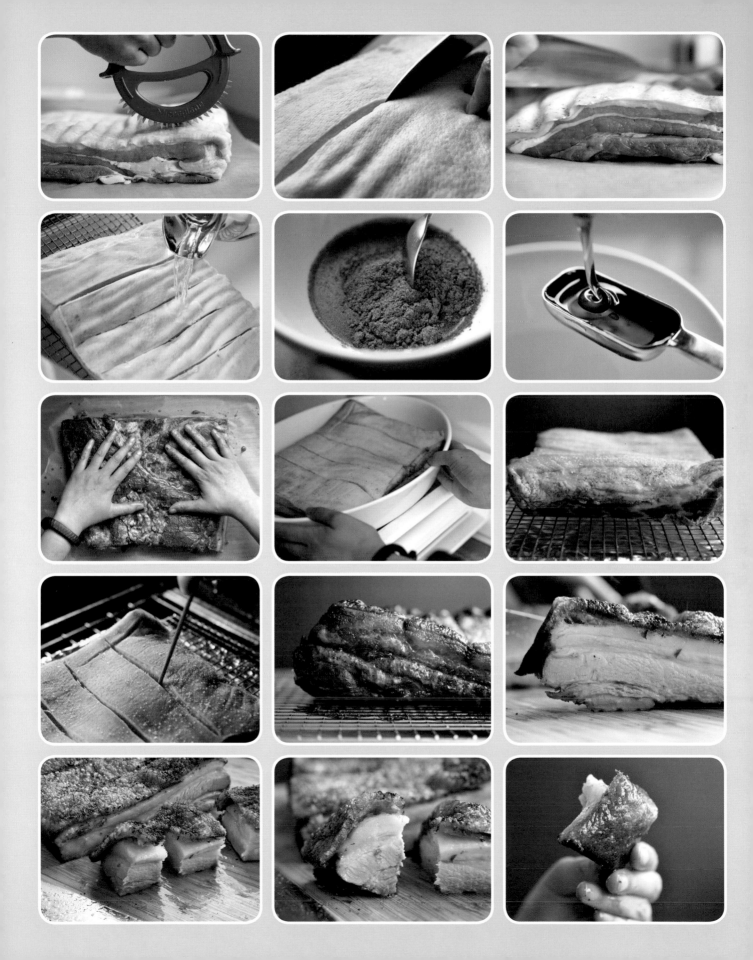

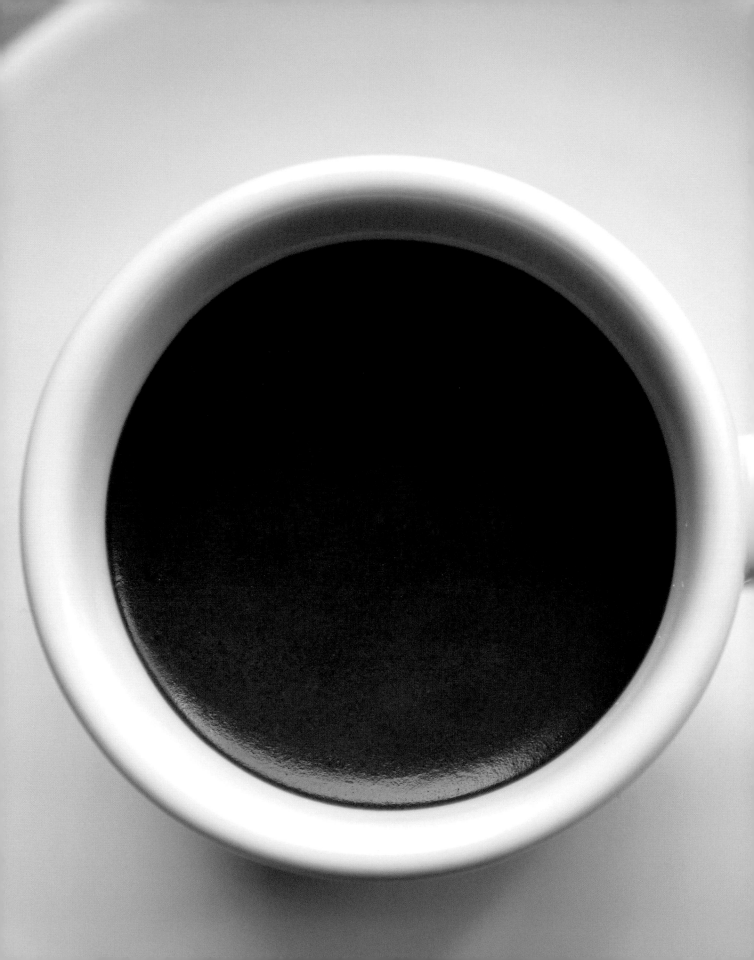

CHAPTER NINE:
TREATS

CINNAMON APPLE SCONES

I'm glad I'm no longer addicted to pastries, but to be honest, I still feel an occasional twinge of nostalgia for scones—tender and crusty, with just a touch of fruity sweetness. My husband's to blame for this grain-free recipe; after trying one of his scones, I had to banish the rest from the house, fearing I'd eat the entire batch in one sitting. (Of course, since then, I haven't been able to stop thinking about them. Argh.)

Makes 6 scones
Hands-on time: 10 minutes
Total time: 40 minutes

3 cups blanched **almond flour**
1½ teaspoons **baking soda**
½ teaspoon **fine sea salt**
4 tablespoons **butter**, as cold as possible (preferably frozen), cut into small pieces
1 teaspoon ground **cinnamon**
2 large **eggs**
2 tablespoons **apple cider vinegar**
2 tablespoons **honey**
1 small Granny Smith or Fuji **apple**, peeled, cored, and cut into thin tiles

BONUS RECIPE!

IN THE MOOD FOR DARK CHOCOLATE CHERRY SCONES INSTEAD? FOLLOW THE SAME RECIPE, BUT LEAVE OUT THE CINNAMON AND APPLE. ADD 1 TEASPOON OF VANILLA EXTRACT IN STEP 3. THEN, IN STEP 5, ADD 3 OUNCES OF SUPER-DARK CHOCOLATE, CUT INTO BITE-SIZE CHUNKS, AND ¼ CUP OF DRIED CHERRIES.

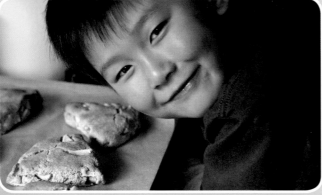

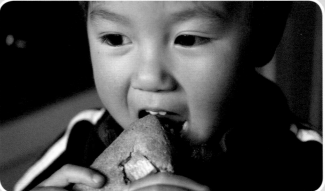

DO THIS:

1. Preheat the oven to 350°F with the rack in the middle position, and line a rimmed baking sheet with parchment paper.

2. In a large bowl, combine the almond flour, baking soda, and fine sea salt. Use your hands or a pastry cutter to work the pieces of cold butter into the dry ingredients until a crumbly mixture is produced. Then, mix the cinnamon into the almond flour mixture.

3. In a separate bowl, thoroughly whisk together the eggs, apple cider vinegar, and honey.

4. Make a well in the middle of the dry ingredients, and pour the egg mixture into it.

5. Gently mix with a spatula until a wet, chunky dough forms, and then throw in the apple. Combine the ingredients with your hands, and form a ball of dough.

6. On a sheet of parchment paper or a nonstick surface, gently flatten the ball with your hand. The round of dough should be about ¾ inch thick. Using a pastry cutter or a sharp knife, cut the dough into 6 equal-sized wedges, and arrange them on the parchment-lined baking sheet.

7. Bake for 20 to 25 minutes, rotating the tray halfway through. The scones are ready when they're golden brown, and an inserted toothpick comes out clean. Transfer the scones onto a wire rack to cool slightly before serving.

THIS ISN'T JUST ANOTHER SUBPAR SUBSTITUTE FOR THE REAL THING. IT'S BETTER THAN SCONES MADE WITH WHEAT FLOUR!

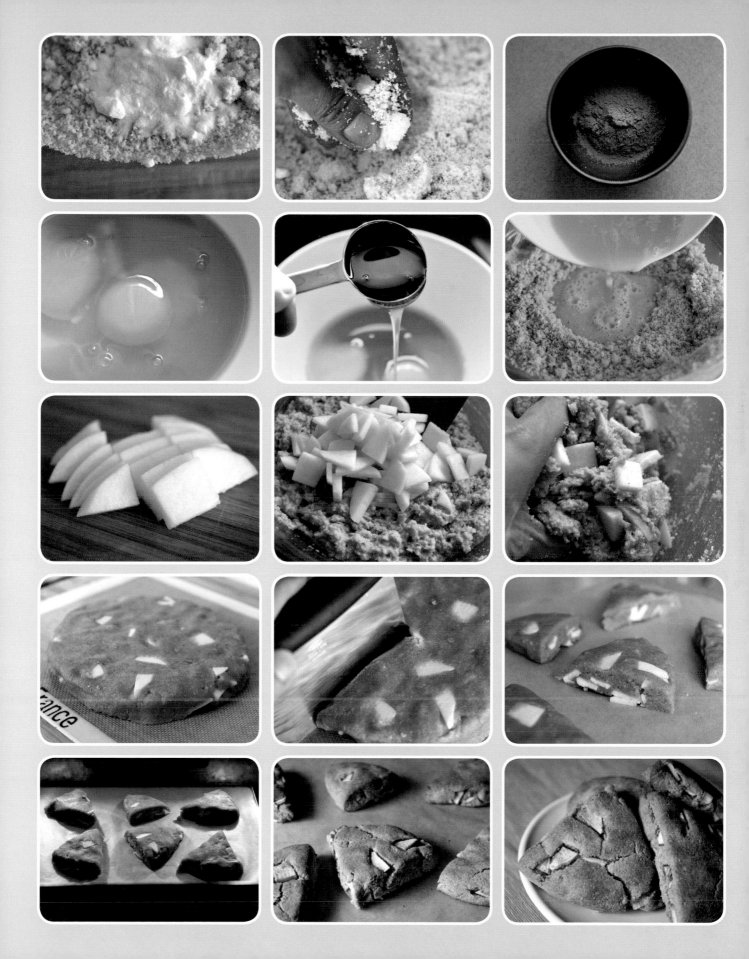

LIAR BARS

There are a growing number of Paleo-friendly snack bars on the market, but they're not cheap, and we're not made of money. So naturally, I make my own version. With the addition of macadamia nuts, I think these are even better than the bars available at the grocery store, but my boys like to remind me that they're knock-offs. "Those are Liar Bars, Mommy." True, but these Liar Bars are honestly good.

Makes 6 bars
Hands-on time: 10 minutes
Total time: 10 minutes

1 cup unsweetened **coconut flakes**
⅓ cup dry-roasted and salted **macadamia nuts**
10 large **Medjool dates**, pitted and chopped (about 1 cup)

DO THIS:

1. Preheat the oven to 300°F. Toast the coconut flakes in a single layer on a parchment-lined rimmed baking sheet for 3 to 5 minutes or until golden brown. Cool the flakes.

2. Toss the macadamia nuts in a food processor, and pulse until finely chopped. (Don't go overboard and process them into a nut butter.) Transfer the chopped nuts to a separate bowl and set aside.

3. Put the chopped dates into the empty food processor, and pulse until they form a sticky ball. Add the toasted coconut flakes, and pulse until the mixture holds together when you squeeze it between your fingers. (But don't stick your fingers in the work bowl until you've unplugged the food processor, genius.) Be careful not to pulverize the coconut flakes; you don't want to purée them.

4. Transfer the mixture to the bowl with the macadamia nuts, and thoroughly combine the ingredients. The result should be a loose, sticky mass. Using your hands, form the mixture into a ball.

5. Place the ball between two sheets of parchment paper, and flatten it with your hand, a rolling pin, or a heavy book. Remove the top sheet of parchment, and form the flattened mixture into a square. Cut it into equal-sized bars. Store them in an airtight container for up to 3 days—or just eat 'em up!

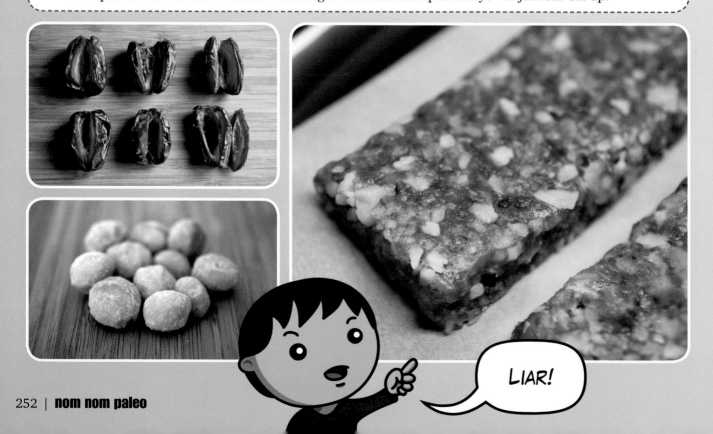

LIAR!

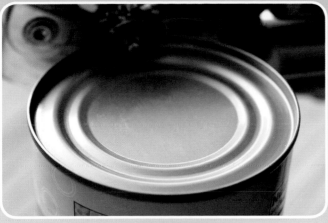
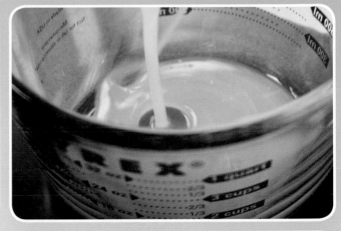
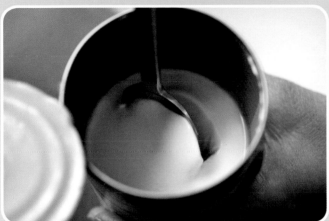
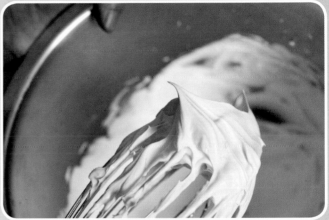

WHIPPED COCONUT CREAM

Before going Paleo, my desserts were often served with dollops of freshly whipped crème chantilly, a rich vanilla-infused embellishment that elevated even the most ordinary treat. These days, I get the same results using the thick layer of cream that rises to the top of a chilled can of coconut milk. Want to see how I do it?

Makes 1 cup
Hands-on time: 5 minutes
Total time: 8 hours

1   (14-ounce) can full-fat **coconut milk**
1   tablespoon **coconut sugar** (optional)
½   **teaspoon vanilla extract**

DO THIS:

1. Turn a can of coconut milk upside down, and refrigerate overnight. This will cause the coconut cream to separate from the liquid and rise. Chill a mixing bowl and a wire whisk in the fridge, too.

2. Take the can out of the fridge, and turn it right-side up. The coconut cream will now be on the bottom of the can. Using a can opener, cut two slits on the top of the can, and pour out the liquid (coconut water—yum!), leaving only the thick layer of coconut cream in the can.

3. Open the can, and transfer the stiff coconut cream to the chilled bowl. Add the coconut sugar (if desired) and vanilla extract, and whisk the ingredients until medium peaks form.

4. Pipe onto your favorite desserts, or just spoon some into a bowl with a handful of fresh berries.

 COCONUT SUGAR IS *STILL SUGAR*, SO WHEN I'M TOPPING AN ALREADY-SWEET DESSERT WITH THIS WHIPPED CREAM, I PREFER TO LEAVE OUT THE EXTRA SUGAR.

SUMMER BERRY SOUP

On a muggy summer evening, after a hearty family barbecue, the last thing I want to do is spend more time in the kitchen. Instead, I prefer to finish with a refreshingly cool berry soup 'cause it's a breeze to make and a crowd-pleaser to boot. Use sweet, chilled, in-season berries, and you won't even need to add honey.

Makes 4 servings
Hands-on time: 10 minutes
Total time: 10 minutes

GET:

1   cup red seedless **grapes**
1   cup fresh or frozen **blueberries**
1   cup fresh or frozen **raspberries**
1   cup fresh or frozen **strawberries**
1   tablespoon fresh **lemon juice**
1   tablespoon **honey** (optional)
1   cup **Whipped Coconut Cream** (page 253)

DO THIS:

Put all the ingredients except the whipped coconut cream in a high-speed blender, and purée until smooth. Strain through a fine-mesh sieve. Top with a dollop of whipped cream before plating. Serve immediately.

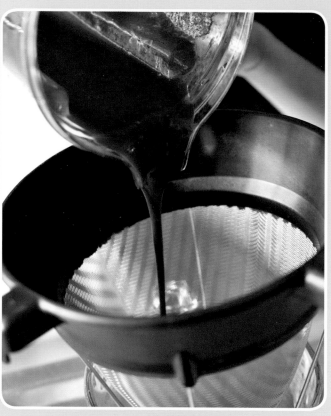

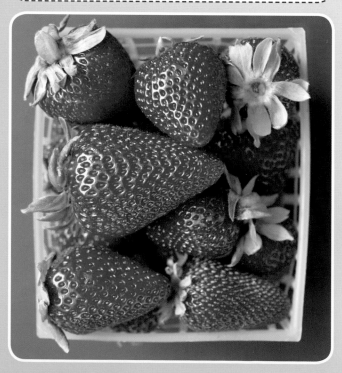

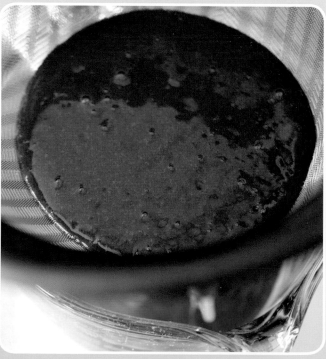

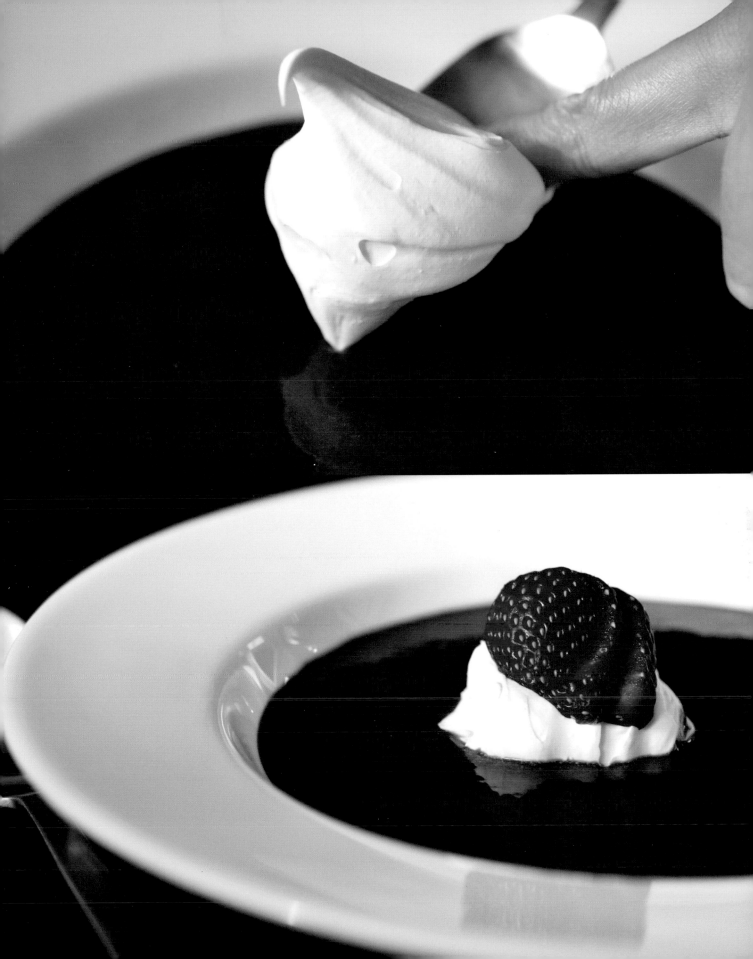

MEXICAN CHOCOLATE POTS DE CRÈME

When it comes to chocolate pots de crème, there's no messing around. These dense little cups of smooth, dark chocolate don't pretend to be delicate or airy, and you'll never mistake them for bland-tasting instant pudding or low-fat chocolate mousse. With just one bite, you'll taste the message loud and clear: these bittersweet pots de crème are intensely chocolatey, decadently full-fat, and proud of it.

My favorite way to amp up the intensity of this special treat is with a touch of cinnamon, vanilla, and ancho chile powder—a flavor combination inspired by the rich, spicy kick of traditional Mexican hot chocolate.

Makes 8 servings
Hands-on time: 30 minutes
Total time: 4½ hours

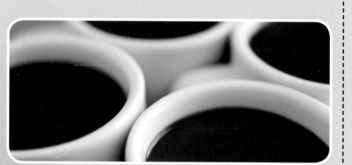

7	ounces **dark chocolate** (70% cacao or higher), finely chopped
1	(14-ounce) can full-fat **coconut milk**
2	large **egg yolks**
¼	teaspoon **ancho chile powder**
⅛	teaspoon **kosher salt**
1	**cinnamon stick**
1	tablespoon **vanilla extract**
1	cup **Whipped Coconut Cream** (page 253)
1	tablespoon **ground cinnamon**

DO THIS:

1. Place the chocolate in a bowl and set aside. In a saucepan, whisk to combine the coconut milk, egg yolks, chile powder, and salt. Drop in the cinnamon stick.

2. Heat the mixture over medium-low heat, stirring constantly until it thickens and forms a smooth custard that coats the back of a spoon, 10 to 15 minutes. Watch the custard like a hawk—you don't want to overcook it. Remember: steaming is good, but simmering and boiling are bad. When in doubt, use an instant-read thermometer to ensure the final temperature is about 175°F.

3. When the custard is ready, take the pot off the heat, and fish out the cinnamon stick. Position a fine-mesh sieve over the bowl of chocolate, and pour the custard through to catch any lumpy bits.

4. Let the chocolate-and-custard mixture sit undisturbed for 5 minutes. Seriously: set a timer and walk away. Staring at the chocolatey goodness is just going to drive you bonkers.

5. When your timer goes off, grab a spatula and stir ever so gently to mix the melted chocolate into the custard base. If you stir like crazy, the temperature will drop too quickly, and you'll end up with grainy chocolate. (Mexican chocolate is traditionally coarse-ground and can be crumbly in texture, but I prefer my pots de crème to be sinfully smooth.) Steady, slow stirring is essential for ensuring a stable emulsion. Once you've achieved a smooth mixture, stir in the vanilla extract.

6. Divide the mixture evenly among eight 2-ounce espresso cups or ramekins, and cool to room temperature. Cover the cups with plastic wrap and refrigerate for at least 4 hours.

7. When you're ready to serve, remove the pots de crème from the fridge, and spoon a dollop of the whipped coconut cream onto each cup—or if you're feeling particularly fancy, use a pastry bag fitted with a star tip to pipe the cream on top.

8. Dust with a shower of cinnamon, grab a spoon, and dig in.

AFTER TASTE-TESTING MY LITTLE CHOCOLATE POTS, JAMES BEARD AWARD-WINNING CHEF MICHAEL MINA DECLARED THEM TO BE "DELICIOUS!" I COULDN'T STOP SMILING FOR DAYS.

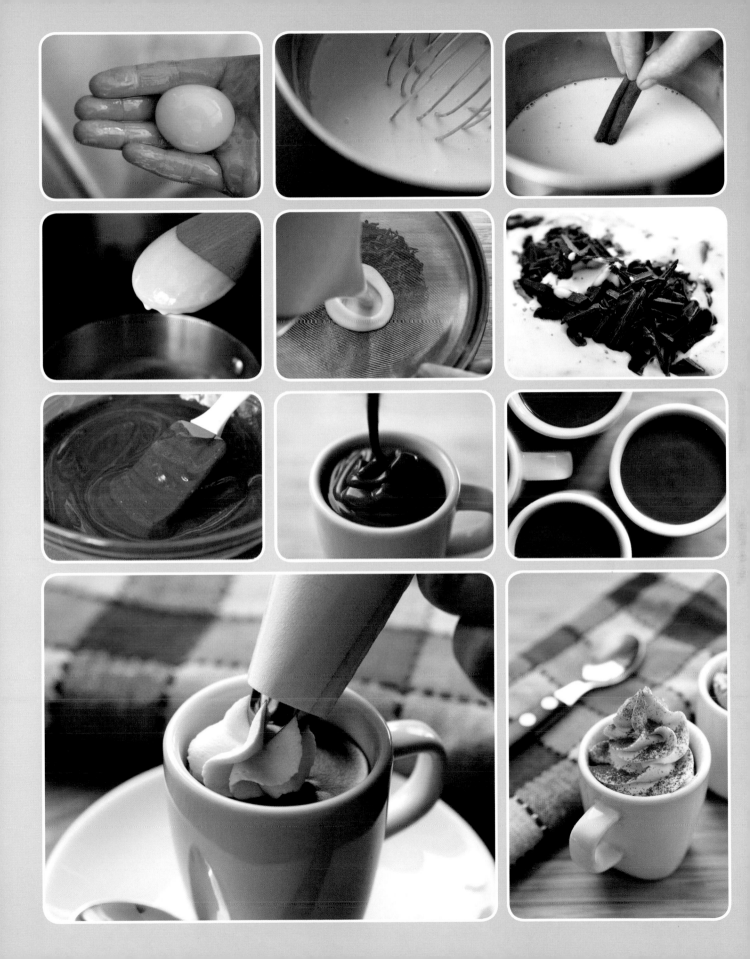

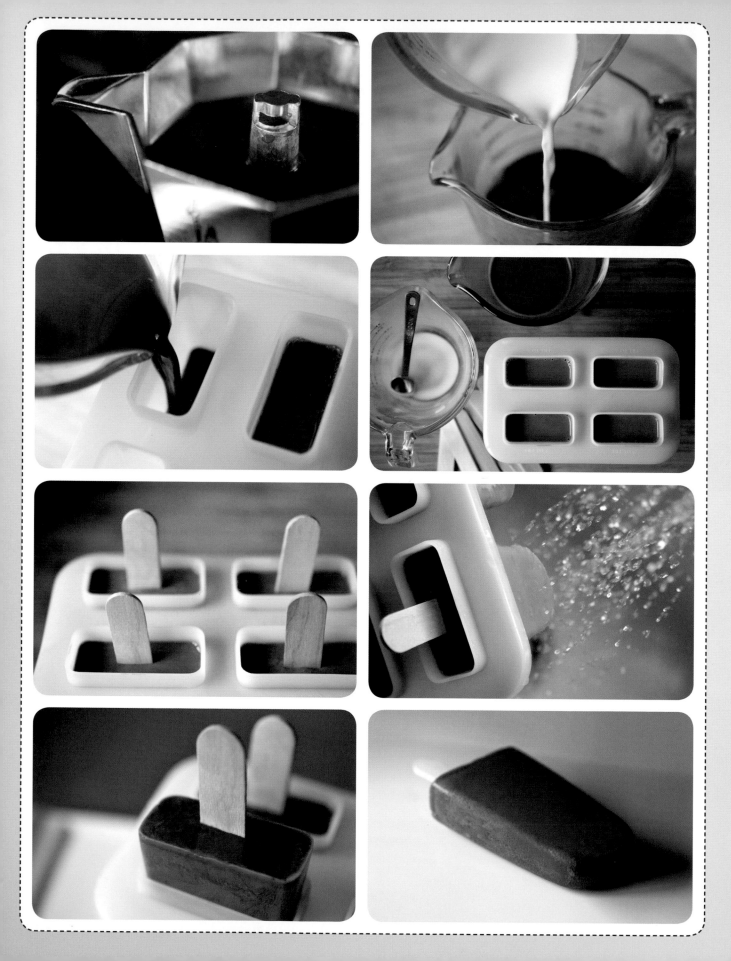

MOCHA ICE POPS

To make it through my graveyard shifts at the hospital, I allow myself two vices: a nightly square of super-dark chocolate and a shot of espresso. But during the sweltering summertime months, scalding-hot coffee and mushy chocolate aren't my idea of a good time. To help me beat the heat, my husband concocted this frosty, chocolatey, caffeinated treat. The only catch? I can't indulge too close to bedtime.

Makes 4 popsicles
Hands-on time: 15 minutes
Total time: 4 hours

1   cup **espresso** or strong coffee
2   tablespoons **honey** or **maple syrup**
1   tablespoon unsweetened **cocoa powder**
½   teaspoon **vanilla extract**
    Pinch of **salt**
½   cup full-fat **coconut milk**

DO THIS:

1. Make the espresso, and cool it slightly. (No espresso maker? Then just brew the strongest coffee you can. I'm talking coffee so strong that your neighbors start growing chest hair. Even the girls.)

2. Stir the honey, cocoa powder, vanilla extract, and pinch of salt into the coffee while it's still warm.

3. Add the coconut milk, and mix well. Taste and adjust to the desired sweetness.

4. Pour the mixture into ice pop molds, add popsicle sticks, and freeze until solid. (This will take anywhere from 2 to 4 hours, depending on the size of your molds and the temperature of your freezer). Run a little warm water on the outside of the molds, and the pops will slide right out.

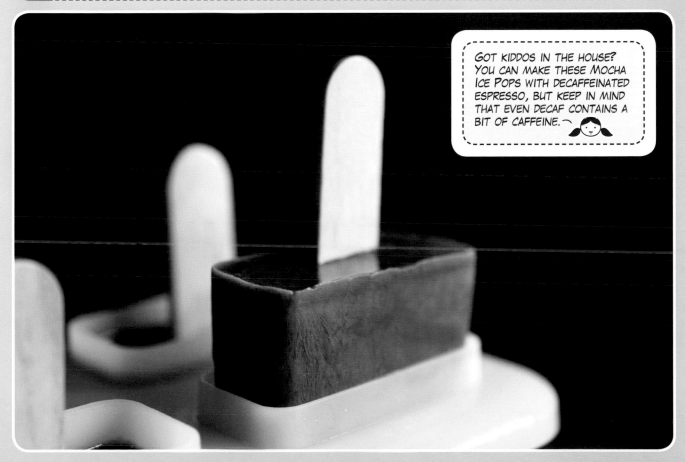

GOT KIDDOS IN THE HOUSE? YOU CAN MAKE THESE MOCHA ICE POPS WITH DECAFFEINATED ESPRESSO, BUT KEEP IN MIND THAT EVEN DECAF CONTAINS A BIT OF CAFFEINE.

~ TRUTH BE TOLD, A SUBSTANTIAL PORTION OF THIS COOKBOOK WAS WRITTEN UNDER THE INFLUENCE OF COFFEE AND CHOCOLATE.

STRAWBERRY BANANA ICE CREAM

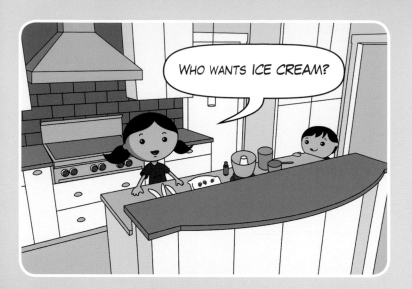

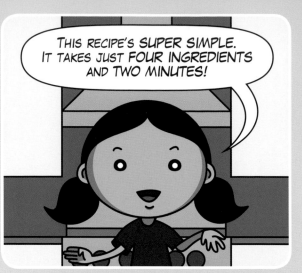

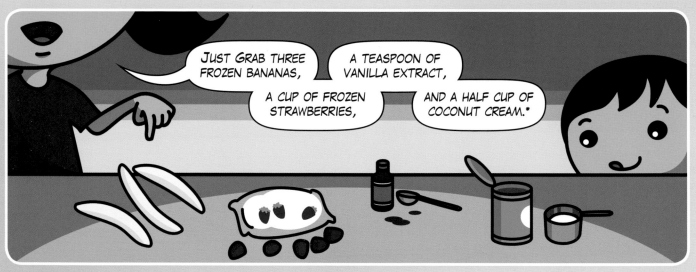

*OR FULL-FAT COCONUT MILK

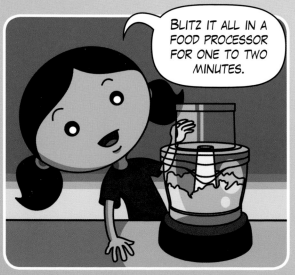

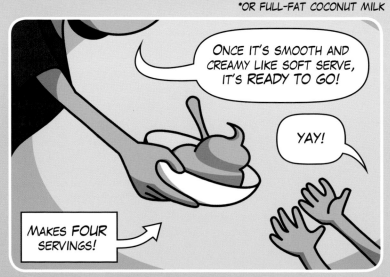

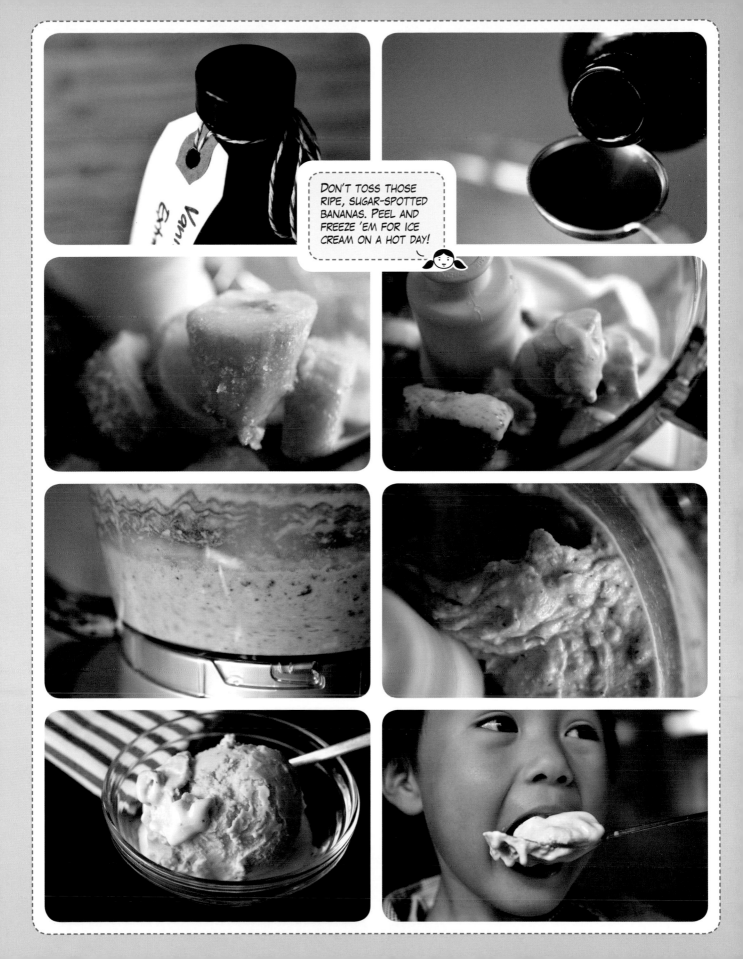

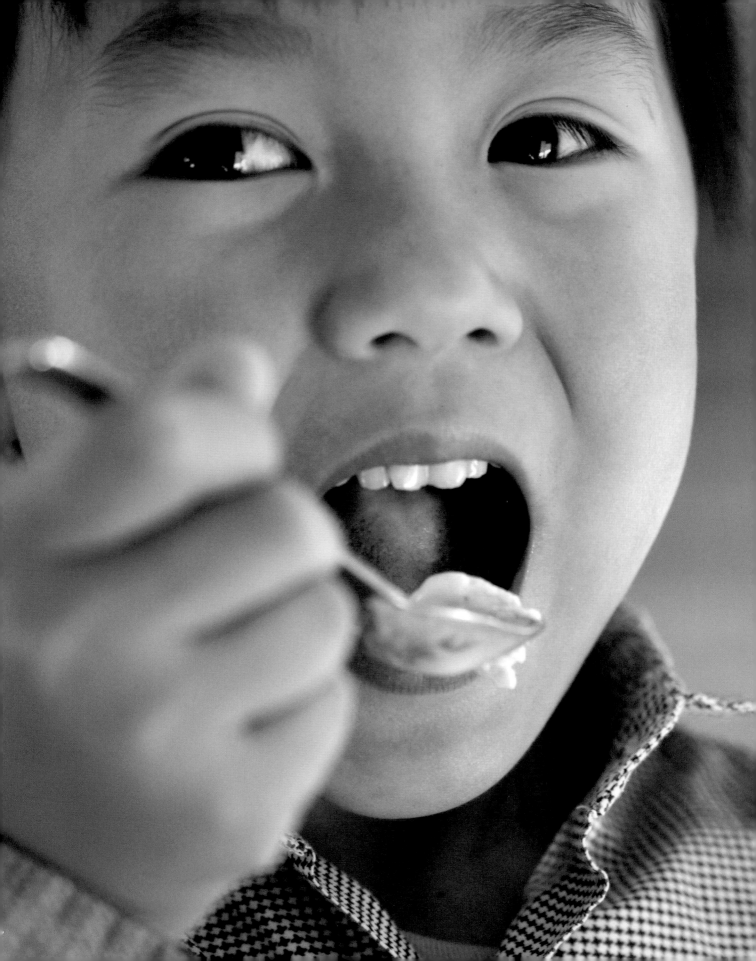

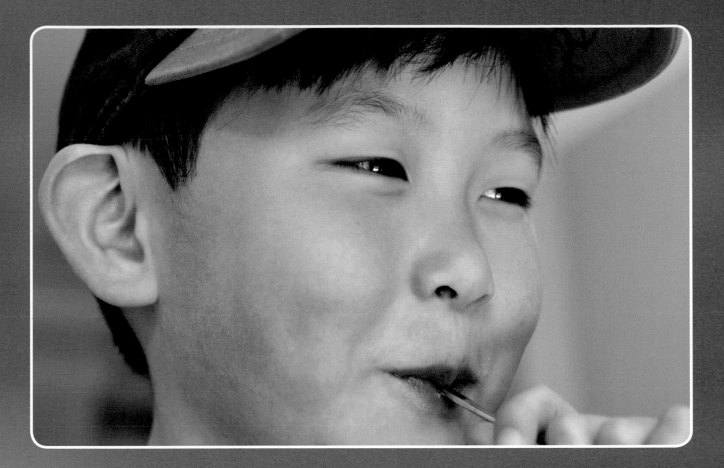

A PARTING NOTE ABOUT SWEETS

I know what you're thinking: *That's it? That's the end?!? No more dessert recipes? Don't you have recipes for Paleo sugar cookies or Paleo candy canes or Paleo triple-decker chocolate fudge brownies? I can't believe I read this entire book and have no Paleo cake pops to show for it. Grrr.*

Here's the thing about desserts: this book reflects the way I cook for my family. And these days, I rarely whip up sugary treats—"Paleo" or otherwise.

It wasn't always this way. Growing up, if you waved something bready and/or sugary in front of me, I'd gladly chomp your hand off to get at it. I was a dessert junkie.

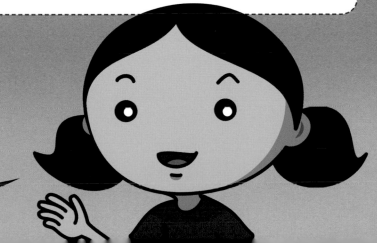

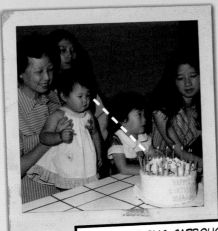

I'M A LIFELONG CARBOHOLIC.

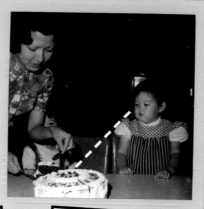

IN FACT, AS A KID,

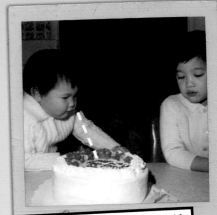

I HAD EYES ONLY FOR ONE THING.

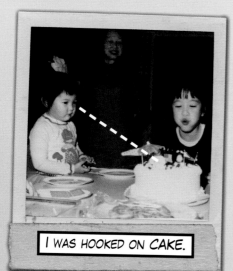

I WAS HOOKED ON CAKE.

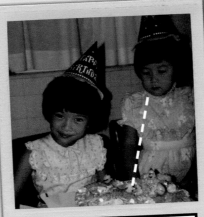

AND WHEN I SAY "HOOKED,"

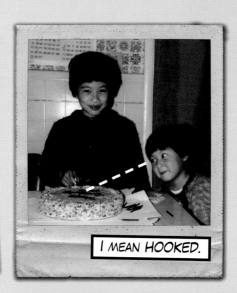

I MEAN HOOKED.

THIS OBSESSION WITH SWEETS CONTINUED INTO ADULTHOOD,

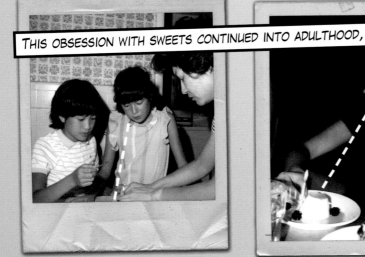

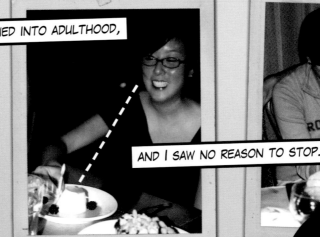

AND I SAW NO REASON TO STOP.

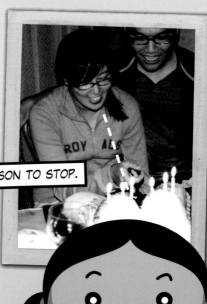

⸝YEESH!⸜

I didn't stop stuffing my face with sweets even after I adopted a so-called "healthier" diet of whole grains and low-fat fare. *There's no reason to ditch dessert*, I told myself. *I can always bake pastries with whole wheat flour instead of all-purpose flour. And those food scientists employed by the industrial flavor industry are doing amazing things with artificial sweeteners these days, don't you think?*

Too bad my agave-nectar-drenched whole-grain pastries tasted gross, and made me feel even worse.

After adopting a real-food lifestyle, I finally took a serious look at my relationship with treats. I realized I was addicted to sugar, and that switching out processed ingredients for almond flour and natural sweeteners wasn't going to fix the problem. Just because treats can be made "Paleo-friendly" doesn't make them a healthful choice. So I made a conscious decision to make a break from dessert. And as I transitioned into a real-food approach, I found that my cravings for sweets subsided. Now, when I want something sweet, I find that a bowl of fresh berries or sliced fruit usually hits the spot.

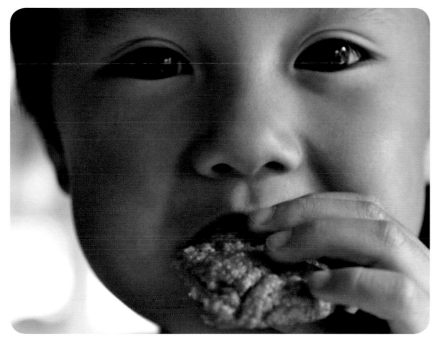
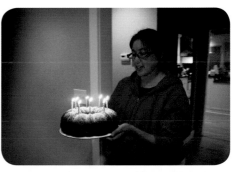
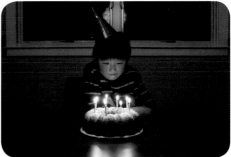

Don't get me wrong: I still love dark chocolate, and we always peek at the dessert menu after dining out with friends. The treats in this book are perennial favorites in our house, and our kids literally dance around the house on "S" days (Saturday and Sunday) because it means they can have a bowl of berry soup or a grain-free cookie after supper. But that feels right to me. For us, treats are celebratory foods—not everyday fare.

Nowadays, I indulge in sugary treats only on occasion—when it's really worth it. To me, the candy from the jar at the receptionist's desk is not worth it. Nor is the fruitcake at the neighborhood holiday party. And certainly not the endless boxes of dessicated factory-processed cookies on supermarket shelves.

But that sinfully decadent chocolate layer cake that your mom baked for your birthday? The freshly fried beignet from that cute little mom-and-pop joint in New Orleans? That hand-churned gelato from the stand at the farmer's market? You only live once, so when any food is *that* insanely good, go ahead and enjoy it—regardless of whether it's Paleo-friendly or not. (Unless you're deathly allergic, in which case never mind.) Just be mindful of your food choices instead of gobbling up every "Paleo" donut that crosses your path.

Your mileage may vary, but now that I've gotten the upper hand in my dysfunctional relationship with sugar, I tend to make treats only on rare special occasions, which explains the pared-down selection of sweets on these pages. Besides, if I included more dessert recipes, this book would be even longer, and I desperately need to wrap this up before you get too sick of me.

WHERE CREDIT'S DUE

This book owes its existence to the support of our friends, family, and mentors. We especially want to thank:

- Kirsty Melville and Jean Lucas, for braving uncharted waters with a couple of hapless numbnuts and saving us from ourselves. Same goes for Lynne McAdoo, Andrea Colvin, Kathy Hilliard, Andrea Shores, Tim Lynch, Carol Coe, Dave Shaw, Kristen Liszewski, Julie Bunge, and the entire AMP family.

- Fiona Kennedy, for contributing recipes to this book and helping me troubleshoot mine. Not only are you my kitchen guru and secret weapon, you'll always be my favorite sister, too.

- Melissa Joulwan and Dave Humphreys, for their generosity and friendship. You inspired us to chart our own path and to accept no compromise. Let's close down a few more restaurants together.

- Melissa and Dallas Hartwig, not just for spreading the good food gospel, but for planting the seed of this cookbook in our heads in the first place.

- Our pals in the Paleo and food blogging communities, who are too numerous to individually name (but you know who you are). Thank you for being our sounding boards, dining companions, housemates, mentors, and friends. Your support means the world to us.

- Tori Ritchie, for teaching me how to write about food. You are my Yoda, but way prettier.

- Elise Bauer, for opening my eyes and cleaning out my mouth. It was a game-changer, and you are, too.

- Sidney Majalya and Jory Steele, for meals and conversations here, there, and everywhere. We're incredibly fortunate to have you (and Matthew!) in our lives.

- Rebecca Katz and Kevin Walters, for the pork belly and belly laughs. Thank you for taste-testing even my foulest concoctions (and for not spitting anything out).

- Diana and Andrew Rodgers, for your passion. I'm really glad I didn't burn down your farmhouse.

- Jackie and Ben Linder, for the matzoh balls, business advice, and the greatest lunch containers in the universe (available at *lunchbots.com*).

- Lauren Ratcliff, Mark Bartels, Heidi Peckover, and David Dick, for making us come alive.

- Sarah Wilson of Fashletics (*fashletics.com*), whose handiwork adorns the very first page of this book.

- Will Moy, for being a patient and understanding Work Husband. Please do not stroke out.

- The Five Tribe and Women's Class at CrossFit Palo Alto, for all the heavy lifting.

- Jennifer Yue, for letting me be the boss of the shoe store. You're the little sister I never had.

- Eliot Adelson, for being like a brother to Henry, even after he broke your nose.

- Chris Kennedy, for turning my sister Irish, and for the best smoked turkey known to humankind.

- Our parents, Gene and Rebecca Tam and Kenny and Wendy Fong, for sharing with us their love of good food, and for their incredible sacrifices through the years. (Including the free babysitting.)

- Our kids, Owen and Ollie, for letting Mommy and Daddy have extra computer time so we could write this cookbook. We're sorry if this book embarrasses you when you're older, but as your parents, it's our job to mortify you in front of your friends. We love you more than you will ever know.

- Lastly, the readers of Nom Nom Paleo, for sticking with us through the years. You make it all worthwhile.

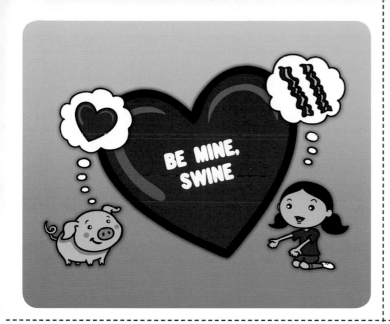

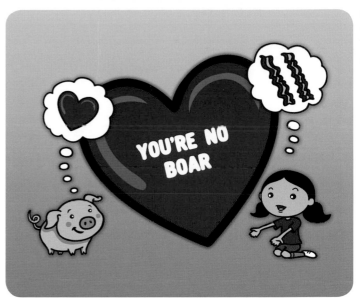

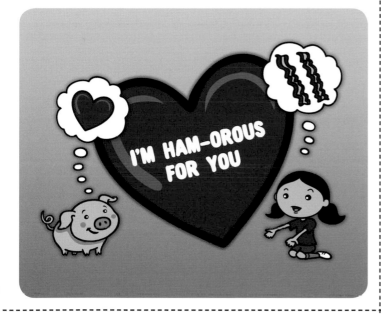

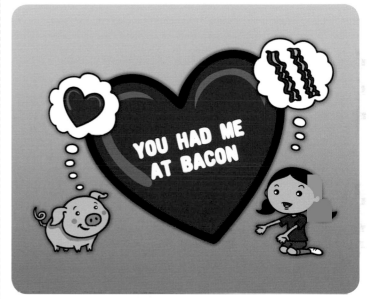

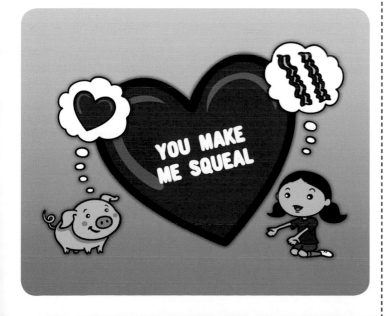

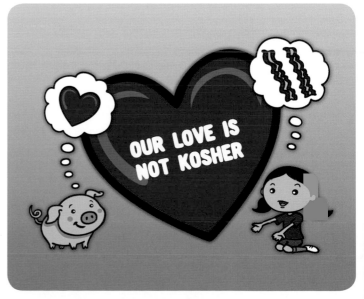

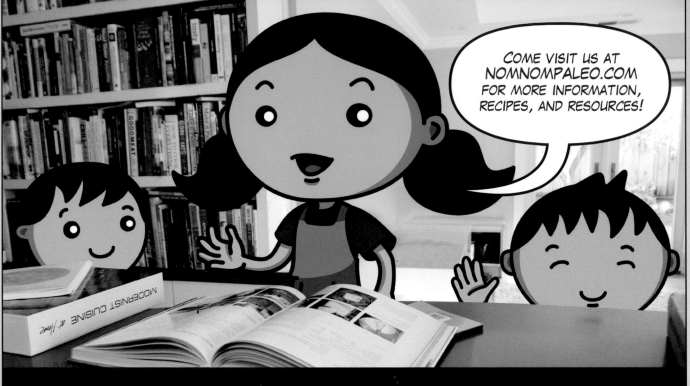

BIBLIOGRAPHY

- Aidells, Bruce. *The Great Meat Cookbook: Everything You Need to Know to Buy and Cook Today's Meat*. New York: Houghton Mifflin Harcourt, 2012.

- Farr, Ryan, and Brigit Binns. *Whole Beast Butchery: The Complete Visual Guide to Beef, Lamb, and Pork*. San Francisco: Chronicle Books, 2011.

- Hartwig, Dallas, and Melissa Hartwig. *It Starts with Food: Discover the Whole30 and Change Your Life in Unexpected Ways*. Las Vegas: Victory Belt, 2012.

- Madison, Deborah. *Vegetarian Cooking For Everyone*. New York: Broadway Books, 1997.

- McGee, Harold. *Keys to Good Cooking: A Guide to Making the Best of Food and Recipes*. New York: The Penguin Press, 2010.

- McGee, Harold. *On Food and Cooking: The Science and Lore of the Kitchen*. New York: Scribner, 2004

- Page, Karen, and Andrew Dornenburg. *The Flavor Bible: The Essential Guide to Culinary Creativity, Based on the Wisdom of America's Most Imaginative Chefs*. New York: Little, Brown and Company, 2008.

- Ruhlman, Michael. *Ruhlman's Twenty: 20 Techniques 100 Recipes A Cook's Manifesto*. San Francisco: Chronicle Books, 2011.

- Sanfilippo, Diane. *Practical Paleo: A Customized Approach to Health and a Whole-Foods Lifestyle*. Las Vegas: Victory Belt, 2012.

- The Editors at America's Test Kitchen, and Guy Crosby. *The Science of Good Cooking: Master 50 Simple Concepts to Enjoy a Lifetime of Success in the Kitchen*. Brookline, MA: America's Test Kitchen, 2012.

- Wolf, Robb. *The Paleo Solution: The Original Human Diet*. Las Vegas: Victory Belt, 2010.

OVEN TEMPERATURES

To convert Fahrenheit to Celsius, subtract 32 from Fahrenheit, multiply the result by 5, then divide by 9.

Description	°F	°C	British Gas
Very cool	200°	95°	0
Very cool	225°	110°	¼
Very cool	250°	120°	½
Cool	275°	135°	1
Cool	300°	150°	2
Warm	325°	165°	3
Moderate	350°	175°	4
Moderately hot	375°	190°	5
Fairly hot	400°	200°	6
Hot	425°	220°	7
Very hot	450°	230°	8
Very hot	475°	245°	9

WEIGHT

¼ ounce	7 grams
½ ounce	14 grams
¾ ounce	21 grams
1 ounce	28 grams
1¼ ounces	35 grams
1½ ounces	42.5 grams
1⅔ ounces	45 grams
2 ounces	57 grams
3 ounces	85 grams
4 ounces (¼ pound)	113 grams
5 ounces	142 grams
6 ounces	170 grams
7 ounces	198 grams
8 ounces (½ pound)	227 grams
16 ounces (1 pound)	454 grams
35¼ ounces (2.2 pounds)	1 kilogram

LENGTH

⅛ inch	3 millimeters
¼ inch	6 millimeters
½ inch	1¼ centimeters
1 inch	2½ centimeters
2 inches	5 centimeters
2½ inches	6 centimeters
4 inches	10 centimeters
5 inches	13 centimeters
6 inches	15¼ centimeters
12 inches (1 foot)	30 centimeters

VOLUME

¼ teaspoon	1 milliliter
½ teaspoon	2.5 milliliters
¾ teaspoon	4 milliliters
1 teaspoon	5 milliliters
1¼ teaspoons	6 milliliters
1½ teaspoons	7.5 milliliters
1¾ teaspoons	8.5 milliliters
2 teaspoons	10 milliliters
1 tablespoon (½ fluid ounce)	15 milliliters
2 tablespoons (1 fluid ounce)	30 milliliters
¼ cup	60 milliliters
⅓ cup	80 milliliters
½ cup (4 fluid ounces)	120 milliliters
⅔ cup	160 milliliters
¾ cup	180 milliliters
1 cup (8 fluid ounces)	240 milliliters
1¼ cups	300 milliliters
1½ cups (12 fluid ounces)	360 milliliters
1⅔ cups	400 milliliters
2 cups (1 pint)	460 milliliters
3 cups	700 milliliters
4 cups (1 quart)	0.95 liter
1 quart plus ¼ cup	1 liter
4 quarts (1 gallon)	3.8 liters

METRIC CONVERSION FORMULAS

To Convert:	Multiply:
Ounces to grams	Ounces by 28.35
Pounds to kilograms	Pounds by .454
Teaspoons to milliliters	Teaspoons by 4.93
Tablespoons to milliliters	Tablespoons by 14.79
Fluid ounces to milliliters	Fluid ounces by 29.57
Cups to milliliters	Cups by 236.59
Cups to liters	Cups by .236
Pints to liters	Pints by .473
Quarts to liters	Quarts by .946
Gallons to liters	Gallons by 3.785
Inches to centimeters	Inches by 2.54

Information compiled from a variety of sources, including *Recipes into Type* by Joan Whitman and Dolores Simon (Newton, MA: Biscuit Books, 2000); *The New Food Lover's Companion* by Sharon Tyler Herbst (Hauppauge, NY: Barron's, 1995); and *Rosemary Brown's Big Kitchen Instruction Book* (Kansas City, MO: Andrews McMeel, 1998).

INDEX

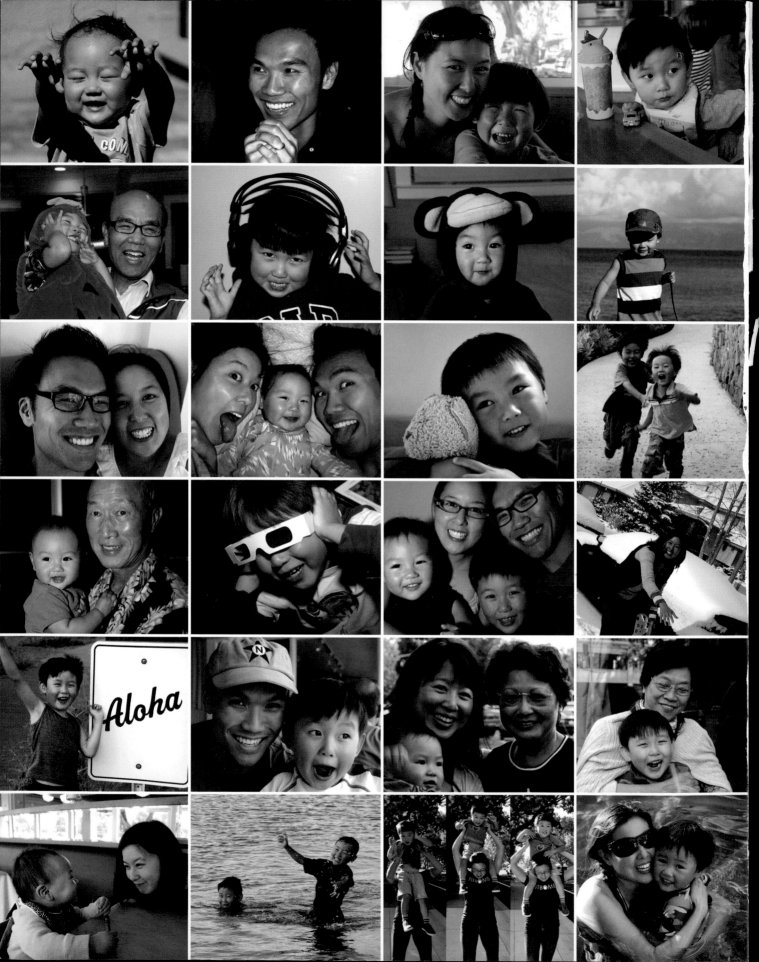

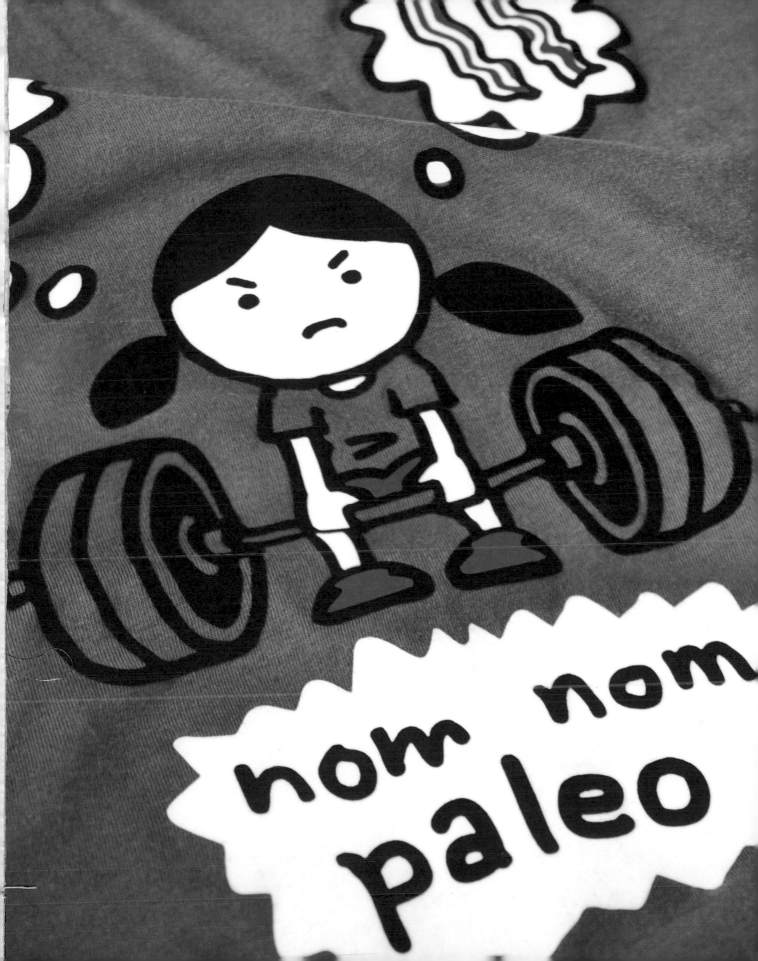